SECOND EDITION

Language Disorders in Children

Fundamental Concepts of Assessment and Intervention

Joan N. Kaderavek
University of Toledo

PEARSON

Boston   Columbus   Indianapolis   New York   San Francisco   Upper Saddle River
Amsterdam   Cape Town   Dubai   London   Madrid   Milan   Munich   Paris   Montreal   Toronto
Delhi   Mexico City   Sao Paulo   Sydney   Hong Kong   Seoul   Singapore   Taipei   Tokyo

Vice President, Editor in Chief: Jeffery W. Johnston
Acquisitions Editor: Ann Davis
Project Manager: Annette Joseph
Program Manager: Joseph Sweeney
Editorial Production Service: Jouve North America
Operations Specialist: Linda Sager
Electronic Composition: Jouve North America
Interior Design: Jouve North America
Cover Design: Bruce Kenselaar
Cover Image: © Monkey Business Images / Shutterstock

Credits and acknowledgments borrowed from other sources and reproduced, with permission, in this textbook appear here and on the appropriate page within text. Chapter opener image: By Adr/Fotolia

Many of the designations by manufacturers and sellers to distinguish their products are claimed as trademarks. Where those designations appear in this book, and the publisher was aware of a trademark claim, the designations have been printed in initial caps or all caps.

10 9 8 7 6 5 4 3 2 1

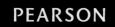

ISBN 10: 0-13-335202-1
ISBN 13: 978-0-13-335202-3

With love and gratitude to my husband, Dave

About the Author

Joan Kaderavek, Ph.D., began her professional life as a clinical speech-language pathologist; she worked with children with language disorders in a community nonprofit clinic and Head Start early childhood programs. In recent years, she has been named a Distinguished University Professor at the University of Toledo for her work teaching speech-language pathologists, early childhood educators, and special educators about children's language development and language disorders. Dr. Kaderavek is a Fellow of the American Speech-Language Pathology Association and has been awarded Honors of the Ohio Speech-Language-Hearing Association.

Dr. Kaderavek is a frequent presenter and author in the area of language development, early literacy, and teacher–child classroom interactions. She has had more than 50 peer-reviewed articles in leading journals. Her research considers the effects of educational interventions on children's language development and educational achievement. She has examined the effects of a teacher-provided book-reading intervention on children's literacy development and currently is conducting research on the impact of classroom science instruction on the language development of young children. She is a co-investigator on a large-scale, 5-year grant to support this work, funded by the National Science Foundation.

This book considers issues of assessment and intervention for children with language impairments. It is written for undergraduate students who are just beginning to think about how to work with children who are language impaired. The assumption is that a student who uses this book will have already completed a course on normal language development.

I have developed the principles used in this book over a number of years of teaching undergraduate speech-language pathology and special education students. Many undergraduate books provide an overview of terminology and describe a broad range of assessment and intervention approaches. As a teacher, I discovered a problem with using such books. The books (and the way I was teaching—primarily with lectures) allowed students to stay in a passive learning mode. Students were able to successfully pass tests at the undergraduate level; but these "good students" were not prepared to begin the analytic thought and problem solving that I expected (and they needed) in graduate-level training. I decided the problem was not with the students but with the way I was teaching! My efforts to become a better teacher are reflected in the first overarching theme of this book.

I decided that rather than just expect students to memorize terms and answer short-answer questions (e.g., *List three communication characteristics associated with autism spectrum disorder*), I wanted to begin to train students to "think like a clinician." I wanted to change my focus to an emphasis on the processes that highly skilled speech-language pathologists (SLPs) and educators use to make assessment and intervention decisions. I realized that I couldn't give students all the facts they needed to know at the beginning level of training. However, I could provide multiple activities that would motivate students to think deeply, ask questions, and solve problems. I also realized that students need to "talk through" a particular problem or process. If I described a problem (and the solution), students nodded wisely and wrote down what I said. When I asked if anyone had any questions, no one raised a hand. But when I asked the students to explain to a small group or a peer what they had just learned, they could not verbalize the issue that had seemed so clear just a moment before.

I began a different kind of teaching. I started each day with a mini-lecture that I tried to keep under a half hour. Then I had students work in groups. I varied the activities. I found that this approach worked very well in face-to-face classes and also when I taught courses via distance learning. Rather than having the students only demonstrate knowledge with objective tests, I set up weekly activities during class time. I asked students in a distance learning class to complete the activities individually, with a partner, or in a small group (depending on the weekly project). I began to include activities such as these:

- I gave the students a decision tree and asked them to put a few descriptive words in each of the decision tree boxes, capturing the communication behaviors they might expect to see at each point in the decision-making process. Students explained the decision tree to a partner. I provide decision trees throughout this book.
- I gave the students simplified versions of assessment tools (trying to capture the essential elements of the decision-making process) and asked students to view videotapes

and begin to classify behaviors using the assessment tools. I realized that students' administration might not be highly accurate! However, the emphasis was on having students verbalize *why* they choose to classify behaviors in a particular way. I provide simplified versions of assessment tools in this book.

- I realized that students needed to "put words into their own mouths." I used activities in which students had to role-play an explanation to a teacher or parent. (A student could write out a script if the course was taught via distance learning.) Information that seemed easy to students during a lecture suddenly presented challenges when the students were asked to teach someone else! I include many suggestions for role-playing in the chapter activities.

- I began to iteratively come back to major points and have students explain to each other (or to the class as a whole, or write down and submit to me) how the fundamental principle applied to the current issue. So, instead of only teaching information on the theories of language development at the beginning of the course, I wanted students to retain old information and apply it to their new learning. For example, in a discussion on intellectual disability, I said, "Working with the person next to you, write down how social interaction theory, behaviorism, and systems theory might apply to our work with an individual with an intellectual impairment." As I walked around the classroom, students asked many questions and actively engaged in solving "the problem." I mirror this technique in many of the "Focus" boxes and "Discussion and In-Class Activities" assignments that occur in each chapter. I also iteratively present information on language theory, form–content–use, and typical development throughout this book and link theoretical information to assessment and intervention decision making.

- I developed a "numbered" system for talking about language subdomains. Previously, I had typically presented the concepts of form, content, and use in the parallel form (as it was taught to me). However, I was frustrated that during case example problem-solving activities, students didn't know where to start; they appeared to "randomly" focus on a domain (e.g., syntax for a child who was at the beginning language learning stage). I wanted students to move sequentially through a thought process that first considered an individual's beginning pragmatic skills and then single words and word combinations, then syntax, and so forth. I created subdomain numbering (introduced in Chapter 2 of this book) to provide a scaffold for this problem-solving task. The communication subdomains and information about four theories of language development are now introduced in Chapter 2 in this second edition of the textbook.

- I began talking to students about *connections* when I introduced new topics. I linked new information to previous information and also discussed how the information might apply more broadly across disorder types. I used the educational principle of helping students move from the known to the unknown. I mirror this approach in this book by including a section called *Connections* in many of the chapters. The *Connections* sections are linkages to previously learned concepts (e.g., applying the form–content–use model to children with autism spectrum disorder) or include discussions of information that can be applied broadly across disorder types (e.g., counseling families).

- Finally, and most importantly, I began to explicitly teach "meta" problem-solving skills. I tried to always explain why an SLP or educator might choose one approach over another or clarify the underlying analytic process fundamental to the task. I gave examples and then asked students to discuss possible solutions to the problem *and* provide a rationale for their decision. I told students: "Right now it is not important if you are wrong or right with your clinical decisions. I might make a different clinical decision than you. But what I want from you right now is to give me a *reason* (based on language theory or researched evidence or family concerns) to support your decision. That is your task at this early stage in professional training." With this approach, students started to take chances and hypothesize about a particular assessment or intervention strategy for a specific child. At the end of a discussion, I typically shared my thoughts and explained why I might make a different clinical decision than a student. But, before giving my opinion, I wanted students to begin to make decisions about intervention approaches that might work, based on their current knowledge. Throughout this book, I provide examples, case studies, and ideas for class discussion to stimulate this process. Chapter 4, which is about clinical decision making, grew out of my efforts to teach "meta" processes.

In sum, I began to be a better and more effective teacher for undergraduate students. This book is the result.

I am pleased that other instructors find that using these techniques helps students learn. After publication of the first edition, I was gratified to receive enthusiastic endorsement from instructors who had adopted the textbook for their courses on language disorders. Instructors wrote and shared that students "read this textbook closely" and that "the communication subdomain model is referred to throughout the academic semester."

A second overarching theme of this book is current issues central to speech-language pathology and special education. This includes discussions of evidence-based practice (EBP), response to intervention RTI, classroom-based assessment and intervention, use of iPads and apps during treatment for communication disorders, and connection building between oral language and literacy learning.

To this end, I give specific attention to each issue in one section of the book but come back to each topic in other chapters. My intent is not to be redundant but to make it clear that certain topics affect broad aspects of service delivery and decision making. My emphasis on EBP is also represented in my decision to present only two or three intervention approaches for each of the disorder groups. Rather than present a full range of possible intervention approaches (without a detailed discussion), I wanted to discuss relevant research for select exemplary approaches and explain how they represented "levels of evidence" within EBP.

I used to wait until graduate-level training to expose students to primary research. I now believe, with the emphasis on EBP, that students need exposure to primary research at the beginning training level. I hope instructors will supplement my discussions of intervention by providing examples of primary intervention research. Students need to begin to evaluate the quality of primary research.

NEW TO THIS EDITION

- **EBP is introduced in a newly organized Chapter 1**; the concepts of EBP are then referenced in discussions of high-quality interventions throughout the book.
- **Elimination of a separate chapter on multicultural issues**; multicultural issues are now is integrated throughout the textbook. The connections to multicultural issues are clinically relevant and practice oriented. Instructors can use this information to help students become more sensitive to nonmajority students and their families.
- **Updated information and research throughout the text** ensures that students are learning the most current information about language disorders.

- Information and implications of DSM-5 is included throughout the text, specifically as it relates to children who are on the autism spectrum.
- **A revised approach to teaching students about language theories** (Chapter 2) consolidates language theories into four basic theoretical approaches: social interactionist, behaviorist, cognitive constructivist, and emergentist. This streamlined presentation allows students to focus on the underlying theoretical principles impacting language intervention and assessment.
- **Two new appendices** provide step-by-step tutorials to T-unit analysis and language analysis of children who demonstrate African American English.
  - The new appendices add to the clinically practical and instructor-friendly appendices from the First Edition (i.e., standardized scoring tutorial, form for language analysis of children with early developing language, example of a language assessment report).
  - The appendices allow instructors to easily incorporate practical hands-on activities into their distance-learning or face-to-face course on language disorders.
- **Chapter 7 provides a balanced description of challenges and opportunities for children with hearing loss** who are learning to speak and listen as well as rationale for introduction of sign language for some children with hearing loss.
  - Research and interventions for children with hearing loss has been updated with the most current data.
- **Chapter 10 focuses on reading, writing, and spelling interventions** for young emergent readers as well as for older school-age students.
  - A model of literacy intervention also is described for students with significant levels of language disability.
- **Chapter 11 on Augmentative Communication has been updated** to include information on iPads and software "applications" (i.e., apps) and their use for students with complex communication needs.

I have enjoyed my years as a practicing SLP, and I am committed to teaching students to "think like a clinician." My greatest hope is that this textbook helps that occur for the students who use it!

ACKNOWLEDGMENTS

Thank you to my husband, Dave (who helped prepare the permission requests for the second edition of this book); to my children, Megan Kaderavek Tsai and Brian Kaderavek; and to my granddaughter, Natalie, who keeps me optimistic about the future!

I'd also like to thank the reviewers of this edition: Valerie Boyer, Southern Illinois University; Deborah C. Cook, Springfield College; and Stephen D. Oller, Texas A&M University—Kingsville.

Contents

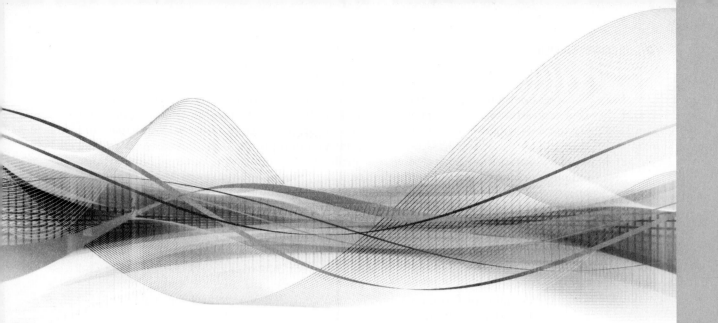

1 The Foundations of Language and Clinical Practice

Chapter Overview Questions

1. What are the differences between a language disorder, a language difference, and a language delay?

2. What are the three levels of communication described in the speech chain? Which level is the focus of this book?

3. What are examples of communication behaviors that represent form, content, and use?

4. What differentiates Level I, Level II, Level III, and Level IV research in evidence-based practice (EBP)? How does an interventionist use EBP to guide intervention?

Welcome to this book about language disorders. The language disorders course in which you are now enrolled is probably your first course focusing on children with communication deficits. Up to this point, your training has concentrated on communication development in children who are developing typically. It is an exciting professional turning point when you begin to consider how to guide assessment and interventions for individuals with language disorders.

This book's goal is to help you think like a practitioner. I focus on underlying theories and fundamental principles guiding clinical decision making. The ability to synthesize information, weigh scientific evidence, and see connections between basic principles will prepare you to work with children who have language impairments.

One book on language disorders cannot teach you everything you need to know to be a successful speech-language pathologist (SLP) or special educator. This book does not try to teach you everything! Instead, I have chosen to (a) emphasize basic principles and then (b) discuss selected assessment and intervention protocols as illustrative examples. I believe that at this early point in your professional training, it is better to provide more extensive information and examples for some exemplary assessment and intervention approaches (and clarify why they are exemplary) than to briefly describe many different approaches.

To help you become a decision maker, I include many examples, case studies, and opportunities for you to practice problem solving. By working through the examples, you will learn important analytic processes. In this chapter, I introduce four important cornerstones of the profession: (a) definitions for and background on language and language disorders; (b) a model of communication (i.e., the speech chain model); (c) the language domains of form, content, and use; and (d) a clinical decision-making model called evidence-based practice.

Definitions and Background Information: Language Disorders

Understanding the difference between definitions is an important cornerstone of the field of communication disorders; specifically, there are differences between the terms *language, speech,* and *communication.* **Language** is a complex and dynamic system of conventional symbols used for thought and expression. Language can be expressed orally, through writing or pictured symbols, or manually (e.g., sign language).

Speech is not the same thing as language. Whereas language involves a symbol system, **speech** is the articulation and the rate (i.e., fluency) of speech sounds and the quality of an individual's voice. **Communication,** in contrast, includes symbolic *and* nonsymbolic information (i.e., facial expressions, body language, gestures, etc.). As an example, if I frown and cross my arms, although I am not using symbolic communication, I am communicating! A communication disorder may be evident in the process of hearing, language, speech, or in a combination of all three processes.

In U.S. schools, children with speech and language disorders (as a specific diagnostic category) make up 2.9% of the total school population. In addition, there are other subgroups of children who are not counted in this group who also have language disorders. Practitioners serve children who have hearing loss (0.2% of schoolchildren), multiple disabilities (0.3%), intellectual disabilities (0.9%), and learning disabilities (4.9%; NCES, 2012). Each of these subgroups demonstrates language impairments. Eighty-three percent of the SLPs who work in schools report that they regularly work with students with language disorders (American Speech-Language-Hearing Association [ASHA], 2012).

A **language disorder** is impaired comprehension and/or use of spoken, written, and/or other symbol systems. A language disorder can represent a deficit in receptive language, expressive language, or a combined expressive–receptive deficit. **Receptive language** refers to an individual's ability to understand and process language; **expressive language** refers to an individual's ability to express and communicate meaning with language. Typically, an individual's receptive language abilities are better than his or her expressive language abilities.

Sometimes a young child (2 to 3 years old) who exhibits a developmental lag in language is said to have a **language delay**, be a **late talker**, or have **late language emergence**. This terminology is used because experts state that a language disorder cannot be reliably diagnosed in young children in the absence of a primary disorder (e.g., intellectual disability, autism; Bishop, Price, Dale, & Plomin, 2003; Rescorla, 2009).

An individual with a language disorder is different from someone with a language difference. **Language difference** results from a variation of a symbol system used by a group of individuals that reflects and is determined by shared regional, social, or cultural/ethnic factors. It is essential that professionals distinguish between aspects of language production representing dialectal patterns (i.e., language difference) and true disorders in speech and language (ASHA, 2003b). For example, a teacher may say to her students, "*I've got y'all's assignments here.*" This is a form of dialect associated with the southern United States; although it may be an unfamiliar expression to some U.S. speakers, it does not represent a language disorder. Information regarding language difference associated with dialect use is presented throughout this book.

As a final important point, I want to underscore that much of what you will learn about language disorders applies across disability categories. Rather than focusing on a child's diagnostic category (e.g., autism, specific learning disability), skilled practitioners use a descriptive-developmental framework to guide intervention. A **descriptive-developmental approach** focuses on a student's language development and function in a variety of natural contexts (Zipoli & Kennedy, 2005). A practitioner who uses a descriptive-developmental approach works to understand an individual's communication strengths and limitations rather than focusing on his or her diagnostic label. This is a particularly important point, because I have organized the chapters in this book by disability category. There is, for example, a chapter on autism, a chapter on intellectual disability, and so forth. I organize chapters by disability categories because, in my teaching experience, I have found that beginning practitioners learn most easily with this organizational strategy. However, to counterbalance my organizational strategy, I continually clarify descriptive and developmental similarities between disability groups and highlight connections between intervention approaches across disability types. Read more about categorical versus descriptive approaches in Focus 1.1.

The Speech Chain

The **speech chain model** is a basic model of communication used to explain the processes of communication from the speaker's production of words, through transmission of sound, to the listener's perception of what has been said (Denes & Pinson, 2001). I present this model to point out how language fits into an individual's communication system. The speech chain model is visually presented in Figure 1.1.

The first point I want to emphasize is that the speech chain model reminds us that language has both a receptive and expressive component. The speaker/listener role is visually represented in Figure 1.1 with the left-to-right nature of the diagram. A good communicator speaks *and* listens. Within a conversation, a person alternates between listening (using receptive language) and speaking (using expressive language). A competent communicator effortlessly comprehends the listener and produces meaningful language output. Remember that language output can be represented by spoken language, writing, or manual communication (i.e., sign language).

FOCUS 1.1   *Learning More*

The categorical model organizes language disorders on the basis of an individual's syndromes of behavior; it is fundamentally a medical model. Its advantages are that it (a) is easily understandable, (b) often is necessary in qualifying a child for educational services, and (c) provides a basic explanation of how a particular child may be different from other children. The limitations of the categorical model are the following:

- There is not always a cause–effect relationship between an individual's diagnosis and his or her language impairment. Does a hearing loss mean that a child will automatically have a language delay? (You will read more about this in Chapter 7.)

- Children with different diagnostic labels may be quite similar. A child with a pragmatic disorder may be classified as having autism, intellectual disability, or specific language impairment.
- Children's degree of impairment may vary dramatically within a diagnostic category. For example, a child with autism may be very mildly impaired; the diagnostic label may unfairly prejudice teachers or communication partners with regard to the child's abilities.
- Knowing a child's diagnostic classification may not be very helpful in planning an intervention program. SLPs, instead, use a decision-making process based on an individual's communication strengths and limitations.

The second point about the speech chain is that the communication system requires a number of mechanisms to occur. Acoustic information must be transferred (Level 1 in Figure 1.1), motor activity must take place (Level 2), and the brain is activated at Level 3 to create meaningful symbolic (i.e., linguistic) information. All three levels of the system must be operating effectively for communication to occur. I elaborate on each of the three levels below.

Level 1 represents the acoustic level of communicative function: the external or environmental system. This level describes how physical energy is transferred between communication partners. In its simplistic form, Level 1 represents the molecular vibration forming sound waves and transferring physical energy from the speaker to the listener. It is very likely that you studied the external physical component of communication in a course called Speech Science or Physics of Sound.

Level 2 represents the internal physical/motor system required for communication. In the listener, the physical system consists of the hearing mechanism and the transfer of neural messages to the brain's language center. In the speaker, Level 2 represents the speech system, including respiration, articulation, and phonation. The physical speech systems must be coordinated to produce intelligible speech. It is likely that you studied aspects of Level 2 motor communication in a course called Anatomy and Physiology. You will learn about disorders occurring in the speech system in coursework covering articulation disorders, motor-speech disorders, and voice disorders. You will learn more about Level 2 (i.e., physical) hearing problems in your audiology coursework.

Level 3 of the speech chain model represents the linguistic component of communication. Level 3, the linguistic component, is the focus of this book. The linguistic level is the ability of the listener to receive incoming Level 2 energy (i.e., neural signals) and turn the

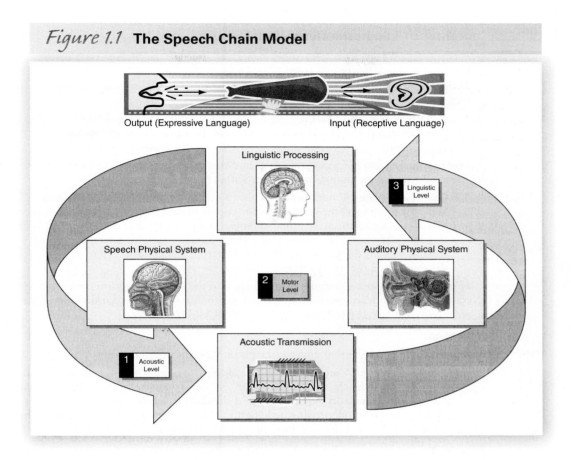

Figure 1.1 **The Speech Chain Model**

physical energy into meaningful information via receptive language. The speaker creates meaningful linguistic information at Level 3.

The speech chain model emphasizes the complexity of the communication system and helps you integrate what you are learning in this course with other coursework. As you progress through your professional training program, continue to frame new knowledge within this basic model of communication functioning.

Let's now move beyond the speech chain model and consider the three fundamental language domains of form, content, and use.

Form, Content, and Use: The Cornerstones of Language

To become an effective linguistic communicator, a speaker must master three language areas: the *form* of the message, the *content* of the message, and the message *use*, or function. Language form includes phonology, morphology, and syntax (i.e., the structure of language). Language content consists of semantics (i.e., meaning of language); language function consists of pragmatics (i.e., how language is used within social contexts). See Table 1.1 for formal definitions and examples of each of these terms.

Table 1.1   **Language Definitions**

Form

Morphology is the system that governs the structure of words and the construction of word forms.

> Example: At age 13 months a child says, "*Two birdie!*" and by 24 months says, "*Two birdie*s!" The child has learned to add the *s* morpheme to indicate a plural form.

Syntax is the system governing the order and combination of words to form sentences and the relationships among the elements within a sentence.

> Example: At age 24 months a child asks a question by saying, "*Doggie outside?*" With this utterance, the child omits the copula verb *is* needed for a question form; this is a typical error at 24 months. However, by 36 months the child says, "*Is the dog outside?*" In the second instance, the child demonstrates understanding of English word order by placing the copula verb *is* at the beginning of the sentence, demonstrating the use of interrogative reversal syntax form.

Phonology is the sound system of a language and the rules that govern the sound combinations. To learn more about phonology and phonological disorders, go to the ASHA website: www.asha.org/public/speech/disorders/ChildSandL.htm.

Content

Semantics is the system that governs the meanings of words and sentences.

> Example: At age 11 months the child calls out, "*da-da*" whenever she sees a male. But by 15 months she only calls "*da-da*" or "*daddy*" for her father; she says "*man*" for unfamiliar men. In the first example, the child overgeneralizes the meaning of *daddy,* using it to refer to any male figure. This is a common early semantic pattern. As semantic knowledge develops, the child learns the meaning of the word *daddy* and uses this word only for her father.

Use

Pragmatics is the system that combines the language components described above in functional and socially appropriate communication.

> Example: A child tugs on his father's pants and points to the TV. This is an example of a nonverbal request.

Source: Based on information from *Definitions of Communication Disorders and Variations [Relevant Paper],* 1993, American Speech-Language-Hearing Association (ASHA). Available from www.asha.org /policy.

Lois Bloom and Margaret Lahey (1978) developed the form–content–use language model and demonstrated how the three language areas intersect during communication (see Figure 1.2). The interlocking circles in the diagram are a reminder that (a) vocabulary (i.e., semantics) is used to produce (b) sentences involving the use of syntax structure and morphology, and that sentences are meaningless without (c) proficiency in language use. Lahey (1988) proposed that language disorders are caused when there is a disruption in language form, content, or use or a combination of disordered components. The inter-locking circles (i.e., Venn diagram) representing form, content, and use remind us that the three domains are interdependent and that an effective communicator demonstrates

Figure 1.2 **Form, Content, and Use Diagram**

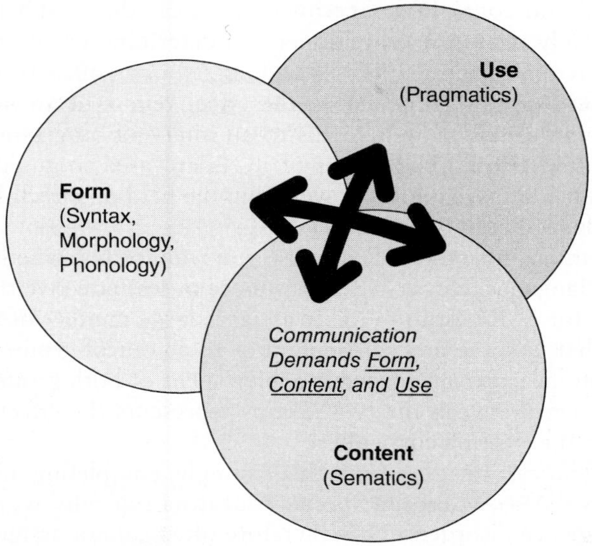

Source: Lahey, Margaret, *Language Disorders and Language Development*, 1st, © 1988. Printed and Electronically reproduced by permission of Pearson Education, Inc., Upper Saddle River, New Jersey.

proficiency in all three domains. The form–content–use model is used widely in the communication disorders literature. You will learn about an elaborated version of the form–content–use chart, something I call the **communication subdomains**, in Chapter 2.

Evidence-Based Practice: A Cornerstone of Clinical Practice

Just as form, content, and use are the cornerstones of how language specialists think about language, there is another approach that has dramatically changed how practitioners think through clinical questions and make decisions about language intervention. This approach is called evidence-based practice (EBP). EBP refers to the process that practitioners use to evaluate whether a clinical practice, a strategy, a program, a curriculum, or an intervention is backed by rigorous evidence of effectiveness and whether a practice is appropriate for a particular individual.

EBP: INTERNAL AND EXTERNAL EVIDENCE

SLPs use both internal and external evidence in their EBP decision making. **Internal evidence** is provided by (a) an individual client's perspective and beliefs and (b) an SLP's clinical expertise. The contribution of internal evidence is part of ASHA's definition of EBP: "An approach in which current, high-quality research evidence is *integrated with practitioner expertise and client preferences and values, into the process of making clinical decisions*" (ASHA, 2005, p. 1).

But internal evidence is not enough to guide EBP: As you can see from the first part of ASHA's definition (i.e., "An approach in which *current, high-quality research evidence . . .*"), EBP also requires external evidence. **External evidence** consists of well-designed and controlled experimental studies that result in experimental data; by analyzing study results, a practitioner can determine whether a particular clinical practice is effective (Dollagen, 2007). Randomized controlled trials (RCTs) are considered the "gold standard" for evaluating the effectiveness of an intervention. RCTs are studies that randomly assign individuals to an intervention group or control group to measure intervention effects. The results of RCTs are used to guide clinical practice in medicine, education, and psychology, as well as in the field of speech-language pathology (Coalition for Evidence-Based Policy, 2003).

As an example of RCT, suppose you want to test whether a particular curriculum for English language learners (ELLs) is more or less effective than your school's existing curriculum for ELLs. You randomly assign a large number of ELLs to either an intervention group that uses the new curriculum or to a control group that uses the existing curriculum. You measure the academic achievement of both groups over time. The difference in achievement between the two groups represents the effect of the new curriculum compared to the existing curriculum.

As you can imagine from this example, completing an RCT is time-consuming and expensive. Also, SLPs and special educators typically work with individuals who have low-incidence disorders. They therefore often cannot assign large numbers of students to one intervention or another. Consequently, in the EBP decision-making process, practitioners evaluate a range of experimental designs to determine whether a particular clinical practice meets the definition of *high quality*. We call this a tiered approach to evaluating external evidence the **levels of evidence** in EBP.

EBP: EVALUATING RESEARCH QUALITY

Because not all experiments consist of an RCT, an SLP evaluates the experimental studies that are available regarding a particular clinical practice and considers the study's experimental level of evidence. The levels of evidence are on a continuum from the highest level (Level I) to the lowest level of clinical evidence (Level IV). As previously stated, the best research is produced by an RCT; **Level I** evidence resulting from randomized experimental research is considered the best research design. Level I evidence also includes meta-analyses. A **meta-analysis** is a specialized form of systematic review in which the results from several studies are summarized using a statistical technique resulting in a single weighted estimate of the results' findings. **Level II** research reflects high-quality, but nonrandomized, experiments. **Level III** evidence reflects well-designed nonexperimental studies and case studies. A nonexperimental design is typically a description of clinical results implemented with a small group of students without the use of a comparison treatment. **Level IV** represents expert opinion. (See Table 1.2 for a summary of the levels of evidence.)

EBP: FACTORS CONTRIBUTING TO RESEARCH QUALITY

Now that you know about the levels of evidence, let's consider how practitioners evaluate a study's research quality. Let's start with Level I. Remember that Level I research reflects the most rigorous investigation standard because studies assigned to Level I (a) compare performance of two or more groups of students (i.e., control group design) and (b) randomly assign students to one group or the other.

Table 1.2   **Levels of Evidence for Scientific Studies**

Level	Criteria
Level I	• Evidence from one well-conducted randomized clinical trial.
	• Systematic review or meta-analysis of high-quality randomized controlled trials.
Level II	• Similar findings demonstrated from nonrandomized experiments (with good experimental design) from several different researchers.
Level III	• Well-designed nonexperimental studies (i.e., correlational and case studies).
Level IV	• Expert committee report, consensus conference, clinical experience of respected authorities.

Source: Information from ASHA, www.asha.org/members/ebp/assessing.htm.

Comparison of the effects of different treatments is the "heart and soul" of Level I research; in the best-case scenario, two different *interventions* (also called *treatments*) are compared. The ELL curriculum study described above is an example of two comparison treatments.

Sometimes, however, instead of comparing the effects of two different treatments, researchers compare students in a treatment condition with students who receive no treatment (i.e., treatment vs. no-treatment design). In the no-treatment group, students continue with their regular school or home activities but do not receive any special intervention. Although comparison between treatment and no-treatment groups is an acceptable Level I design, it is not as strong as comparison of two different treatments. Consider that in the treatment vs. no-treatment design, students in the treatment group may improve because they receive regular, positive interaction with an attentive adult; student gains may not be directly attributable to specific characteristics of the intervention. Comparison of two different treatments solves this problem.

Subject randomization also is an important component of Level I research. In a randomized research design, a group of students consent to participate in a study. After the researchers obtain consent, they randomly assign the students to the treatment group or the comparison group. Randomization adds certainty to the interpretation of results. If randomization is not used, there is a possibility of bias. For example, imagine that I say, "I would like you to participate in a study on the effects of exercise. You can choose to be in a group in which you will exercise four times a week, or you can choose to be in a group that exercises two times a week." In this situation, it is likely that individuals with specific character traits (perhaps highly motivated individuals) will choose to be in the group that gets more frequent exercise; less motivated individuals may choose the two-times-per-week group. Study results would then potentially represent variations in motivation levels rather than compare exercise effects. Random assignment increases the validity of experimental results.

Other factors contribute to the evaluation of research quality. An overall goal of high-quality research is to (a) limit any extraneous factors that could potentially contaminate the results, (b) determine that participants in the group are similar except for treatment exposure, (c) document results with highly reliable and valid measures of performance, and (d) provide statistically significant and meaningful data (Gillam & Gillam, 2008). These factors are described in more detail below.

One goal of high-quality research is to document that reported effects are not contaminated by unintended variables. One factor that causes contamination is research bias. Research bias occurs when an examiner unconsciously inflates a student's abilities because he or she knows the student participated in an intervention and "should" improve. Potential for research bias is reduced when blinding is used. **Blinding** means that the individual who assesses the students is not the same individual who provides the intervention or directs the study. Without blinding, there is potential for contamination of outcome data.

Contamination also occurs when the individual providing the treatment fails to implement the treatment as planned. To counter this possibility, high-quality studies include measures of treatment fidelity. **Fidelity** refers to the degree to which an intervention is carried out as described. One way to document intervention fidelity is to videotape intervention sessions and count or code the interventionist's behaviors.

A second factor impacting research quality is documentation of group similarity prior to the intervention. As I have already pointed out, randomization makes it more likely that the groups do not differ. However, in communication disorders research, investigators must also demonstrate prior to the study that subjects in treatment and comparison groups are relatively the same. Without this assurance, it can be argued that the participants' ability level or environmental circumstances influenced the results. For example, consider that I am completing a study, and I find that my comparison-group students are significantly more impaired than my treatment-group students. My results are affected because I cannot be certain treatment-group improvement is due to my intervention. Because the treatment group was (on average) less impaired, improvement may represent natural development and may not represent change due to the intervention. To minimize this factor, prior to implementing an intervention, researchers document participants' age, communication ability, socioeconomic status, classroom environment, intellectual ability, ethnicity, etc. Documentation and analysis clarify group equivalency prior to the treatment implementation.

A third factor in research design relates to assessment. Good research studies use highly reliable and valid measures to document change in students' behaviors. You will learn how to judge the reliability and validity of assessment measure in Chapter 4.

The final factor to be considered when evaluating a research design is the need for study results to be statistically significant as well as clinically meaningful (Schuele & Justice, 2006). To determine significance, the (most basic) process is to compare mean performance between treatment and comparison groups. Significance tests reflect the probability that the reported outcome being due to chance, or random fluctuation, is adequately small. When interpreting intervention research, statistical significance demonstrates that the intervention made a *real* difference in student performance.

Although statistical significance is important, by itself it is not sufficient. It is possible for a study to produce statistical significance, but the degree of change may not be clinically meaningful. To overcome the limited interpretability of statistical significance, high-quality research studies report effect sizes. **Effect-size estimates** are numerical values designed to characterize results in functional and meaningful ways. Effect-size data indicate the magnitude of an effect in addition to estimates of probability (Schuele & Justice, 2006). Typically, effect-size estimates are interpreted with two processes. The first process uses a commonly accepted benchmark to differentiate small, medium, and large effect sizes (Cohen's *d:* .2 = small effect, .5 = medium effect, and .8 = large effect; Cohen, 1988). In a second process, the researcher compares his or her effect size to effect sizes achieved in similar studies.

Now that you understand the factors used to determine a research design's quality, consider the steps I followed when evaluating one study (Figure 1.3). As you can see, I evaluated an RCT that compared the language gains between three groups of students with language impairment following an intervention. Students were randomly assigned to receive either a specialized computer intervention (i.e., Fast ForWord) or two alternative group assignments (a generic computer program and a no-treatment group). With your classmates, consider each factor in the left-hand column and identify the study characteristics that align with each factor (in the right-hand column). Hopefully, by examining one RCT in detail, you will gain an appreciation of how the EBP process works. At the end of the chapter, I provide several suggestions of additional RCTs that could be analyzed in a similar fashion.

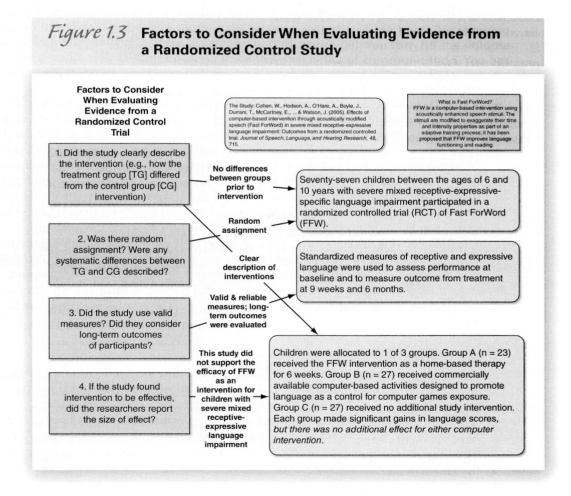

Figure 1.3 **Factors to Consider When Evaluating Evidence from a Randomized Control Study**

Although in this example I evaluated a Level I study, remember that Level II, III, and IV studies also can be of very high quality even though they are not randomized comparison-group studies (Fey, 2006; Justice & Fey, 2004). High quality at Levels II to IV is documented with similar factors as described for Level I studies: careful description of subject characteristics, the use of valid and reliable measures to document change, minimization of contamination of results, and reporting of outcome data to document significant and meaningful results.

EBP: EVALUATING THE QUANTITY OF DATA AND USING DATA TO MAKE CLINICAL DECISIONS

When professionals use EBP decision making to guide intervention selection, they also consider the quantity of supporting evidence (ASHA, 2005; Justice, 2006). Interventions with a body of documentation have more evidence supporting their use. Many commonly used speech-language pathology interventions have not yet been evaluated by RCT studies. In such cases, a professional examines the body of evidence across all levels, including nonrandomized research studies, case studies, and expert opinion.

Interventionists develop skills to assess research results and judge the accumulated body of research on a proposed intervention. Professionals use searches to access peer-reviewed research, such as the one available with Google Scholar (http://scholar.google.com). In contrast to regular Google access (which typically does not represent peer-reviewed research), Google Scholar allows a professional to access peer-reviewed research (Nail-Chiwetalu & Ratner, 2006).

In addition to searching for research studies on Google Scholar, today's SLPs have many additional resources to help locate high-quality research studies. For example, in 2005, ASHA began to compile research on intervention effectiveness. This database is called the Compendium of EBP Guidelines and Systematic Reviews, and if you are a NSSHLA member, you can access the site at www.asha.org/members/ebp/compendium/. As a classroom activity, go to this site and look at the systematic reviews under the category "Language disorders." As you can see, there are many different reviews; as you progress through the chapters in this book, go back and search for topics that are covered (e.g., hearing loss, autism, specific language impairment, literacy and reading).

After looking at the possible reviews, begin to consider how evaluating the research will help you select the appropriate intervention approach for students with communication disorders. To help in this process, whenever possible I include a description of the level of evidence for each intervention approach I present in this book. By threading this information throughout the book, my intent is to help you become more comfortable with EBP concepts.

EBP: FINAL THOUGHTS

EBP is very important to the field of speech-language pathology and education. However, it may take some practice and thought before you feel comfortable evaluating the quality of clinical and educational research. Remember that practitioners across many professions use EBP to help guide their clinical decisions. Using EBP helps them answer the question; "Is there clear evidence that the approach I am recommending will be effective?" Understanding the principles of EBP will set you on the path to becoming a successful professional.

Summary

- A language disorder is impaired comprehension or use of spoken, written, or other symbol systems. An individual with a language disorder is different from someone with a language difference. Language difference is a variation of a symbol system used by a group of individuals that reflects and is determined by shared regional, social, or cultural/ethnic factors. Sometimes a young child (2 to 3 years old) who exhibits a developmental lag in language is referred to as having late language emergence; experts use this terminology because language impairment cannot be reliably diagnosed in young children in the absence of a primary disorder.
- Receptive and expressive language occurs at the linguistic level of the speech chain. Other communication processes that are within the motor/physical and the acoustic levels contribute to the communication system.
- Language consists of three overall domains: form (syntax, morphology, phonology), content (semantics), and use (pragmatics). The three domains are interdependent, and an effective communicator demonstrates proficiency in all three domains.
- Evidence-based practice (EBP) refers to the process that practitioners use to evaluate whether a clinical practice, strategy, program, curriculum, or intervention is backed by rigorous evidence of effectiveness and whether a practice is appropriate for a particular individual. Research studies are evaluated according to four levels of evidence. Level I refers to randomized comparison-group studies; this is considered the "gold standard" of research evidence. Level II represents research from nonrandomized experiments but with good experimental design from several different researchers. Level III represents research from correlational studies or case studies, and Level IV refers to expert opinion.

Discussion and In-Class Activities

1. In groups, give examples of communication behaviors in children's morphology, pragmatics, semantics, and syntax that will be demonstrated as the child matures.
2. Explain the speech chain model to an individual who is not in your class. Draw a simple diagram to illustrate your explanation. Role-play this explanation in class.
3. Go to the video library at the Colorado Department of Education: www.cde.state.co.us/resultsmatter/RMVideoSeries.htm. Watch several of the child-interaction videos and discuss the behaviors or language that illustrate the domains *form, content,* and *use.* How do these domains overlap in the communication that you see?
4. Using the process outlined in Figure 1.3, evaluate the following research studies:

   Gillam, S. L., Gillam, R. B., & Reece, K. (2012). Language outcomes of contextualized and decontextualized language intervention: Results of an early efficacy study. *Language, Speech, & Hearing Services in Schools, 43,* 276–291.

   Justice, L. M., Mashburn, A., Pence, K. L., & Wiggins, A. (2008). Experimental evaluation of a preschool language curriculum: Influence on children's expressive language skills. *Journal of Speech, Language, & Hearing Research, 51,* 983–1001.

Ruston, H. P., & Schwanenflugel, P. J. (2010). Effects of a conversation intervention on the expressive vocabulary development of prekindergarten children. *Language, Speech, & Hearing Services in Schools, 41,* 303–313.

Discuss in class whether you feel these studies would qualify as Level I or Level II in the levels-of-evidence hierarchy.

Chapter 1 Case Study

Consider each of the descriptions of a child with a language delay or disorder. Discuss in class whether you think the child has a disorder of form, content, or use. Sometimes more than one domain is impacted. Remember that the goal in this first case assignment is for you to begin talking and discussing the concepts of form, content, and use. I provide many more details about the domains in Chapter 2.

- Olivia is 29 months old. She plays with toys in age-appropriate ways, points at objects she wants, and interacts socially with her brother and parents. She has three words she uses to communicate: *mama, kitty,* and *Bob* (her brother).
- Gina is 10 years old. She has difficulty reading and makes many grammatical errors in her writing. Her sentences are short and unelaborated. She is well liked by her peers and is a very good soccer player.
- Colton is 8 and has difficulty making eye contact. Although he can talk, he rarely initiates communication with others. When he does communicate, he wants to talk about his passion—trains—to the exclusion of other topics.

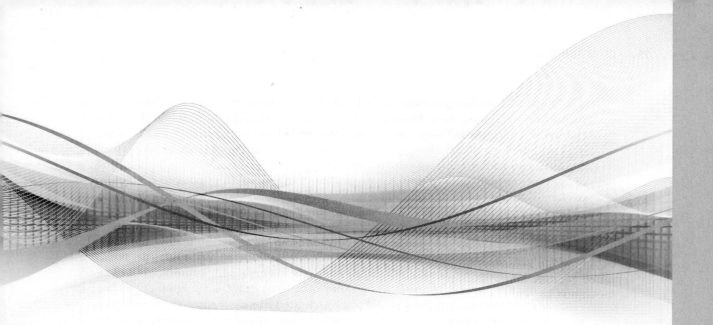

2 Language Theory and the Communication Subdomains

Chapter Overview Questions

1. What are the primary differences between the *nature* and *nurture* perspectives of language development?

2. What are the four different theories of language development as described in this chapter?

3. How does each theory influence intervention approaches?

4. What are the five different communication subdomains?

5. What is the most important communication characteristic associated with each subdomain?

6. How do practitioners use information regarding the subdomains to guide clinical interventions?

The first two chapters of this book introduce you to important fundamental concepts. I build on these foundational concepts in future chapters that focus on language disorders. In Chapter 1, you learned important terminology associated with language disorders and read about the foundational clinical principle *evidence-based practice*. This chapter continues to build on that information by (a) introducing four major theories of language development and (b) discussing how children move through the language domains of form, content, and use with the communication subdomains model.

I hope you are not groaning inwardly at the mention of language theories! This book focuses on explaining how language theories are important principles used to identify children's language challenges and to develop intervention programs. I will be referring back to language theory throughout this book when I discuss intervention options for children with communication impairments.

It is important to recognize that no single theory can explain the complex process of communication, but each theory makes a contribution toward understanding how language develops and how intervention helps children who struggle to communicate. To help you understand the contributions of language theory, I first provide an overview of the debate between the nature and nurture theories of language development. Then I present more detailed information on four theories of language development: behaviorism, constructivist theory (i.e., Piagetian cognitive theory), social interactionist theory, and emergentist theory. You will learn about other important language theories later in your clinical training, but the four theories presented in this chapter are foundational. I will refer to these theories in later chapters when I present information on specific clinical interventions.

Language Development: Nature versus Nurture

Perhaps the most fundamental issue in language development focuses on the question "How and why does a child develop language?" Many theorists have debated this question, and the popularity of various theories has changed over time. It is important for a language practitioner to understand the underlying issues regarding these debates, because strong intervention approaches are linked to language theory. When a skilled practitioner chooses an intervention approach, she must understand its theoretical base.

A historical debate centers on whether language is an innate ability of humans or a function of an individual's environment. This debate is often referred to as *nature* versus *nurture*. Theories favoring the contribution of nature to language development began with Plato in classical Greece and evolved into a viewpoint supported by Noam Chomsky in the 1950s. A summary of the nature-supported position is that certain fundamental language skills are innate, and language capacity is present from birth. Theorists who favor the role of nature are sometimes referred to as *nativists* or (historically) as *rationalists*.

On the opposite side of the theoretical debate are those who favor the environment as the critical factor in language development. Theorists who support this position are sometimes referred to as *empiricists*. In an extreme interpretation of the empiricist viewpoint, a newborn is a "blank slate" on which the environment shapes language development. The empiricist viewpoint has shaped many language theories, including the behavioral theories of B. F. Skinner (1957), and it has played an important role in the Piagetian perspective (1926/1952). I will be discussing behaviorism and Piaget's cognitive constructivist approach in the sections below.

It is important to remember that there is no simple answer to the question of how children learn language so quickly and so uniformly across many different cultures. However, for now, remember that the theories presented in this chapter—behaviorist, constructivist, social interactionist, and emergentist—represent different viewpoints along the nature-versus-nurture continuum.

BEHAVIORIST THEORY

Behaviorist theory that suggests that learning occurs when an environmental stimulus triggers a response or behavior. As mentioned previously, this theory is strongly influenced by the empiricist viewpoint. Behavioral principles suggest that when we reward or punish behaviors, we can either increase the frequency of positive behaviors or decrease or alter negative behaviors. B. F. Skinner (1957) is the individual most closely associated with behaviorism.

Skinner proposed that language, like other behavior, is produced because caregivers selectively reinforce words. For example, the parent says the word "*cracker,*" and the child responds by saying "*ka-ka.*" The parent says, "*Yes, this is a cracker!*" and gives the child a cracker. The parent's positive response and the cracker both provide reinforcement.

The word *ka-ka* gradually is shaped to match the adult production of the word. **Shaping** occurs when an individual is expected to produce closer approximations to the behavioral target prior to reinforcement. In this example, the parent eventually expects the child to say "*cracker*" before providing the desired item.

A number of important concepts used in speech-language pathology and special education are based on behaviorist theory:

- *Reinforcement:* Reinforcing a child's behavior makes it more likely that the behavior will occur in the future. **Positive reinforcement** is a stimulus using pleasant rewards that increases the frequency of a particular behavior. In contrast, **negative reinforcement** is unpleasant to the child. An example of negative reinforcement is an adult frowning, nagging, or making disapproving comments to a child and continuing to do so until the unwanted behavior ends. The child stops the unwanted behavior (presumably producing a more desirable behavior) to avoid the negative stimuli. Reinforcement can be social ("high-fives," smiles, encouragement, or praise), activities (participating in a pizza party following successful completion of therapy activities), or material (allowing the child to have favorite foods or earn points for toys).
- *Extinction:* Extinction is based on the behavioral principle that when a child's response is not reinforced, the ignored behavior will decrease or disappear. An example of extinction is ignoring a child's negative behavior.
- *Antecedent:* An antecedent event is a stimulus that precedes a behavior. The child's behavior (with reinforcement) can be linked to the antecedent event. For example, a child sees a cookie (the antecedent event) and says, "*Want cookie!*"
- *Punishment:* Punishment is a negative response that a child views as undesirable. It follows a behavior that the adult wishes to eliminate. Punishment makes it less likely that the negative behavior will occur; an example of punishment is placing a child in a "time-out chair" following the child's misbehavior.
- *Chaining:* **Behavioral chaining** occurs when an activity requires a number of linked steps; a complex behavioral sequence is broken down into smaller units so the child can be trained to complete a multistep task. For example, if a child is being trained to wash his hands, he is first taught to turn on the water, then to use soap and engage in hand washing, then to turn off the water, and then to dry his hands. Individual components are rewarded in successive steps.

Clinical Implications of Behaviorist Theory. Behaviorism has influenced educational practice in many ways. First, drill-and-practice activities within intervention sessions are based on behaviorist theory (Fey, 1986). The goal in drill-and-practice sessions is to stimulate many child behaviors that can be shaped and rewarded by the interventionist. Drill-and-practice also tends to focus on discrete, isolated aspects of language, with the idea that small skills are sequentially linked in a step-by-step approach to form more complex communication behaviors. The step-by-step principle underlies many intervention programs for children with more significant levels of disability (e.g., intellectual disabilities, autism; Pelios, MacDuff, & Axelrod, 2003).

Second, behaviorist theory principles underlie the practitioner's focus on observable and measurable behaviors. Behaviorism demands that a child's responses be documented and that change in language performance be demonstrated by ongoing progress monitoring. A skilled practitioner documents a child's performance and progress toward achieving long-term goals.

All language theories have limitations and strengths in explaining language learning. The limitation of behaviorist theory is that it is not a comprehensive theory; it does not explain how an individual produces complex and novel behaviors. For example, children produce utterances they have not heard, without reinforcement. Behaviorism does not explain this phenomenon. However, behaviorist theory helps explain how children learn discrete behaviors. As a result, the application of behaviorist principles is useful in certain intervention programs.

CONSTRUCTIVIST THEORY

Cognitive constructivist theory is based on the numerous writings of Jean Piaget (e.g., Piaget, 1952). Piaget examined children's logical reasoning abilities (i.e., problem solving) and proposed a sequence of progressively sophisticated cognitive skills, from primitive thinking (at the beginning of the sensorimotor stage) to advanced cognitive ability (in the formal operations stage). Piaget was influenced by empiricist theory because—while he believed that the cognitive processes underlying language (e.g., the mental processes that allow one to recognize, recall, create, and evaluate) are innate—like the other empiricists, he believed language itself is not innate. However, Piaget differed from other empiricists in that he proposed that children actively contribute to the language-learning process. He emphasized that children use the symbolic properties of language to represent conceptual knowledge about the world and that specific cognitive achievements are required for linguistic development. He believed that linkages exist between children's motor ability, play behavior, and language development. Characteristics of Piaget's four stages of cognitive development are summarized in Table 2.1. Figure 2.1 illustrates a child at play who is developing her problem-solving skills at the sensorimotor stage of development.

The parallel development of motor, play, and language milestones is summarized in Table 2.2. There is a very practical need for language interventionists to understand cognitive constructivist theory: Practitioners use Piagetian principles to evaluate cognitive skills needed for language development and often observe children's play behavior with a Piagetian perspective. A detailed description of a play-focused observational protocol is provided in Chapter 6. The following important concepts are based on Piaget's cognitive theory:

- *Schema:* A schema is a concept, mental category, or cognitive structure; children form many different schemata as they interact with their environments. (*Schemata* is the plural form of *schema.*)
- *Assimilation:* A child evidences assimilation when he takes in new information and incorporates it into his existing schemata. When a child sees an unfamiliar animal, such as a camel, and says "*horse,*" he is evidencing assimilation.

Table 2.1 **Piaget's Cognitive Stages**

Age	Stage	Characteristics
Birth to 2 years	Sensorimotor	Begins with reflexive and motor learning. Progresses rapidly, learning object permanence, means–end, etc.
2 to 7 years	Preoperational	Most rapid stage of language learning. Child learns to solve physical problems.
7 to 11 years	Concrete operations	Child learns to categorize and organize information; begins to be a logical thinker.
11 to 15 years	Formal operations	Learns to be an abstract thinker, tests mental hypotheses.

Figure 2.1 **An Infant's Exploration of Her Physical Environment Facilitates Cognitive Development**

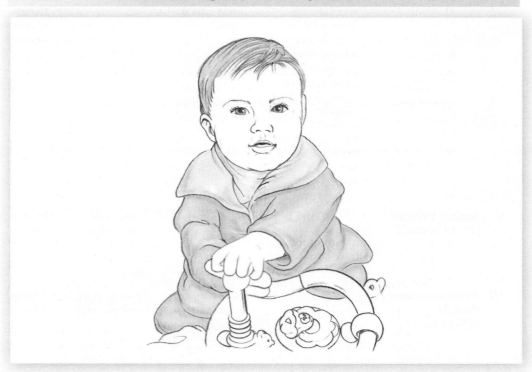

Table 2.2 **Linkages between Piaget's Sensorimotor Substages and Motor/ Cognitive, Play, and Communication Behaviors**

Substage (age)	Motor/cognitive	Interactions and imitation	Play	Communication
I Reflexive (Birth–1 month)		• Interactions are caregiver initiated		
II Primary circular (1–4 months)		• Child repeats own behaviors	• Grasping, looking at object	• Cries, laughs, coos
III Secondary circular (4–8 months)	• Behaves as if he or she is cause of all actions (early causality)	• Imitates behaviors that he or she has produced before • Child begins to initiate interactions	• Begins to interact with people with gestures and vocalizations	• Babbles (child actively interacts) • Beginnings of semantic understanding (6–8 months)
IV Causality (8–12 months)	• Looks for object if sees it being hidden (object permanence) • Knows other people can cause activities (more developed causality) • Evidence of planning of intentional behaviors (means–end)	• Imitates behaviors not produced before		• Links gestures and vocalization • Expansion of semantic function
V Tertiary circular (12–18 months)			• Figures out how to make toys work (cause and effect)	• First meaningful words
VI Representational thought (18–24 months)		• Imitates actions that are stored mentally	• Progresses to symbolic play	• Multiple-word utterances

- *Accommodation:* A child evidences accommodation when he adjusts his schemata on the basis of new information. In the preceding example, the child eventually accommodates new information and uses the word "*camel.*"
- *Equilibrium:* Piaget believed that children attempt to find a balance between assimilating new information into old schemata and developing new schemata through accommodation. This balance is called equilibrium.
- *Disequilibrium:* As a child recognizes that two schemata are contradictory, disequilibrium occurs. Reorganization to higher levels of thinking is motivated by this disequilibrium. Disequilibrium is evidenced in the preceding example when the child recognizes that the word "*horse*" fails to capture the camel's unique characteristics.
- *Symbolic play:* Symbolic play is evidenced when a child uses one object to represent another. For example, a child might tie a towel around his neck and say the towel is a cape and that he is Superman.
- *Object permanence:* A child evidences object permanence during the sensorimotor stage of development when he realizes that an object exists even when he cannot see it. Very young children cannot understand that objects continue to exist even when they can't be seen or felt. For example, prior to achieving object permanence, a child will quickly lose interest in (and not search for) a hidden toy.
- *Object constancy:* Object constancy is another concept of the sensorimotor stage; a child learns that he is viewing the same object, regardless of distance, light, or different viewing angle.
- *Means–end:* Means–end behavior is evidenced when a child demonstrates intentionality; it occurs when the child identifies a problem and makes a plan to solve the problem. An example of means–end behavior is a child pushing a button or pulling a string to make a toy move. A child calling out "*Mama!*" and waiting for his mother to appear also demonstrates means–end behavior.

Practice your clinical problem-solving skills by considering the information in Focus 2.1. What Piagetian concepts are the children demonstrating in each example?

Clinical Implications of Cognitive Theory. Practitioners observe children's play behaviors to gauge children's general cognitive ability and level of representational thought. I provide an example of this decision-making process in Figure 2.2. Representational

---

FOCUS 2.1 *Clinical Skill Building*

Use what you know about Piaget's sensorimotor stages. What cognitive process (or processes) is each child demonstrating?

- Child pulls off his sock, gleefully throws it on the ground, and then looks down to see where it has fallen.

- Child pulls a toy toward herself, using a string tied to the toy.
- Child waves good-bye as he leaves his father; his father is waving and saying "*bye-bye!*"
- The child's mother walks around a corner, and the child immediately starts to cry.

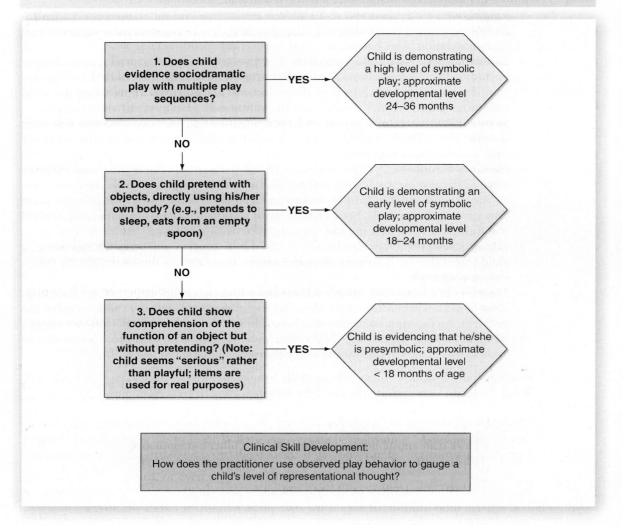

Figure 2.2 **Observing Children's Play to Understand Levels of Representational Thought**

1. Does child evidence sociodramatic play with multiple play sequences?

YES → Child is demonstrating a high level of symbolic play; approximate developmental level 24–36 months

NO ↓

2. Does child pretend with objects, directly using his/her own body? (e.g., pretends to sleep, eats from an empty spoon)

YES → Child is demonstrating an early level of symbolic play; approximate developmental level 18–24 months

NO ↓

3. Does child show comprehension of the function of an object but without pretending? (Note: child seems "serious" rather than playful; items are used for real purposes)

YES → Child is evidencing that he/she is presymbolic; approximate developmental level < 18 months of age

Clinical Skill Development:
How does the practitioner use observed play behavior to gauge a child's level of representational thought?

thought is the child's ability to represent one object with another. An example of high-level symbolic play (the first step in Figure 2.2) is a child pretending to cook dinner, setting the table, placing dolls and stuffed animals around the table, and pretending to serve dinner. Practitioners look for evidence of representational thought to gauge a child's readiness for symbolic language.

The limitation of cognitive constructivist theory is the proposal that children (a) move through discrete and qualitatively different stages of development and (b) work through the stages sequentially. A child at the sensorimotor stage is thought to solve problems by using qualitatively different strategies than a child at a later stage of development. However, children do not always follow this linear and step-by-step developmental progression. Sometimes children solve surprisingly difficult problems (i.e., problems seemingly beyond their cognitive stage) within certain contexts and with the right support. On the other hand, the strength of cognitive constructivist theory is that it helps practitioners understand how children use physical exploration to increase their problem-solving abilities.

SOCIAL INTERACTIONIST THEORY

Social interactionists view language as a means of making social connections and communicating ideas (Nelson, 2010). Social interactionists favor the role of nurture in the nature–nurture debate. An early advocate for this position was Lev Vygotsky (1934). Vygosky was a Russian psychologist; his work was translated into English and began to influence modern language theory in the 1970s.

Vygotsky viewed a child's interactions with adults and more able peers as being key to their overall development. Like Piaget, Vygotsky believed that children construct their own knowledge. However, whereas Piaget believed that cognitive development occurs primarily through children's interaction with physical objects, Vygotsky believed that cognitive development is socially mediated—that is, that a child's interactions with others influences cognitive understandings (Bodrova & Leong, 2007).

Vygotsky proposed that initially a child and a more capable partner (an adult or older child) solve problems together, but eventually the child internalizes the process and is able to carry out the function independently. There has been an explosion of research exploring Vygotskian principles in recent years (Winsler, 2003).

Vygotsky also asserted that language plays a critical role in shaping learning and thought. For example, he proposed that **private speech** plays a role in cognitive development. Private speech occurs when children speak aloud as they are engaged in play. Vygotsky's view was that private speech is a step that allows children to internalize important concepts. One of the most important Vygotskian principles is the notion of the **zone of proximal development (ZPD)**. The ZPD is the competence that a child demonstrates with minimal assistance. The ZPD is the area between the zone of competence (what a child can do independently) and the zone of incompetence (what a child is unable to do, even with assistance; Baroody, Lai, & Mix, 2006). Vygotsky proposed that teaching children within the ZPD (at the point where children can *just* perform a task with some assistance) is the key to maximizing child learning. Using the ZPD principle has prompted practitioners to introduce tasks to young children even when the tasks are difficult (Kaderavek & Justice, 2004). For example, preschool children are engaged in early literacy activities with adult support. You will learn more about this concept in Chapter 10.

Social interactionists believe that parents play a critical role in children's language development. Parents provide support for their child's learning by introducing names for objects and actions in meaningful contexts, by responding to a child's utterances, and by finding ways to show or tell children when there are linguistic confusions. For example, if a child says, "*You drinking juice,*" the adult typically says, "*Mommy is drinking coffee; this coffee is hot!*" When parents expand their child's utterances, they are providing subtle feedback about the child's language. Vygotsky's social interactionist theory was made prominent in the Western world by Jerome Bruner (1983), who emphasized the role of adult–child interaction in children's language learning. Additional important concepts in social interactionist theory include:

- *Infant-directed talk:* Infant-directed talk (also called **motherese;** Baldwin & Meyer, 2007) describes the characteristics of child-directed communication that enhance an infant's ability to learn language. Characteristics of infant-directed talk include the use of content words (i.e., nouns, verbs) in isolation, placement of content words at the end of sentences ("*A doggie, see the doggie?*"), increased pitch on content words, and talking about objects and events in the "here and now." It has been theorized that these facilitating characteristics help infants extract the important information and make linkages between speech and objects or events.
- *Coordinating attention:* Adults follow an infant's focus of attention and match their communication to the child's eye gaze. Also, in Western cultures, adults try to direct infants' attention to specific objects by pointing or showing (Baldwin & Meyer, 2007).
- *Scaffolding:* Scaffolding refers to adult support that allows a child to engage in a challenging activity. Scaffolding techniques can include simplifying a task, providing directions and clarifying a task, reducing a child's frustration, modeling a correct response, and motivating and soliciting a child's task engagement. When used effectively, scaffolding is faded from levels of high support to minimal levels of guidance.
- *Mediation:* The term *mediation* is related to scaffolding. In scaffolding, the focus is on the adult's manipulation of the task to increase the learner's success. In mediation, the goal is to provide the learner with insights in order to teach the learner "how to learn." During a mediated learning task, the student is encouraged to accept responsibility so that he or she can function more independently. When mediating a task, the practitioner might say, "*Tell me the steps you are going to follow to finish this project.*" The practitioner's goal is to increase the student's awareness of the steps required for task completion.
- *Parent–child communication routines:* Adults structure infant play routines in systematic patterns sometimes called scripts. **Scripts** involve predictable patterns of action that facilitate infant participation. The interaction familiarity allows the child to anticipate his or her role in the interaction, building pragmatic communication skills (Baldwin & Meyer, 2007; Bruner, 1981). Examples include "*How big is baby? SO big!*" (the child is encouraged to lift his or her arms overhead); "*Peek-a-boo!*" (the child anticipates the "*boo!*" by laughing and eventually initiates hiding); repeated book-reading routines (parent repeats familiar vocabulary or prompts actions); and waving while saying "*bye-bye.*"

Clinical Implications of Social Interactionist Theory.   Speech-language pathologists (SLPs) and special educators frame many of their assessments and interventions based on social interactionist theory. Social interactionist theory encourages practitioners to incorporate children's caregivers into intervention programs and to work with children in their homes and classrooms to build social interactions. I describe strategies to enhance child–caregiver language interactions in Chapter 6.

The limitation of social interaction theory is that, taken on its own, it does not explain everything about language development. For example, in some cultures caregivers do not use infant-directed speech, yet children still develop language. Again, we are reminded that one language theory, by itself, is not sufficient to explain the complex behavior of language development.

EMERGENTIST THEORY

While the theories discussed so far have been discussed for decades (and even centuries), there is a relative newcomer to language theory: emergentist theory. Proponents of emergentist theory believe that debates on whether language ability is based on nature or nurture are overly simplistic and reflect a time when researchers lacked access to sophisticated computer modeling programs and brain imaging procedures (e.g., functional magnetic resonance imaging [fMRI]). Enhanced technology allows language researchers to explore language development in ways not possible in the past (MacWhinney, 1998, 2010). Learn more about how emergentist research uses current technology in Focus 2.2.

In the emergentist position, language learning is an interconnected system that involves more than a person's genetic makeup, his or her environment, or the neural connections that develop as a child is exposed to a language. It is a complex, open system in which a child's biology adapts to his or her environment. Importantly, emergentist theory underscores the need for children to be actively engaged in their environments (Evans, 2008). In order for a system to adapt and change, the child must be an active user and processor of language input.

Emergentist theory guides many current research programs focusing on children's language acquisition. One research approach uses computer simulations to model how the brain develops neural linkages that support language learning. It is hypothesized, for example, that children learn to extract specific language features because they detect consistent patterns (i.e., cues). For example, it has been estimated that a human hears more than 15 acoustic sounds in every speech syllable (Anderson, 2000). However, very quickly a toddler learns that some acoustic differences are important and others are not. Think about the subtle but important distinction between "*spot*" and "*stop*" (especially if the toddler is running toward the street!). At an early age, the child's recognition of an acoustic pattern increases survival (an evolutionary rationale for the cognitive skills needed to develop a language system). Linguistic cues are also provided by a child's understanding of a situation (i.e., pragmatic cues) or can be provided by word order or meaning. Using acoustic, pragmatic, semantic, or syntax cues to detect language patterns is biologically efficient because it reduces the child's cognitive load and has the previously described evolutionary function. Computer simulations are used to understand how cue recognition streamlines language comprehension and use.

FOCUS 2.2   *Research*

Emergentist research is data driven. The computer simulations critical to emergentist research require transcribed child language; a source of these language samples is the *Child Language Data Exchange System* (CHILDES). CHILDES was established in 1984 to serve as a repository for language data. Its earliest transcripts date from the 1960s, and CHILDES now has language samples (transcripts, audio, and video) in more than 20 languages. During the early 1990s, CHILDES researchers developed software programs capable of analyzing language transcripts. To date, more than 3,000 published studies cite the CHILDES database or transcription software as a source of their data or data analysis. You can learn more about the CHILDES repository at http://childes.psy.cmu.edu/intro/.

Clinical Implications of Emergentist Theory. An emergentist perspective can be used to guide language assessment and intervention. A practitioner who uses an emergentist perspective is likely to attend to the inconsistencies in a child's language and carefully note emerging features. Intervention with this theoretical base would engage the child with targeted features to foster systemwide change. The emergentist approach is consistent with two intervention approaches discussed in later chapters: language recasting and focused stimulation (Poll, 2011).

The Five Communication Subdomains

Experts have developed and debated the theories discussed above; these theories are critical to our understanding of the field. This section of the chapter is not about language theory—rather, it discusses the five communication subdomains, a model of language development that I have created to help students understand how children move through the language domains form, content, and use. In my teaching, I find that many beginning clinicians struggle to understand where to start with a child who has communication impairments. An experienced SLP can assess a child and fairly quickly determine whether the child needs to work primarily on social language (i.e., pragmatics) or word combinations (i.e., semantics), or whether the communication impairment involves the child's use of grammar and sentence complexity (i.e., syntax). To help students learn clinical decision-making skills, I train them to consider sequentially each of the subdomains when analyzing a child's communication behaviors. So, after you review the information in Focus 2.3, let me introduce you to the communication subdomains.

To understand the five communication subdomains, consider Figure 2.3. This figure presents form, content, and use in parallel boxes aligned in relation to four age groups: infant, toddler, preschool, and school-age children. Form, content, and use are represented by the left-to-right columns in Figure 2.3. The age groups are shown from top to bottom. Form, content, and use are subdivided into five communication subdomains: early pragmatics, vocabulary, early word combinations, morphosyntax, and discourse. Practice your clinical decision-making skills regarding form, content, and use by reading and thinking about the information in Focus 2.4.

FOCUS 2.3 *Clinical Skill Building*

As you learned in Chapter 1, form, content, and use are typically presented in a Venn diagram as three linked circles. The linked circles remind us that the three domains interact with each other and that no single domain functions in isolation. Keep this important relationship in mind as you read about the communication subdomains. I present the subdomains in linear fashion—to help students understand how the domains develop—but it is important not to lose sight of the critical relationships between the domains. It is the relationship between form, content, and use that allows an individual to be an effective communicator.

Figure 2.3   **Diagram Demonstrating Form, Content, and Use and the Five Communication Subdomains**

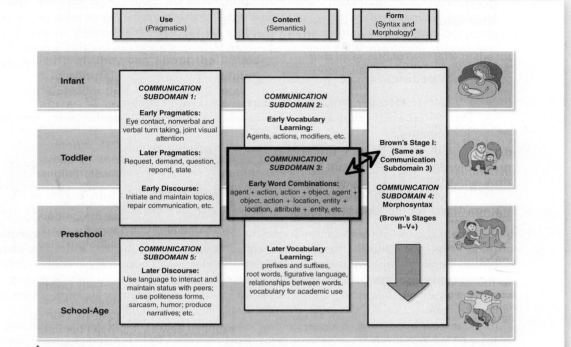

*Phonology also is an important component of the form domain, although it is not a focus of this text.

FOCUS 2.4   *Clinical Skill Building*

Consider the following case examples and decide whether the deficits reflect form, content, or use. Remember that sometimes a deficit impacts more than one domain.

- A fourth-grade student is having difficulty comprehending his reading, especially in science and geography. He is very social and gets along well with his peers.
- A sixth-grade student who has been diagnosed with a learning disability does not appear to understand when other students are using sarcasm; he takes their statements literally. This situation is causing problems at school.
- A 2-year-old has 50+ words, but almost all of the words are nouns. He is not making 2-word combinations.
- An eighth-grade student is getting poor grades in writing composition. His teacher says his writing is "immature" and that he does not write with enough complexity.

The five subdomains are presented in the following pages in this order: (1) early pragmatics, (2) vocabulary, (3) early word combinations, (4) morphosyntax, and (5) discourse. This order parallels the thinking process of a skilled practitioner. When a skilled practitioner observes an individual's communication, he or she mentally "checks off" specific language abilities that are (or are not) observed. The process is not hit or miss; on the contrary, the important communication behaviors are identified, deliberately observed, and sequentially documented. As mentioned earlier, to train students to use this process, I ask them to consider each subdomain one step at a time. During a child language observation, I ask each student to answer the following questions:

- Do you see the early pragmatic skills associated with Subdomain 1?
- Do you see the beginning use of vocabulary in the young speaker associated with Subdomain 2?
- Do you see the word combinations expected in Subdomain 3?
- Is the student developing the advanced vocabulary expected at later stages of Subdomain 2?
- Do you see the morphosyntax features associated with Subdomain 4?
- Do you see the sophisticated discourse skills typically seen with Subdomain 5?

When the student answers each question, he or she focuses attention on the sequential process of communication development. Through this step-by-step process, students' critical-thinking skills become more deliberate and focused. I hope this overview is helpful as you read about each of the communication subdomains. As you read about each of the communication subdomains, merge this model with all your prior knowledge of language development.

It is also important that you connect the subdomains with your understanding of Brown's stages of language development. Roger Brown (1973) traced children's syntax acquisition by considering their mean length of utterance (MLU; i.e., average sentence length) and documenting the morphemes occurring at varying levels of MLU. Brown's Stage I is demonstrated in children between 12 and 26 months of age; it describes children prior to their use of morphemes. In contrast, Brown's Stages II–V+ describe children with MLUs of 2–4+ words per utterance. Brown's Stages II–V+ occur in children developing typically between the ages of 27 and 46 months (2 to 4 years of age).

At Brown's Stages II–V+, children demonstrate an increasing use of morphological forms. I will be describing children's morphosyntax development in the section on Communication Subdomain 4. More background on Roger Brown and his stages of language acquisition are provided in Focus 2.5. An overview of Brown's stages of syntax development and his morphological features associated with each stage is provided in Table 2.3.

Following the discussion of each communication subdomain, I cover briefly the implications of the subdomain skills in relation to assessment and intervention. I will refer back to the five communication subdomains in upcoming chapters.

Subdomain 1: Early Pragmatic Skills

Communication Subdomain 1 begins at birth and is observed in children's prelinguistic communication. Figure 2.4 is a visual graphic for Communication Subdomain 1. At the earliest stages, children make sounds, movements, and gestures, and they give visual attention without communication intention. However, communication partners attribute meaning to these actions, with the result that children developing typically eventually

FOCUS 2.5 *Learning More*

In 1962, Roger Brown and his associates at Harvard began a long-term study of syntax and morphological development. They followed the language development of three children they called Adam, Eve, and Sarah. Researchers observed and transcribed the children's speech every week for a period of 1 year (for Eve) to 5 years (Adam and Sarah). Observations lasted from 30 minutes to over 2 hours. Brown partitioned the children's increasingly longer utterances into five stages, according to the children's MLU.

Brown noted that during Stage II, the children's utterances typically became longer than two words and other linguistic forms (morphemes) emerged. Brown analyzed intensively 14 of the morphemes; he suggested that morphemes emerge in a specific sequence in most children: (1) the present progressive *ing* inflection on verbs; (2 & 3) the locative prepositions *in* and *on* (these develop at the same time); (4) the plural *s* inflection on nouns; (5) past irregular verbal inflections such as *did, went,* and *came* (Brown looked at a large set of irregular past tense verbs); (6) the possessive *'s* inflection on nouns; (7) the uncontractible copula *be* (In sentences such as "*Here I am*" and "*There it is,*" the copula cannot be contracted.); (8) the definite and indefinite articles *a* and *the*; (9) the past regular *ed* inflection on verbs; (10) the third-person present tense regular verb inflection *s* ("*He talks*"); (11) the third-person present tense irregular verb inflections *does, doesn't,* and *has*; (12) the uncontractible auxiliary *be* (The past tense form cannot be contracted; we must say "*He was going.*"); (13) the contractible copula ("*It's red*"); and (14) the contractible auxiliary *be* ("*He's going*").

Source: Information based on Segal, E. F. (1975), "Psycholinguistics discovers the operant: A review of Roger Brown's 'A first language: The early stages.'" *Journal of the Experimental Analysis of Behavior, 23,* 149–158.

Table 2.3 Brown's Stages of Language Development

Age/Brown's stage	Morphemes	Examples
18–24 months/*Stage I MLU 1.0–2.0*	Semantic combinations: two-word utterances	See Communication Subdomain 3 (Morphological development has not yet emerged.)
24–30 months/*Stage II MLU 2.0–2.5*	*ing* verbs Prepositions (*in, on*) Plural *s*	"*Boy runn*ing." "On *box*." "*See two kitties*."
30–36 months/*Stage III MLU 2.5–3.0*	Irregular past tense verbs Possessive *'s*	"*I went home.*" "*That Daddy's car!*"
36–42 months/*Stage IV MLU 3.0–3.75*	Uncontractible copula Articles (*a, the*) Regular past tense Regular 3rd-person verbs	"*He is.*" "The *toy broke.*" "*Grandpa cooked dinner.*" "*She likes it.*"
42–60 months/*Stage V–V+ MLU 3.75–4+*	Irregular 3rd-person verbs Uncontractible auxiliary Contractible auxiliary Contractible copula	"*The dog has a bone.*" "Is *he going?*" "*Kitty's eating.*" "*He's little.*"

Figure 2.4 **Communication Subdomain 1**

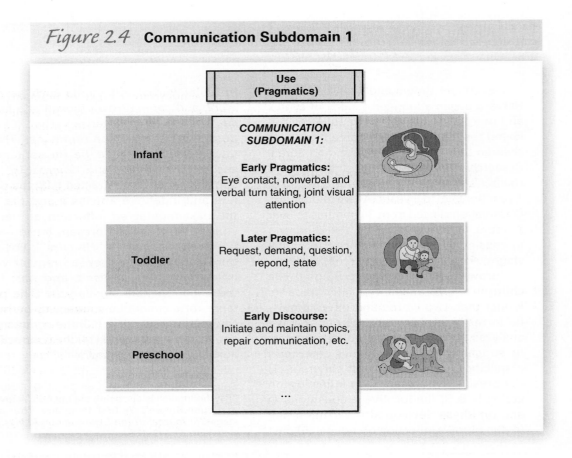

produce these same behaviors with communication intent. Children are thought to have **communication intent** when they exhibit a collection of behaviors including (a) producing gestures, vocalization, and/or eye contact to direct the attention or actions of a communication partner; (b) exhibiting joint visual attention; (c) waiting after a communication attempt (i.e., expecting the partner to respond); or (d) persisting in a communication attempt that is not understood. The frequency and rate of early intentional communication behaviors are associated with more advanced language during the child's later years (Calandrella & Wilcox, 2000).

JOINT VISUAL ATTENTION

Joint visual attention (JVA) is a particularly important early communication skill. The child demonstrates the ability to respond to JVA when he follows the visual direction of an adult's gaze (i.e., looks where the adult is looking). The child initiates JVA when he points or shows an object with the intention of drawing his partner's attention to the object or event. JVC is one of the first interactive communication acts. Children reliably produce JVA between 10 and 12 months of age. It is important to remember that there will be cultural variation with respect to children's use of eye gaze, along with differences in other aspects of early pragmatic function resulting from cultural communication patterns (Ochs & Schieffelin, 2001).

DEVELOPMENT OF EARLY PRAGMATIC FUNCTIONS

Between 8 and 15 months, children begin to demonstrate a range of pragmatic functions. These functions include requesting objects or activities, refusing, and commenting. Between 16 and 23 months, new pragmatic functions are added, including requesting information, answering questions, and acknowledging a response (Chapman, 2000). It is important to remember that children's pragmatic functions can be demonstrated using varying communication means. For example, a child can demonstrate a request by pointing, gesturing, using a word and a gesture, or producing one- or two-word utterances (*"Want cookie"*). In all cases, the child is producing a request, although the way he or she is requesting varies from nonlinguistic to linguistic.

EARLY DISCOURSE SKILLS WITHIN COMMUNICATION SUBDOMAIN 1

As children become more adept communicators, they begin to actively participate in communication exchanges demonstrating the skills associated with discourse. **Discourse** is the connected and contingent flow of communication between two or more individuals. At the beginning stages of Communication Subdomain 1, a child's conversational turns will be nonverbal (e.g., pointing, gesturing). Discourse skills include the following conversational rules that are required to complete a successful communication (Hegde & Maul, 2006):

- Initiating a conversation rather than always depending on the communication partner to initiate a new topic
- Taking turns during a conversational exchange rather than monopolizing the conversation
- Maintaining the ongoing topic of conversation rather than making overly abrupt topic changes
- Using language or nonverbal indicators to indicate when a conversational topic is being switched
- Indicating when the conversation is not understood and/or sensing when the communication partner does not comprehend the conversation (i.e., conversational repair)
- Using language appropriate for the context and situation (i.e., code switching)

The ability to use and request conversational repair is an important discourse skill. **Conversational repair strategies** are verbal behaviors exhibited by a speaker or listener during a communication breakdown. A listener uses conversational repair to indicate that he or she has not understood the speaker's message. A repair can be as simple as *"What?"* or indicated by a more formal request, such as *"I don't understand what you just said."* A speaker uses conversational repair when he or she realizes there has been a communication breakdown. Preschoolers use an early level of communication repair when they repeat their message verbatim. More sophisticated conversational repairs are evidenced when the speaker restates or elaborates the utterance.

The term **code switching** refers to an individual's ability to alternate between formal and informal language in conversations. It also to refers to an individual's ability to vary between dialectal language patterns and General American English. See Focus 2.6 to learn more about dialects.

FOCUS 2.6 *Multicultural Issues*

Dialects are variations of a particular language and are spoken by a large group of people who may share ethnic, regional, or national similarities. A dialect, like a language, has distinct syntactic, semantic, and phonetic features. There are at least 24 regional dialects within the United States. African American English (AAE) is one of the most frequently used nonmajority dialects in the United States. Dialects are often mislabeled as regional accents; however, accents reflect regional differences in phonology (e.g., pronunciation of vowels) and semantics (e.g., use of different words to describe the same object, such as "sack" versus "bag"). When one dialect is seen as "superior and proper," the result is **linguistic chauvinism**. Linguistic chauvinism often results in speakers of a particular dialect being scorned. It may ultimately result in a student being afraid to express himself. Children often bear the brunt of linguistic chauvinism and may suffer psychological distress and educational barriers.

As an example of the negative effects caused by linguist chauvinism, imagine a Jamaican American preschooler trying to communicate to his teacher using the dialect he was taught at home. Initially, the child may be surprised to understand that his teacher does not understand him, and he may be hurt if he is told, "*That is not the right way to speak.*" Instead of reprimanding the child, a teacher should repeat the child's comment in General American English (i.e., "Standard English"). Next, the teacher should briefly explain that it is okay to talk differently at home than at school.

The teacher's explanation about "home language" versus "school language" serves two purposes. First, the explanation facilitates the child's meta-awareness of his speech pattern; it introduces the child to the concept of code switching by explaining that one language or dialect is appropriate at home and another is appropriate at school. Second, the teacher's explanation honors the child's home language and acknowledges that the child has the right to speak with varying dialectal patterns.

A child demonstrates conversational code switching when he or she uses one questioning style with a peer ("*Wanna go?*") and switches to a formal questioning style when communicating to a teacher ("*May I please go to my locker right now?*"). Early discourse skills begin in preschool and continue to advance through the school-age years (see Subdomain 5).

CLINICAL IMPLICATIONS FOR COMMUNICATION SUBDOMAIN 1

The beginning pragmatic skills in Communication Subdomain 1 (i.e., joint visual attention, turn taking) underlie all later communication; children developing typically have pragmatic intent before they produce words (Chapman, 2000). This means that, as a skilled practitioner, you may focus on building pragmatic skills in older children with atypical communication. For example, if you are working with an older student with intellectual disability who lacks joint attention, turn taking, and imitation, you would facilitate these basic pragmatic skills in your intervention program. Pragmatic interventions also include helping individuals with social communication deficits join in peer play or group interactions (Timler, Olswang, & Coggins, 2005).

A focus on underlying pragmatic abilities is generally the first aspect of communication that is "checked off" during the observational process. If an SLP or a special educator identifies a weakness in an individual's ability to enter interactions, become a part of interactions, and stay in interactions, Communication Subdomain 1 becomes the focus of intervention (Fujiki & Brinton, 2009).

Subdomain 2: Vocabulary Development

The early stage of Communication Subdomain 2 (vocabulary development) overlaps with early pragmatic development. In fact, it is important to remember that all the stages in the form, content, and use domains co-occur and influence each other.

Vocabulary development begins toward the end of the first year of life and continues to develop throughout one's life. Vocabulary development "takes off" during the early preschool years and then experiences another surge during the school years, when children develop advanced vocabulary associated with content areas (i.e., content words associated with social studies, science) and written language (see Chapters 6 and 10). Figure 2.5 is a visual presentation of Communication Subdomain 2.

Figure 2.5 Communication Subdomain 2

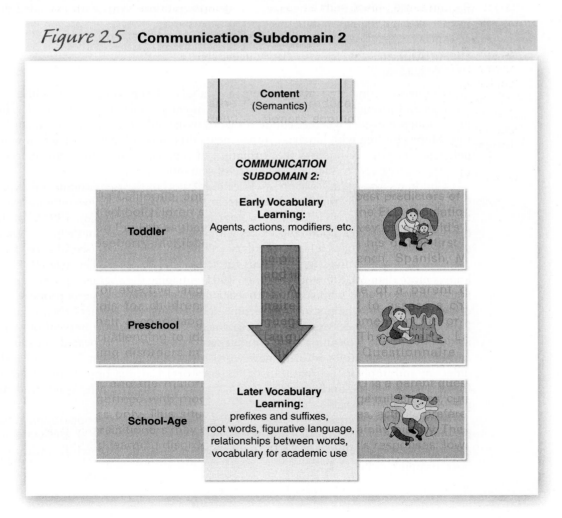

Content
(Semantics)

COMMUNICATION SUBDOMAIN 2:

Early Vocabulary Learning:
Agents, actions, modifiers, etc.

Toddler

Preschool

School-Age

Later Vocabulary Learning:
prefixes and suffixes, root words, figurative language, relationships between words, vocabulary for academic use

A child's first words are typically produced between 10 and 16 months. First words usually describe:

- Appearance/disappearance/recurrence (*"more," "all gone," "hi," "bye-bye"*)
- Names of people, pets, and interesting objects (*"Mama," "Dada," "kitty," "light"*)
- Affective attitudes (*"hug," "no"*) (Chapman, 2000)

Fillmore (1968) proposed that children's semantic use of words precedes syntax and is guided by universal concepts. He named his theory *case grammar*.

Children's vocabulary development progresses quickly: By the time they are 2 years old, children typically produce 200 to 500 words and understand many more words than they produce (Fernald et al., 2001). By 30 months, children's vocabulary consists of approximately 54% common nouns, 7% verbs, and 5% adjectives. Other categories include function words (*the, a, and, mine*) and sound effects (Caselli, Casadio, & Bates, 2001). Semantic deficits are characteristic of many language disorders, including developmental delay, autism spectrum disorder, hearing impairment, and specific language impairment. During the school years, students with language-learning disabilities continue to demonstrate semantic problems. For example, students with language impairments have difficulty comprehending stories in both spoken or written form, have difficulty with figurative (i.e., nonliteral) language, and demonstrate problems with extended discourse (McGregor, 2009).

CLINICAL IMPLICATIONS FOR COMMUNICATION SUBDOMAIN 2

Practitioners continually evaluate whether vocabulary levels can support a child's communication and promote academic achievement. At early stages in vocabulary development, practitioners consider whether children's word usage reflects a variety of semantic categories. Many children with language impairments do not develop enough action words; this deficiency negatively impacts the formation of sentence production. An interventionist may train caregivers to facilitate a variety of semantic forms.

Children's vocabulary use often varies in relation to their environmental experiences. Consider, for example, that first-graders from families of high socioeconomic levels know twice as many words as children from poor families (Hart & Risley, 1995). An interventionist takes this into account and works with some families to train them in book-reading strategies and implement other vocabulary-enhancing approaches (see Chapter 5).

Vocabulary continues to be a focus for school-age students. The average 17-year-old knows more than 60,000 words (Bloom, 2001); imagine the challenges for a student with language impairment who struggles to learn new vocabulary! Experts propose a number of best practices to help students become successful word learners (National Reading Panel, 2000; Nelson & Van Meter, 2006). Successful vocabulary interventions should (a) integrate new word meaning with familiar words; (b) provide repeated, meaningful, and contextual opportunities to learn new words; (c) provide explicit (i.e., teacher-directed, didactic) and implicit (i.e., naturalistic, exploratory) learning opportunities; (d) aim for fluent and automatic understanding and use of new words; and (e) teach students to be more independent word learners.

A concept associated with word learning is called syntactic bootstrapping. **Syntactic bootstrapping** occurs when a child is able to glean the meaning of a novel word from the surrounding function words. I provide more details and research regarding syntactic bootstrapping in Focus 2.7.

FOCUS 2.7   *Research*

Syntactic bootstrapping occurs when a child is able to glean the meaning of a novel word from the surrounding function words. For example, if I say, "*He saw a bleeper,*" you are likely to guess that the word *bleeper* is a noun because it follows the article *a.* Research has confirmed children's use of syntactic bootstrapping at a very young age. For example, Mintz and Gleitman (2002) showed that 36-month-old children identify a word as an adjective from its position in a sentence. In their experiment, a puppet described an object using a nonsense adjective. For example,

"*Look at this* stoof *horsie! This horsie is very* stoof." After presenting the training items, an experimenter showed the children two test objects side by side and asked, "*Look at these two things. Can you give the puppet the stoof one? Can you show the puppet which of these two things is stoof?*" The results indicated that preschoolers identified objects with shared descriptive characteristics (i.e., the same color or size), showing that preschoolers use syntax to make deductions about word characteristics. Syntactic bootstrapping helps children learn the meaning of new words.

Figure 2.6   **Communication Subdomain 3**

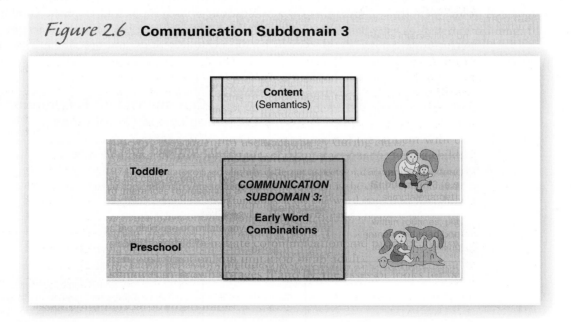

Subdomain 3: Multiple-Word Combinations

Once an individual produces approximately 50 individual words, word combinations begin to emerge. Figure 2.6 visually demonstrates the word combination stage, Communication Subdomain 3. Early word use is not categorized by syntax terms such as *noun* or *verb*. Consequently, Communication Subdomain 3 (early word combinations) and Communication Subdomain 4 (morphosyntax) are qualitatively different. I elaborate on what I mean by "qualitatively different" in the next two paragraphs.

Remember that Brown's stages of language acquisition are framed around syntax and morphological acquisition. Therefore, Communication Subdomain 1 (early pragmatics), Communication Subdomain 2 (early vocabulary learning), and Communication Subdomain 3 (beginning word combinations) all occur *before* a child demonstrates the use of syntax and morphology. I demonstrate this visually in Figure 2.7.

This concept can be confusing for a beginning practitioner. It is important to clear up any confusion, however, because (unfortunately) some interventionists focus on syntax and morphology too soon. So—at the risk of repeating myself—the foundational skills demonstrated within Communication Subdomain 1 (i.e., joint visual attention, turn taking, imitation, early pragmatic skills), the one-word productions uttered at the early stages of Communication Subdomain 2, and the semantic word combinations produced within Communication Subdomain 3 *precede* an individual's readiness for Communication Subdomain 4 (morphosyntax). In the first three subdomains, children are not using syntax and morphology. However, the communication skills characteristic of the first three subdomains are always noted; delayed or nonexistent skills within the first three subdomains are targeted for intervention.

So, to return to the issue of "qualitative difference," Communication Subdomain 3 is qualitatively different from Communication Subdomain 4 because, at this early word combination level, children are not governed by adult syntax rules and do not use morphological forms. Instead, in Communication Subdomain 3 children create combinations of words by naming objects or people of interest, stating the actions objects or people perform, describing the object's or person's characteristics, and describing who owns or

Figure 2.7 **Relationship between Communication Subdomain 3 and Brown's Beginning Use of Morphemes**

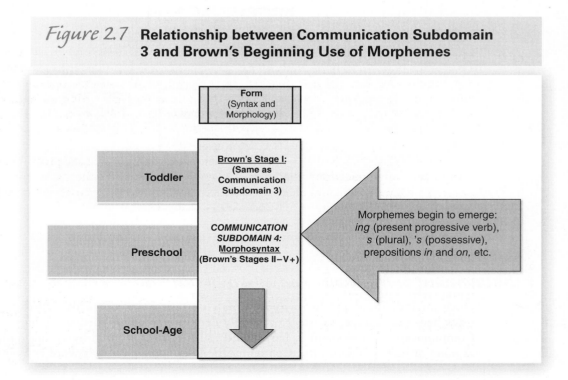

Table 2.4 **Examples of Two-Word Combinations**

Semantic combinations	Examples
Agent + action	*"car go," "kitty bye-bye"*
Action + object	*"kiss dolly," "need juice"*
Agent + object	*"kitty ball"*
Action + location	*"put in"*
Entity + location	*"Sam outside"*
Possessor + possession	*"my doll"*
Demonstrative + entity	*"that doggie"*
Attribute + entity	*"wet sock"*

possesses an object. Practitioners use semantic terms to describe these productions: *agent* (the "doer" of the action), *object* (the receiver of the action), *action, location, possession,* and *object attribution.*

Children's early word combinations must be judged within the contexts in which they occur. For example, a child might say *"Doggie house"* and mean *"The dog is in his doghouse"* or *"That is the dog's house"* or *"I want the dog to come in my house."* Table 2.4 provides examples of early word combinations and demonstrates how the word combinations are described using semantic terminology.

CLINICAL IMPLICATIONS FOR COMMUNICATION SUBDOMAIN 3

Once a child is able to demonstrate Communication Subdomain 1 (early pragmatic skill) and has more than 50 single words (developed during early-stage Communication Subdomain 2), practitioners target early word combinations (Communication Subdomain 3). Interventionists engage children in early play activities (e.g., playing with building blocks or trucks, sociodramatic play with dolls) to facilitate multiple-word combinations. A child's caregivers also are trained to facilitate these semantic combinations.

For older individuals with significant communication impairments, practitioners also may target Communication Subdomain 3. Communication may either be verbal or incorporate an augmentative and alternative communication (AAC) approach. You will learn more about AAC in Chapter 11.

Subdomain 4: Morphosyntax Development

Communication Subdomain 4 coincides with Brown's stages of language acquisition II–V+. At this point children's utterances begin to demonstrate characteristics of syntax and morphological development (i.e., language form). The emergence of syntax and morphemes occurs between 24 and 36 months for children developing typically. Examples of early-developing morphological structures include the present progressive *ing* verb form and the initial occurrence of the plural *s*. (Review Table 2.3 for the list of Brown's morphemes.)

By the time children are age 5, their sentences evidence complex syntax, including the use of embedded phrases and clauses. Figure 2.8 is a visual presentation of Communication Subdomain 4.

I use the term **morphosyntax** to avoid wordiness throughout this book and because the lines between syntax and morphology are blurred. For example, when a speaker asks the question "*Are you going to the party?*" she uses several morphemes (e.g., the auxiliary verb *are* and the *ing* verb). However, the speaker also uses syntax rules to sequence the morphemes into an interrogative reversal sentence. The term *morphosyntax* captures this combination of features. However, you should also keep in mind that the three components of language form (morphology, syntax, and phonology) have distinct properties that can independently challenge children who have language impairments. In Chapter 6, I describe particular morphological challenges of children with specific language impairments.

Morphology by definition involves the smallest unit of linguistic meaning. Some morphemes are considered to be free morphemes. Free morphemes can stand alone, as in the example of unmarked verbs (*walk, drive, go*) and unmarked object names (*boy, tree, street*). A bound morpheme carries meaning but must occur with a free morpheme. Bound morphemes include the plural *s* (*boys*), possessive *'s* (*girl's*), verb tenses (*walked*), and so forth.

An interesting feature of bound morphemes is their morphophonologic features. **Morphophonology** refers to the phonological variations occurring with morpheme use. For example, when creating a plural form, speakers sometimes use an *es* and sometimes an

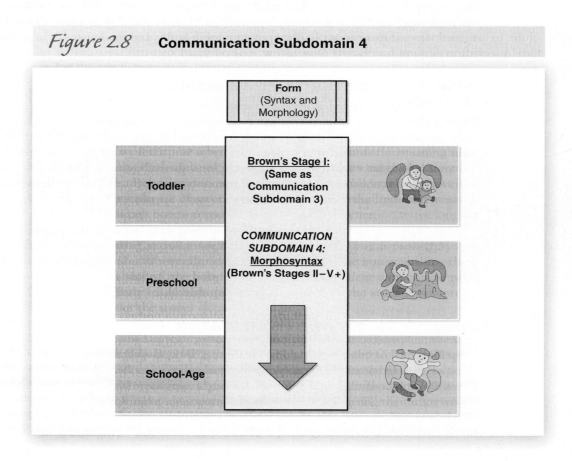

Figure 2.8   Communication Subdomain 4

Form
(Syntax and Morphology)

Toddler

Brown's Stage I:
(Same as Communication Subdomain 3)

COMMUNICATION SUBDOMAIN 4:
Morphosyntax
(Brown's Stages II–V+)

Preschool

School-Age

s, depending on the final phoneme in the word. To illustrate, speakers produce the plural of *bus* with *es* (*bus*es) but produce the plural of the word *hat* with *s* (*hat*s). In another version of plural form, speakers produce the plural of a word with a final /f/ (*leaf*) with *ves* (*lea*ves).

Morphophonologic variation also is demonstrated by different pronunciations of the past tense *ed* morpheme. Speakers produce a voiceless /t/ when the root verb ends with a voiceless phoneme (*push*ed, *walk*ed, *bounce*d) but use a voiced /d/ when the root verb ends with a voiced phoneme (*play*ed, *carri*ed, *show*ed).

CLINICAL IMPLICATIONS FOR COMMUNICATION SUBDOMAIN 4

Once an individual (a) demonstrates the ability to use foundational pragmatic functions (Communication Subdomain 1) and (b) produces multiword combinations using a variety of semantic categories (Communication Subdomain 3), practitioners typically evaluate a speaker's use of morphosyntax using the framework developed by Brown (1973). In Chapter 3, I describe the process used to complete a language analysis using Brown's stages.

An individual's syntax competency continues to increase in sophistication during the school years. Consequently, practitioners focus on syntax skills in their interventions with school-age students who demonstrate weaknesses in this area. Often syntax deficits are demonstrated in students' ability to read difficult texts and write at the level required for school success. During the school-age years, syntax analysis and intervention often focus on the speaker's use of sentences with conjunctions (*and, but, then, or, because, after, unless*) and sentences with embedded clauses. I describe assessment and intervention of complex syntax production in Chapters 3, 6, and 10.

Subdomain 5: Advanced Pragmatic and Discourse Development

Although Communication Subdomain 5 is listed last in my ordering system, remember that all the aspects of form, content, and use have been developing side by side since the child began to communicate. In children developing typically, the discourse skills associated with Communication Subdomain 5 have evolved seamlessly from the early pragmatic/discourse skills associated with Communication Subdomain 1. Further, the older child's discourse skills require the vocabulary and syntax competency associated with the other subdomains. Remember that discourse is defined as the connected and contingent flow of language between two or more individuals. Vocabulary, morphologic, and syntax skills are required to have a connected and contingent flow of information! A visual diagram of Communication Subdomain 5 is shown in Figure 2.9.

Between ages 3 and 7, children's developing pragmatic/discourse skills include the ability to use language to reason and to reflect on past experiences, predict events, express empathy, maintain status and interactions with peers, use and understand sarcasm and politeness forms, and code switch in order to adapt communication to the situation and listener (Chapman, 2000).

During the school years, students continue to increase the sophistication of discourse competencies. A successful learner develops communicative behaviors required for school success. High-level pragmatic/discourse skills are needed to (a) gain access to social activities, (b) participate effectively in group learning activities (e.g., science experiments), (c) respond to others' comments by validating their opinions, (d) sustain cooperative group

Figure 2.9 **Communication Subdomain 5**

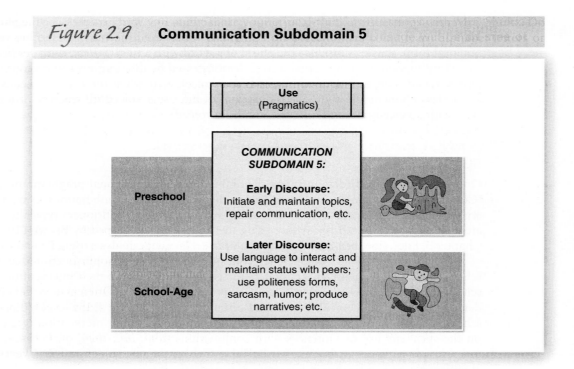

communication, (e) negotiate differences of opinion, (f) offer contradicting opinions with socially acceptable strategies, and (g) respond appropriately to teacher or peer feedback (Fujiki & Brinton, 2009).

Teacher–student communication is a form of discourse called classroom discourse. **Classroom discourse** generally is characterized by the teacher's initiation of a question, the teacher's evaluation of the student's verbal contribution, and the teacher's control of the conversational topic (Moore, 2012). Also, classroom discourse currently is viewed as the mechanism that facilitates students' high-level thinking skills (e.g., problem solving in mathematics, science, social studies; Nilsson, 2008).

Students also have to learn to modify discourse styles for different situations. Some forms of discourse are called narratives. An **oral narrative** is a verbal retelling of past experiences or a telling of "what happened" (Ukrainetz, 2006). An individual's ability to produce narratives is associated with school success (Green, 2009). A different form of narrative is called an **expository narrative**. This is an informational genre; teachers ask for expository narratives when they ask students to describe a scientific experiment or summarize a historical event (*"Describe the events leading up to and causing the Civil War"*). Each discourse and narrative genre places unique demands on the language learner. I provide more information on narrative development and discourse interventions in Chapters 5 and 10.

CLINICAL IMPLICATIONS FOR COMMUNICATION SUBDOMAIN 5

Skilled practitioners track children's abilities to use vocabulary, produce sentences, and use advanced language within sophisticated discourse genres demonstrated in Communication Subdomain 5. SLPs and special educators recognize that very specific discourse demands are placed on students entering school; the challenges are even greater for children with language disorders (Peets, 2009). To obtain a complete picture of a student's discourse abilities, a practitioner must observe the student in the classroom, with peers, during production of narratives, and in response to a variety of stimuli and situational prompts (e.g., story retelling, expository narratives, group interactions).

The accurate assessment of discourse demands careful language analysis skills; I discuss discourse analysis in Chapter 3. Interventions focusing on peer interactions and the sophisticated language abilities needed for reading and writing are discussed in Chapters 6 and 10.

Summary

- Nature versus nurture is a historical debate over whether language is an innate ability of humans or a function of an individual's environment.
- Behaviorist theory suggests that learning occurs when an environmental stimulus triggers a response or behavior.
- Cognitive constructivist theory is based on the writings of Jean Piaget, who proposed that children demonstrate a sequence of progressively more sophisticated cognitive abilities.
- Social interactionist theory is based on the principle that communication interactions play a central role in children's acquisition of language; this theory is often connected to the writings of Vygotsky.
- Emergentist theory views language learning as an interconnected system that is more than one's genetic makeup, or environment, or the neural connections that develop as a child is exposed to a language; it is a complex, open system in which a child's biology adapts to his or her environment.
- Practitioners use behaviorist theory when they use reward systems to train behaviors.
- Practitioners observe children's play behaviors to informally gauge children's general cognitive ability and level of representational thought; this is an example of how cognitive theory has influenced clinical practice.
- Social interactionist theory has influenced many current therapies; practitioners use this theoretical approach to focus on enhancing interactions between communication partners.
- Emergentist theory guides much of the current research on language acquisition; the research often uses computer simulations to understand language development.
- Communication Subdomain 1 encompasses early pragmatic skills, including joint visual attention, imitation, and turn taking.
- Vocabulary (Communication Subdomain 2) progresses from the early one-word level and continues to develop through adulthood.
- Once children have more than 50 words, they typically begin to produce 2-word combinations during the development of Communication Subdomain 3.
- Syntax and morphological development, often described in terms of Brown's stages of language development, are evidenced during Communication Subdomain 4.
- Children's discourse skills continue to develop in Communication Subdomain 5.
- Early pragmatic functioning (Communication Subdomain 1) is fundamental to all communication and may be the focus of intervention for individuals with severe social communication deficits.

- Practitioners may target teaching children a variety of semantic meanings at the one-word level and facilitate advanced vocabulary learning for children with vocabulary deficits (Communication Subdomain 2).
- Practitioners use language facilitation techniques and/or train caregivers to develop children's use of multiple-word utterances. Some children with severe disabilities may use augmentative and alternative forms of communication to communicate at this level (Communication Subdomain 3).
- If children are having difficulty with morphosyntax in Communication Subdomain 4, practitioners use language analysis to determine appropriate linguistic targets.
- Practitioners facilitate social use of communication to enhance a child's social and academic achievement; this is the focus of Communication Subdomain 5.

Discussion and In-Class Activities

1. In groups, brainstorm three activities that you could implement with five different individuals. Each group should focus on an individual with a primary deficit in one of the five subdomains. Share the activities in class. Compare and contrast how the activities differ based on the communication priorities of each communication subdomain.
2. Following the dicussion above, identify a theoretical approach supporting one activity from each communication subdomain.
3. Find a number of catalogs that contain intervention materials and assessments. In small groups, locate materials listed in the catalogs that you believe are based on the following theoretical approaches: behaviorism, social interactionism, and cognitive constructivism (i.e., sensorimotor emphasis). List or underline the words in the item description that support your conclusion. Share what you find with the rest of the class.
4. View video recordings of individuals with communication impairments. If you had to pick only one communication subdomain to target in intervention, which one would it be? Explain your answer.
5. Watch this YouTube clip on African American English (AAE): www.youtube.com /watch?v=Zqohw8nR6qE. One of the speakers discusses how and when he decides to code switch. Does everyone code switch to some degree? Give examples.
6. Listen to American dialects posted on the Internet at http://dare.wisc.edu (select Sample, Audio Samples, and then click one of the samples listed). Have students break into groups and have each group choose an area of the country. The group should then summarize that area's dialect in terms of vocabulary (i.e., word choice), prosody, and phonology. The group should determine what stereotypes are sometimes associated with the dialect it studies.

Chapter 2 Case Study

Sachi is a 4-year-old female attending a preschool program; it is an inclusion program (i.e., some children are developing typically, and others have developmental delays). Although Sachi has not been formally diagnosed, she demonstrates behaviors on the autism spectrum. She is not linguistic, does not interact socially with others, and does not initiate early pragmatic functions. She spends most of her time wandering around the classroom, carrying a small battery-powered fan that she and turns off and on. As the assessor, you have identified goals in Communication Subdomain 1 as the most important communication targets. You have been working with Sachi in the classroom, incorporating her peers in turn-taking games such as "marble raceway" (i.e., the children take turns dropping the marble into the spiral racetrack). Sachi is starting to respond to her name and make eye contact when it is her time to take a turn.

Sachi's parents are Japanese American. They speak some English, but to communicate effectively, you must speak slowly and use simple vocabulary. Sachi's parents have scheduled a conference with you; they are concerned because you are not teaching Sachi "to talk." To explain your intervention goals, you begin by showing video-recorded interactions of young children (toddler age). You turn off the volume so that Sachi's parents will focus on the nonverbal signs of communication. You ask Sachi's parents to identify instances of nonverbal communication. With your help, they identify gestures, pointing, eye gaze, smiling, joint attention, and waiting behaviors. You emphasize the importance of these behaviors as a foundation for later communication.

Finally, you show a video recording of Sachi in her supported classroom interactions. You and Sachi's parents identify instances where Sachi is beginning to demonstrate early pragmatic communication. Together, you and Sachi's parents begin to identify some activities they can do at home to facilitate Sachi's early pragmatic skills.

Questions for Discussion

1. View videotapes of young children; watch while the volume is turned off. Locate instances of behaviors reflecting Communication Subdomain 1.
2. Role-play the interaction with Sachi's parents with other students in your class. Practice explaining your communication goals in simple terms. Draw a simple diagram to help Sachi's parents understand the need to begin with nonverbal pragmatic communication behaviors.

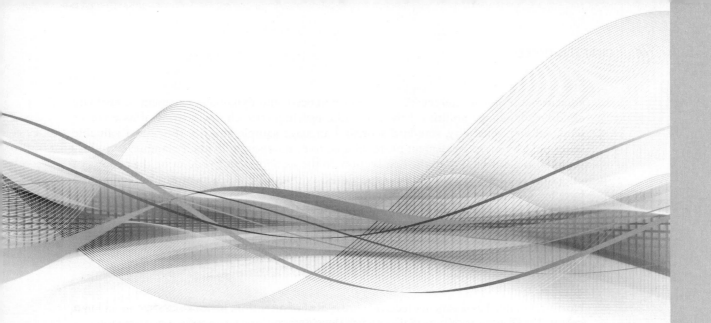

3 *Assessment of Language Disorders*

Chapter Overview Questions

1. What are the characteristics, disadvantages, and advantages of norm-referenced and criterion-referenced assessment? Why would an SLP use dynamic assessment protocols?
2. How do validity and reliability impact assessment tools? How are standard scores interpreted to identify students with language impairment?
3. How does an SLP or educator compute mean length of utterance? How does MLU differ from a T-unit analysis?
4. How does an assessor complete a micro-level analysis for a beginning language learner? For a higher-level language learner? What macro-level analyses are completed for individuals with language impairment?
5. Describe an assessment protocol appropriate for an individual with a primary disorder in Subdomains 1–5.

The information in the first two chapters has prepared you to begin to think about the assessment process in ways that reflect your understanding of language theory, development, and the implications of the three language domains (form, content, and use). I organize this chapter into two major sections. First, I describe the tools of the assessment process. In the first section, I discuss how speech-language pathologists (SLPs) and educators use norm-referenced, criterion-referenced, and dynamic assessment to evaluate children's language abilities. I then describe psychometric characteristics of assessment (e.g., validity, reliability, standard scores). Language sample analysis (LSA) is a valuable criterion-referenced assessment protocol used to evaluate an individual's language production; I also describe LSA in the first section. In the second section, I describe the process of assessment: screening, assessment procedures, synthesizing assessment results, counseling families, and report writing.

Assessment Tools

DEFINING NORM-REFERENCED, CRITERION-REFERENCED, AND DYNAMIC ASSESSMENT

Norm-referenced assessments receive a great deal of attention. School SLPs spend an average of 3.8 hours a week on diagnostic evaluations and use norm-referenced assessments approximately 80% of the time to assess children's receptive and expressive language (ASHA, 2010). Norm-referenced assessments are sometimes also called standardized tests or formal tests (Haynes & Pindzola, 2008). However, assessments that are not norm referenced can be standardized, so I avoid using the term *standardized testing*.

An assessor uses **norm-referenced assessment** to compare an individual's abilities to those of his or her peers. A norm-referenced test provides a "snapshot" of a child's abilities at a point in time. A primary assumption of norm-referenced assessments is that children with language impairment (LI) will demonstrate below-average performance (Oetting & Hadley, 2009). Norm-referenced assessments are used to answer the clinical question "Does this child have language impairment?" Norm-referenced assessments have statistical properties that identify group differences (i.e., that allow the assessor to determine where the child is placed relative to his or her peer group). I discuss the psychometric properties of norm-referenced assessment in the subsection below.

Criterion-referenced assessments are test instruments in which the individual's performance is compared with a prespecified standard or a specific skill. Often, the items in a criterion-referenced assessment are organized in a developmental sequence. Typically, the assessor attempts to observe multiple examples of a skill within a particular domain. The number of items completed correctly reflects a student's mastery of the targeted skill.

A particular kind of criterion-referenced assessment is called a progress-monitoring assessment. Progress-monitoring measures play an important role in the educational process. A student's growth over time is assessed to allow data-based decisions about the effectiveness of specific instructional interventions. Progress-monitoring assessment also is used to identify when children need more intensive and focused educational intervention in order to master specific communication or academic skills. I discuss several kinds of progress-monitoring assessments in Chapter 4 (i.e., individual growth and development indicators [IGDIs]) and Chapter 10 (i.e., curriculum-based measures [CBMs], typically used for reading assessment).

Criterion-referenced assessment answers the clinical question "How does this child perform a particular communicative or academic task?" Criterion-referenced tests can be clinician developed. Like a norm-referenced test, a criterion-referenced assessment documents a student's abilities at a particular point in time. An example of a criterion-referenced assessment is shown in Figure 3.1. In this example, the criterion-referenced assessment is used to document a child's early print abilities, including the ability to recognize print in the environment and enjoy shared book reading.

Figure 3.1 **Early Literacy Print Skills Checklist for 3- and 4-Year-Old Children**

Directions: Observe the child in an array of early literacy activities (for example, during shared-book storybook reading or whole-class writing and reading activities). Check each of the following that you observe.

1. Child recognizes that print runs from left to right.	
2. Child distinguishes scribbles ("writing") from pictures when drawing.	
3. Child knows that words are comprised of letters.	
4. Child uses a print vocabulary such as *word, read, write, letter.*	
5. Child responds to signs in the classroom.	
6. Child recognizes common logos, such as store names or a sports team.	
7. Child shows interest in what items say in the classroom.	
8. Child differentiates between pictures and print on posters and signs.	
9. Child asks for help to "read" signs and words in the environment.	
10. Child understands that print has a different function than pictures on signs.	
11. Child is interested in reading and sharing books.	
12. Child identifies the front and back of a book.	
13. Child holds book correctly (right side up, front side forward).	
14. Child can tell the title of a favorite book.	
15. Child turns pages from front to back when looking at book.	
16. Child knows that print tells the story.	

Source: From "Designing and Implementing an Early Literacy Screening Protocol: Suggestions for the Speech-Language Pathologist, by L. M. Justice, M. A. Invernizzi, and J. D. Meier, 2002, *Language, Speech, and Hearing Services in Schools, 33,* pp. 84–101. Copyright © 2002 by Sage Publications.

Both norm-referenced and criterion-referenced assessments are considered static assessments. Both provide snapshots of an individual's performance at a particular point in time; they document a child's abilities and deficits. However, there are limitations to many static assessments because most norm-referenced tests typically represent the performance of European American children. Because of this limitation, dynamic assessments are particularly valuable when assessing children from a nonmajority culture. **Dynamic assessment (DA)** is considered a nonstatic or process-oriented assessment protocol—it evaluates a child's ability to learn.

Dynamic assessment is a method of conducting an assessment to identify the skills that an individual possesses as well as his or her learning potential. DA is based on Vygotskian theory in that the adult interacts with the student in his or her zone of proximal development; DA has been described as being "fluid and responsive" (Lidz & Peña, 2009). In a dynamic assessment, the assessor demonstrates, and briefly practices, a language task with the child. During the practice session, the assessor observes the child's ability to modify his or her performance. Children who are developing typically usually make significant changes during the short-term teaching session. On the other hand, a child with language impairment often cannot change performance with a brief exposure to the task. Dynamic assessment answers the clinical question "Given exposure and opportunity, can this child perform a particular language or academic task?"

During DA, the *test–teach–retest* approach is taken (Patterson, Rodriguez, Dale, & Philip, 2013). First, children are tested to get a baseline score. Then, in the **mediated learning phase,** the examiner spends time directly teaching the child the skill; the mediated learning phase is followed by a retest (Ukraninetz, et al., 2000).

During the mediated learning phase, children are assessed for learning behaviors, such as attention span, planning, self-regulation, motivation, and their response to the intervention. Children are encouraged to try or to "guess" at an answer even if the task is unfamiliar to them. It is important to be aware of cultural differences when you ask children to "guess." Focus 3.1 explains more about how individuals from different cultural groups may respond to a prompt to guess at an answer. However, with prompting, if a child receives positive scores in the mediated phase, the assessor infers that the low baseline score was likely a result of cultural differences in learning styles or lack of experience with the task.

Consider the following example that demonstrates how DA can be used to assess a child (Gutierrez-Clellen & Peña, 2001). This example focuses on vocabulary learning, but DA can be used to assess a child's ability across language domains (e.g., syntax, semantics, pragmatics):

- First, in the pretest phase, the SLP documents the child's ability to produce specific vocabulary items (e.g., asks the child to name objects or pictures).
- Then, in the mediated phase (i.e., "teach"), the SLP interacts with the child, providing embedded and meaningful definitions during contextually relevant interactions (e.g., "Oh you want to see the girl *skipping*. She is hopping with one leg and then the other. She is *skipping*, isn't she?").
- During the mediated phase, the SLP uses techniques that encourage the child to use the new vocabulary item (e.g., "Good, you used the new word, *skipping*!") and highlights the rationale for using the new vocabulary item (e.g., "When you used the word *skipping*, I knew exactly which picture you were looking at!").
- After completing the "teach" cycle, the practitioner evaluates the child's ability to independently perform the targeted task and the child's learning style (i.e., posttest

---

FOCUS 3.1   *Multicultural Issues*

Dynamic Assessment

- In contrast to using norm-referenced assessment, dynamic assessment has been endorsed as an assessment procedure appropriate for ethnic minority children. In dynamic assessment, the examiner has an opportunity to distinguish disorders from cultural differences due to a child's learning style or exposure.
- Some children may not understand the purpose of the task during dynamic assessment. During the mediated learning phase, assessors typically explain

that the goal of the task is to "try" even if it means guessing (Hwa-Froelich & Vigil, 2004). The assessor must be careful to explain that the child should make a serious guess, not a playful guess. In some cultures, children are only asked to guess when an adult is playing, joking, or teasing. In this context, children may make farfetched guesses, with the intention of maintaining a playful interaction. In contrast, some Asian children may refuse to respond when they are uncertain of the answer (Hwa-Froelich, 2000).

phase). This can be done informally or more formally, using rating scales such as (a) The Modifiability Scale and (b) The Learning Strategies Checklist (Gutierrez-Clellen & Peña, 2001). These ratings scales are shown in Figure 3.2:
- The Modifiability Scale is used to summarize a child's overall modifiability to the test–teach–test sequence. Modifiability is rated using a Likert scale, based on the

---

Figure 3.2   **Utterance-Level Worksheet for Beginning Language Learners with MLU between 1 and 3**

APPENDIX. RATING SCALES

Learning Strategies Checklist

	None of the time	Some of the time	Most of the time
Attention/Discrimination			
• initiates focus with minimum cues	0	1	2
• maintains focus with minimum cues	0	1	2
• responds to relevant cues, ignores irrelevant cues	0	1	2
Comparative Behavior			
• comments on features of task	0	1	2
• uses comparative behavior to select item	0	1	2
• talks about same/different	0	1	2
Planning			
• talks about overall goal	0	1	2
• talks about plan	0	1	2
Self-Regulation/Awareness			
• waits for instructions	0	1	2
• seeks help when difficult	0	1	2
• corrects self	0	1	2
• rewards self	0	1	2
Transfer			
• applies strategies within tasks	0	1	2
• applies strategies between tasks	0	1	2
Motivation			
• persists even when frustrated	0	1	2
• shows enthusiasm	0	1	2

Modifiability Scale

	Extreme	High–Moderate	Moderate	Slight
Examiner Effort	3	2	1	0
Child Responsivity	3	2	1	0

	Low	Medium	High
Transfer	0	1	2

Source: Courtesy of Elizabeth D. Pena.

following components: examiner effort ("How difficult was it to facilitate the new task?"—0–3 points), child responsivity ("How easily did the child demonstrate competence in the new task?"—0–3 points), and transfer ("How well did the child perform on the posttest?"—0–2 points).

- As shown in Figure 3.2, The Learning Scales Checklist consists of 16 ratings ranging from 0 to 2 (none of the time, some of the time, most of the time) in areas assessing the child's attention, self-regulation, planning, etc.

An SLP uses the information from the DA and the rating scales to (a) help identify strategies facilitating or limiting the child's ability to learn and (b) determine whether variations in performance are due to cultural or environmental experience.

ADVANTAGES AND DISADVANTAGES OF ASSESSMENT TOOLS

There are many approaches to assessment; a professional recognizes the advantages and disadvantages of each assessment tool and uses the best tool to answer clinical questions. Typically, a combination of assessment procedures is used to (a) identify whether a child does or does not have a language impairment (via norm-referenced assessment), (b) identify specific targets for intervention (via criterion-referenced assessments, language sample analysis, and developmental checklists), and/or (c) decide whether the child has a language difference or a language disorder (via dynamic assessment).

Advantages and Disadvantages of Norm-Referenced Assessment. Norm-referenced assessments have several advantages. Norm-referenced assessments are efficient to administer, and the guidelines for test administration are very clear. The psychometric properties of norm-referenced assessments allow the assessor to compute standard scores; this allows educators to qualify students for educational services. Norm-referenced assessment also is used at state and national levels to document school performance.

Norm-referenced assessment does, however, have disadvantages and weaknesses (Wiig & Secord, 2006). A primary disadvantage is that norm-referenced assessments typically are administered individually in an unfamiliar context (e.g., the therapy room). Accordingly, a child's performance during a norm-referenced assessment may not capture his or her best performance. Recall from Chapter 2 that social interaction theory suggests that a child's performance should consider his or her everyday context. Norm-referenced assessments are less likely than criterion-referenced measures or dynamic assessment to document communication competency in daily living.

A second disadvantage is that norm-referenced assessment can overidentify children from minority cultures. Normative data (i.e., data collected to compare children with their peer group) usually represent middle-income rather than low-income children, and those data often do not reflect adequate minority representation. As a result, some test norms prohibit fair comparison for children from minority cultures. Sometimes nonmajority children are identified as having a language deficit when in actuality they have a language difference.

A third disadvantage is that norm-referenced tests often have only a few items to assess each language target. On a syntax test, for example, a particular verb form (e.g., *ed* [past tense]; *The dog bark*ed) may be assessed only one or two times. It is possible that a student may use the past tense verb form correctly within conversation but miss the past tense verb during the test administration. In such a case, the assessor may inaccurately identify past tense verbs as an intervention target. Due to the limited number of items per language task, norm-referenced tests should not be used to identify specific intervention targets; criterion-referenced assessments are the appropriate tools for this task.

Norm-referenced assessment also should not be used to document a student's progress in language intervention. Children may begin to use a language skill within familiar contexts but fail to use the developing skill in the more artificial norm-referenced assessment procedure. Norm-referenced tests are not designed to pick up subtle variations in skill.

In Chapter 2, I described five different communication subdomains. Norm-referenced tests are used most frequently when assessing Subdomains 2 (vocabulary; language content) and 4 (morphosyntax; language form). They are less helpful, and used less frequently, when assessing students who are significantly impaired (e.g., older students with difficulties in Subdomain 1 or 2) or for assessment of discourse function (Subdomain 5; language use). Some norm-referenced assessments assess an individual's ability across a variety of language domains. For example, the Clinical Evaluation of Language Fundamentals–Fifth Edition (CELF-5) is made up of a variety of subtests, and the different subtests evaluate different language domains (e.g., semantics, morphosyntax). The American Speech-Language-Hearing Association maintains a directory of speech and language assessments describing the domains assessed within each test; you can view this information at www.asha.org/assessments.aspx.

Advantages and Disadvantages of Criterion-Referenced Assessment. There are a number of advantages to criterion-referenced assessment, particularly in the area of intervention goal setting. SLPs and educators use criterion-referenced assessments to identify targets for intervention because enough items are chosen to meaningfully tap into an individual's skill level. The assessor chooses a criterion-referenced protocol to specifically address the student's communication weakness.

In contrast to norm-referenced assessments in which a student's performance is statistically compared to his or her peer group, during criterion-referenced assessment, the assessor typically uses a raw score (i.e., number of correct responses) to summarize performance. The scoring simplicity is another advantage of criterion-referenced assessment. Criterion-referenced assessment is an appropriate tool for documenting a student's progress during intervention.

A disadvantage of criterion-referenced assessment is that the assessment protocol may not be well defined; this is in contrast to a norm-referenced test, where the administration protocol must be followed exactly. The lack of defined protocol may result in some variation between assessors or between repeated administrations of the criterion-referenced assessment. The variation may result in reduced reliability of the assessment instrument. Variability in test administration can be minimized by carefully describing the procedures used to collect data in a criterion-referenced protocol.

Criterion-referenced assessments are useful across all communication domains and subdomains. Some criterion-referenced protocols are used very frequently; a good example of this is the use of language sample analysis (see the following subsection). I discuss other important criterion-referenced assessments, including play-based observation and curriculum-based language assessment, in Chapter 6.

Psychometric Features of Assessment

Assessment tools differ in their psychometric properties. As mentioned previously, norm-referenced assessments use special statistical techniques to compare the performance of children with that of their peer group. On the other hand, criterion-referenced assessments are documented with raw scores. However, both norm-referenced and criterion-referenced assessments must meet basic standards of validity and reliability. I discuss validity and reliability next, and then the specific statistical properties characteristic of norm-referenced assessment.

Validity. Validity is the most important part of an assessment instrument (Lord & Corsello, 2005). A test has high **validity** if it measures what it says it measures. For example, if a student receives a lower-than-average score on a receptive language test, the SLP or educator expects the student to have difficulty following multipart directions and understanding complex sentences in his or her daily life. Obviously, a norm-referenced test is not useful if the results do not reflect real life!

I discuss four types of validity: construct validity, content validity, criterion-related validity, and predictive validity. Typically, an instrument's validity and reliability are reported in the test's administration manual.

Construct validity refers to the underlying theory on which the instrument is based. In Chapter 2, I discuss fundamental theories of language development. In order for a language test to be useful, a logical theory must underlie the instrument's construction (Zeidner, 2001). For example, imagine that I construct a test to document gender identity. I develop items asking questions such as *Would you rather repair a car motor or knit socks?* I decide that the answer *repair a car motor* will be recorded as a masculine response. If the individual chooses *knit socks,* the answer is assigned as a feminine response. "Wait a minute!" you respond. "Fixing cars or knitting socks has nothing to do with gender identity!" You point out my flawed thinking and suggest that I read peer-reviewed literature on the topic. After educating myself, I admit that my test did not have construct validity; it did not reflect current understandings of gender identity. This example points out an important concept: Even if a test looks sophisticated, the underlying test construct can be flawed. The issue of construct validity underscores the need for professionals to understand the theory underlying clinical procedures.

Content validity is the degree to which test items represent a defined domain. To determine content validity, experts examine the test items and decide whether there are enough items to represent the domain (i.e., area being examined), whether the items logically link to the domain, and whether the items appropriately assess the domain. For example, when an assessor measures receptive language, the test must be constructed so that the individual responds nonverbally. It would not make sense to ask the client to answer verbally; a verbal response taps into expressive language. Therefore, receptive language tests have to allow pointing or other nonverbal actions as a measure of comprehension.

Criterion-related validity considers the degree to which test results for one test align with those of another test measuring the same construct. Test developers report the statistical similarity between the tests in the test manual.

Predictive validity is similar to criterion-related validity. **Predictive validity** refers to how well a test score will predict a student's performance on a future task in the same domain. For example, will a test of syntax ability administered in first grade predict the writing complexity of a second-grader? Will students who scored well in first grade use more complex verbs, clauses, and descriptive language in third grade? This information allows the assessor to make important educational decisions from test results.

Reliability. **Reliability** is the degree to which a test is free from errors of measurement across forms, raters, and time. When an assessor tests or observes a child multiple times, scores reflecting the child's performance may not agree; this would suggest poor test reliability. The focus of reliability measures is to estimate the consistency of scores across repeated observations. Reliability data are reported as correlations; a correlation is a statistical measurement of score similarity. Two sets of scores that are perfectly correlated will have a correlation of 1.00. When making important educational decisions, a norm-referenced test should have a reliability of .90 or better (Webb, Shavelson, & Haertel, 2007). Table 3.1 lists a number of norm-referenced assessments that are often used to document an individual's expressive and receptive language abilities. Reliability is reported in the right-hand column next to each test.

Table 3.1 **Examples of Norm-Referenced Tests**

Test	Domain(s) assessed and description	Age group	Psychometric properties*
Examples of tests that evaluate a specific language domain			
Boehm Test of Basic Concepts–3rd Edition (Boehm, 2000)	Receptive language concepts; 50 basic concepts frequently occurring in kindergarten, first-, and second-grade curriculum. Spanish version available.	5–7:11 years	RELIABILITY: Test–retest reliability estimates ranged from .70 to .89 across forms and grades. Alternate form reliability, based on 216 first-graders, produced a reliability coefficient of .83. VALIDITY: Concurrent validity was based on comparisons with the Boehm–R, the Metropolitan Achievement Tests, the Metropolitan Readiness Test, and the Otis-Lennon School Ability Test, with correlations ranging from .48 to .96, depending on the comparison test.
Test of Pragmatic Language–2nd Edition (TOPL-2; Phelps-Terasaki & Phelps-Gunn, 2007)	TOPL evaluates six subcomponents of pragmatic language: physical setting, audience, topic, purpose (speech acts), visual-gestural cues, and abstraction. Student responds to a visual and verbal prompt illustrating a "dilemma."	6–18:11 years	RELIABILITY: Coefficient alpha for the Pragmatic Language Usage Index range from .82 to .93. The average reliability coefficient is .91. VALIDITY: The correlation between the TOPL-2 index and the WISC-III Full Scale IQ score is .52. This coefficient value is considered "large."

(continued)

Table 3.1   **(continued)**

Test	Domain(s) assessed and description	Age group	Psychometric properties*
Examples of tests that contain a variety of subtests assessing different language domains			
Clinical Evaluation of Language Fundamentals–Preschool 2 (CELF–Preschool 2; Wiig, Secord, & Semel, 2004)	Semantics (e.g., concepts, word classes, vocabulary), syntax (e.g., recalling sentences), morphology, preliteracy (e.g., phonological awareness), and pragmatics.	3–6 years	**RELIABILITY:** Reported test–retest corrected correlations for subtests by age ranged from a high of .94 for expressive vocabulary (ages 5 years to 5 years, 11 months) to a low of .75 for sentence structure (ages 6 years to 6 years, 11 months). Average internal consistency evidence was strong for the clinical groups, with both overall test average alpha coefficient and split-half reliability coefficients at .90 or higher for most of the subtests. The test manual provides acceptable evidence for interrater reliability. **VALIDITY:** Evidence to support the validity of the CELF–Preschool 2 is extensive and adequate.
Structured Photographic Expressive Language Test–3 (SPELT-3; Dawson, Stout & Eyer, 2003)	Morphological use (e.g., preposition, plural, possessive noun and pronoun, present progressive, regular and irregular past, copula, and auxiliary verbs) and syntax skills (e.g., negative, conjoined sentence, *wh-* question, interrogative reversal, relative clause, and front embedded clause).	4–9:11 years	**RELIABILITY:** Test–retest reliability with a median interval of 11 days was .94. Interrater correlations ranged from .97 to .99. Internal consistency estimates on the standardization sample ranged from .76 to .92, with a median reliability estimate of .86. **VALIDITY:** Concurrent validity was established by using the Comprehensive Assessment of Spoken Language (CASL; Carrow-Woolfolk, 1999) as the criterion measure. The correlation between the two measures was .78, indicating substantial overlap between the measures.
Clinical Evaluation of Language Fundamentals–5 (CELF-5; Semel, Wiig, & Secord, 2013)	Semantics, syntax, pragmatics, language memory, written language, and reading comprehension; subtest scores can be combined to compute expressive and receptive language standard scores and compute language composite.	5–21:11 years	**RELIABILITY:** The average reliability coefficients of the CELF-5 tests for the normative sample range from .75 (Structured Writing) to .98 (Pragmatics Profile). **VALIDITY:** The composite scores resulted in a sensitivity of 97% (0.97) and specificity of 97% (0.97). Using the cut score of 80, only 3% of children with LI were missed and 3% of children without language LI were misidentified.

Table 3.1 (**continued**)

Test	Domain(s) assessed and description	Age group	Psychometric properties*
Test of Language Development Intermediate–4 (TOLD-I:4; Hammill & Newcomer, 2008)	Semantics (e.g., picture vocabulary, relational vocabulary, multiple meanings), morphology (e.g., choice between correct/incorrect sentences), and syntax (e.g., word ordering). Subtests can be combined to compute language composite.	8–17:11 years	RELIABILITY: Reliability was assessed by computing coefficient alphas; all subtests were at or above .90 and thus acceptable. VALIDITY: Validity was assessed by demonstrating the ability of the TOLD-I:4 to predict performance on other measures of spoken language (e.g., global measures of spoken language, WISC-IV). The TOLD-I:4 met a general level of acceptability, indicating that the TOLD-I:4 is a reasonably accurate predictor of a student's language ability. The positive predictor ranged from .61 to .71; experts indicate that they should be ≥ .70.
Examples of tests that evaluate reading, writing, or literacy-related skills			
Test of Early Written Language–3 (TEWL-3; Hresko, Herron, Peak, & Hicks, 2012)	Evaluates basic writing (e.g., spelling, capitalization, sentence construction) and contextual writing (i.e., ability to construct a story to a picture prompt).	4–11:11 years	RELIABILITY: Stability reliability of all scores approximates or exceeds .90. Across all forms of reliability, the reliability of the composite index is in the mid to high 90s. VALIDITY: Using the TEWL-3 to predict scores on the Woodcock-Johnson III and the Wechsler Individual Achievement Test–2nd Edition resulted in sensitivity indexes of .86 and .91, respectively.
Lindamood Auditory Conceptualization Test–3rd Edition (LAC-3; Lindamood & Lindamood, 2004)	The LAC-3 measures an individual's ability to perceive and conceptualize speech sounds; the examiner asks the student to use colored blocks to represent changing syllable patterns.	5–18 years	RELIABILITY: Statistics indicate generally high overall reliability. VALIDITY: Evidence presented in the manual indicates that the LAC-3 has acceptable overall validity in terms of its content validity, criterion-related validity, and construct validity.
Test of Phonological Awareness–2nd Edition: PLUS (TOPA-2+; Torgensen & Bryant, 2004)	Phonological awareness (i.e., isolation of individual phonemes in spoken words and understanding the	5–8 years	RELIABILITY: Coefficient alpha values range from .80 to .90. Convincing evidence is presented that the TOPA-2+ has reasonable internal consistency and test–retest reliability.

(continued)

Table 3.1 (**continued**)

Test	Domain(s) assessed and description	Age group	Psychometric properties*
	relationships between letters and phonemes).		**VALIDITY:** Data show median correlation coefficients of .51 and .43 for phonological awareness and .40 and .54 for letter sounds with other similar subtests. Teacher ratings on the Learning Disabilities Diagnostic Inventory correlated the results with TOPA-2+ subscales. Overall, the associations found were moderate.
Test of Narrative Language (TNL; Gillam & Pearson, 2004)	Evaluates a child's ability to use episodic structure during narrative production; evaluates a child's use of literate language features (e.g., temporal and causal adverbs, complex sentences).	5–11:11 years	**RELIABILITY:** Most coefficient alphas for the subtests and all items for the entire norm group, genders, and racial groups exceed the minimum criterion of .80. The test–retest reliability estimates are of concern. **VALIDITY:** Criterion-prediction validity included comparing the TNL and Spoken Language Quotient of the Test of Language Development–Primary: 3rd Edition (TOLD-P: 3) for 47 language-impaired children between the ages of 5 and 10 years. Their scores were similar.

When different assessors give the same test, a reliable test will give very similar results; this is called **interrater reliability**. A second type of reliability, called **test–retest reliability**, documents that a test given to the same individual on different occasions results in the same (or very similar) results. Although measures of reliability are not the only consideration when evaluating a test (and experts suggest reliability is not as important as test validity), it is one consideration in the responsible use and interpretation of tests (Webb et al., 2007).

Norm-referenced and criterion-referenced assessments vary in terms of their validity and reliability. It is generally accepted that criterion-referenced assessments are a more valid measure of performance because the child is provided multiple opportunities to respond and the assessment is generally based on real-life activities. Norm-referenced assessments, on the other hand, have detailed protocols to ensure consistent administration. A skilled assessor recognizes that there is tension between validity and reliability. Making a test more reliable tends to make a test less valid and vice versa; the goal is to use a variety of assessment procedures to account for this variation.

Psychometric Properties of Norm-Referenced Tests. Norm-referenced assessments have special properties because the tests are designed, statistically analyzed, and revised so that the children's scores are distributed along a bell-shaped curve. The **normal distribution of scores** describes any behavior that clusters around the mean. For example, the mean height of a woman in the United States is 5'5". A certain proportion of women will be much taller and some much shorter, but the average woman will be somewhere around 5'5". Similarly, a well-designed norm-referenced test results in most children clustering around an average score; at the same time, the test should discriminate between an average performer and those who are much better or much poorer performers on a particular task (Brown & Hudson, 2002).

When an assessor gives a norm-referenced test, he or she compares the individual's score to the normative sample and identifies whether the individual is within normal limits (i.e., is within the expected range around the mean score). The ability to identify whether an individual is below the normal performance range allows the assessor to identify children with language impairment. As a result, norm-referenced tests are an important part of the process used to qualify students for educational services.

One of the unique properties of norm-referenced assessments is that a child's raw score (i.e., the number of items completed correctly) is converted to a standard score. **Standard scores** are transformed scores measured in standard deviation units. For example, imagine that you test Mary, a 10-year-old female. Mary correctly answers 12 items on a norm-referenced test. Following the test, you check the test manual and find out that the mean score for 10-year-old females is a raw score of 12 (i.e., the average 10-year-old female typically gets 12 items correct on this test). In this case, the standard score is 100. (Note: For the purposes of this example, I am using the standard score of 100 to represent the mean.) The transformed standard score of 100 indicates that Mary is performing within normal limits for her age (in fact, she is exactly at the mean for her age). The **mean** is the statistical average of all the scores in a sample.

If Mary misses many items (e.g., selects only 6 correct answers), when you look up her raw score, you see that she has a standard score of 70. A standard score of 70 indicates a very significant deficit. On the other hand, if Mary correctly selects many items (e.g., 20), you find that her standard score is 125, indicating that she is a higher-than-average performer.

Standard deviation describes the spread of scores around the mean. The average range around the mean is 1 standard deviation above and 1 standard deviation below (the middle part of the bell-shaped curve; see Figure 3.3). In a traditional standard score transformation, 100 represents the mean score and ±15 points above and below the mean is the range for the average performer (a standard score between 85 and 115). One standard deviation below the mean is 100 − 15, resulting in a standard score of 85. One standard deviation above the mean is 100 + 15, resulting in a standard score of 115. Typically, children who are performing at the lowest 10% of the population are considered to be language impaired; the lowest 10% in a normal distribution is represented by children who are 1.25 standard deviations below the mean (i.e., a standard score of 80 or lower).

It is important to remember that there are several possible standard score transformations. I sometimes refer to them as a "family" of standard scores. While educators and SLPs are most familiar with the standard score transformation with a mean of 100, some tests use Z-scores or T-scores to represent an individual's performance in relation to the bell-shaped curve (i.e., document an individual's performance in relationship to same-age peers). Refer to Figure 3.4 to see how the scores in the "family of standard scores" are related.

Understanding the logic behind standard scores is very important: You will need to explain standard scores to other professionals and parents. At the end of the book (see

Figure 3.3 **The Bell-Shaped Curve Representing Normal Distribution of Scores on Norm-Referenced Assessments**

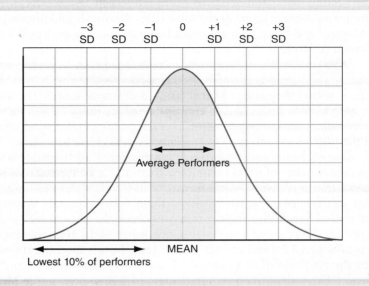

Figure 3.4 **The Family of Standard Scores**

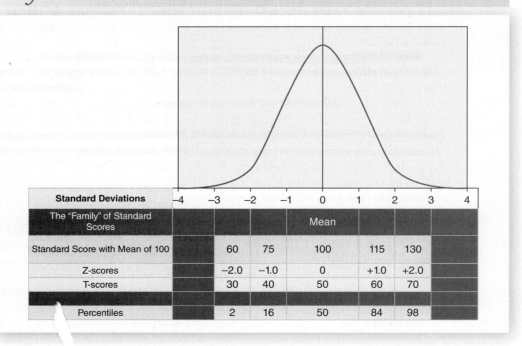

Standard Deviations	−4	−3	−2	−1	0	1	2	3	4
The "Family" of Standard Scores					Mean				
Standard Score with Mean of 100			60	75	100	115	130		
Z-scores			−2.0	−1.0	0	+1.0	+2.0		
T-scores			30	40	50	60	70		
Percentiles			2	16	50	84	98		

Appendix A), I present a tutorial that provides more detail about how standard scores are computed and how they represent a child's abilities. Focus 3.2 gives additional terms relevant to norm-referenced measurement and provides definitions on Z-scores and T-scores.

Language Sample Analysis. Language sample analysis (LSA) is a criterion-referenced task because the child's output is compared to developmental data. LSA evaluates an individual's spontaneous or self-generated speech in naturalistic contexts. Information from LSA provides information needed to develop intervention goals and has been proposed as

---

FOCUS 3.2 *Learning More*

Measurement Terminology and Explanations

A number of terms are used in norm-referenced testing. The following information is summarized from Hegde and Maul (2006):

- *Age-equivalent score:* The chronological age for which a raw score is the average score. Assessors are cautioned against using age-equivalent scores, because reporting that an older student (e.g., age 15 years) achieved an age equivalent of 8 years, 5 months is misleading. It is unlikely that a 15-year-old with a language delay communicates in ways that are equivalent to an 8-year-old student developing typically.
- *Basal:* The specific number of sequential items on a test or subtest that must be answered correctly before a student can continue taking the test. It is assumed that if the student answers three sequential items correctly (if the basal is set at 3), then prior items on the test or subtest would be answered correctly. By establishing a basal, the assessor avoids having to start at the lowest level for all students. Instead, students have varying "entry points" into the test items, depending on chronological age or ability level.
- *Ceiling:* When the student misses a specific number of sequential items on a test, testing is discontinued. It is assumed that the student would miss test or subtest items beyond the ceiling.

- *Composite score:* A total score that consists of the sum or mean score on two or more subtests.
- *Percentile rank:* An indication of an individual's relative standing in terms of percentage; the percentage of people or scores that fall at or below a specific score. If an individual achieves a percentile rank of 60%, it means that 40% in the sample had higher scores.
- *Raw score:* The actual score (number of items correct) on a test. The raw score is the number of items the student answers correctly between the basal and the ceiling items; the assessor then adds in the number of items below the basal (because he or she assumes that all items below the basal would have been answered correctly had they been administered).
- *Standard error of the mean (SEM):* A measure that estimates the distribution of scores for any one person if he or she were repeatedly measured on the same test (assuming that learning did not occur); a boundary of confidence that can be placed around a test score, calculated from the standard deviation and the reliability of the test. SEM is calculated because an individual's performance on a test will vary; there is no one "true" score. SEM is identified to represent the possible range of scores a student might achieve; determining SEM is particularly relevant for students who are near the boundaries for qualifying for services (e.g., at 1.5 standard deviations).

A confidence band (adding or subtracting a certain number of points from the standard score) is used to calculate an individual's SEM. The test developer statistically computes the confidence band; the assessor looks up the SEM in the test manual. If the confidence band is ±3 and a student's standard score is 78, the student's true score could range from 75 to 81.

- *Stanine:* A standard score with a mean of 5 and a standard deviation of 2.
- *T-score:* A standard score with a mean of 50 and a standard deviation of 10.
- *Z-score:* A score calculated by obtaining the difference between the person's actual score and the mean of the normal distribution and dividing that value by the standard deviation. Z-scores are commonly used in educational research.

the best means to identify children with language impairment. Computation of the mean length of utterance (MLU) is the most frequently computed LSA procedure; MLU is a highly reliable and valid index of normal language acquisition and a marker of language impairment (Rice et al., 2010). Experts consider LSA a more sensitive way to identify children with language impairments than using norm-referenced assessments. LSA often is used to confirm and elaborate on the information gained from norm-referenced testing.

LSA has both quantitative (i.e., numerical data) and qualitative (i.e., evaluation of morphosyntax complexity) components. The quantitative analysis answers the clinical question "Is the individual's length of utterance typical for his or her age?" The quantitative protocol varies with regard to the child's length of utterance. For younger children (or beginning language learners), the assessor uses a quantitative protocol called mean length of utterance. For older students who speak in longer utterances (+4 words/utterance), the assessor often uses a quantitative analysis called T-unit analysis.

Following the quantitative analysis, the assessor completes a qualitative analysis of the language sample. In the qualitative analysis, the assessor evaluates the morphological complexity of the child's utterances (for beginning language learners) or evaluates sentence complexity (for later-language learners). The qualitative LSA answers clinical questions such as (a) What sentence constructions occur most frequently? (b) Are there morphosyntax error patterns in the individual's utterances? and (c) Does the student use appropriate levels of sentence complexity (e.g., embedded clauses, gerunds) for his or her age?

LSA is considered a formative assessment. **Formative assessment** is an evaluation of performance in a real-life context; formative assessment allows the assessor to gather information and make adjustments to assist student learning. In contrast, norm-referenced tests are considered summative assessments. **Summative assessments** typically are used to place a child in a particular category (e.g., language impaired versus non-impaired) or as accountability measures (e.g., state reading tests).

Quantitative Analysis in LSA: Beginning Language Learners. An assessor completes four tasks in the first step of LSA. Remember that the clinical question for the first step of LSA is "Is the child's utterance length appropriate for his or her age?" To begin to answer this question, the assessor first obtains a high-quality language sample. The specific steps for obtaining a language sample are provided in Focus 3.3. In general, the assessor engages the student with open-ended questions and encourages the child to talk about pictures or describe an activity. It is best to obtain 50 to 100 child utterances for an in-depth language analysis (e.g., an analysis of the presence of grammatical morphemes, discourse features,

---

FOCUS 3.3   *Clinical Skill Building*

Obtaining a Language Sample

1. The child should be videotaped or audio-taped (or both). Have a familiar adult enter the room with the child.
2. For young children, provide toys that can be used to create a variety of activities, such as eating utensils, dolls, a barn with appropriate animals, a gas station with cars and trucks, people figures, a school-house and bus, a house with furniture, etc.
3. Have the preschooler play with toys while the examiner talks to the adult for approximately 5 minutes; then ask the adult to leave, and play with the child for 15 minutes. The goal is to obtain 50 to 100 child utterances (100 utterances preferred).
4. Avoid questions that can be answered with one-word answers. Instead, manipulate the figures, comment on the actions, pause, and wait for the child to take a conversational turn.
5. After the play session, the familiar adult returns to the room and asks the child about the activities.

6. Older children do not need to be accompanied into the room. Students who are reluctant to talk can be engaged in age-appropriate activities: tiddlywinks, pick-up sticks, or balancing games (e.g., Jenga). Students can be engaged in conversation by asking them (a) to describe a favorite movie, (b) to describe the rules used to play a sport, or (c) questions such as "Did your teacher/friend/brother/sister ever do anything that really bugged you? Tell me about it." Structured interview procedures are more desirable than free play for eliciting stable and consistent language sample measures in school-age children.
7. The assessor can repeat the child's utterances to aid transcription; this is done when the child is difficult to understand. Make sure that exact repetition occurs (e.g., if the child says "*I goed outside,*" the assessor says "*I goed outside.*"

---

mazing). However, shorter samples of child language (1–3 minutes of child talk) can be analyzed for progress monitoring (Heilmann, Nockerts, & Miller, 2010).

Second, the assessor transcribes the sample (i.e., writes down what the assessor and the child say). After transcribing the sample, the assessor separates the child utterances into utterance segments. In young children, utterance segments are determined by (a) voice inflection indicating the end of the utterance, (b) a pause of greater than 2 seconds, (c) inhalation, or (d) sentence structure indicating a "complete" thought (Eisenberg, Fersko, & Lundgren, 2001).

Third, the assessor counts the number of morphemes in the utterance sample. Recall that a morpheme can be a root word (i.e., an unmarked noun or verb) or a grammatical marker that communicates linguistic information (e.g., plural, possessive). Root words are called *free morphemes*; a grammatical marker is called a *bound morpheme*. Table 3.2 provides a set of rules used to count morphemes within a child utterance. Unintelligible utterances are not counted.

Fourth, the assessor computes a child's mean length of utterance in morphemes (MLUm). I describe the procedure for completing MLU in the subsection below. It is important to note that assessors should be cautious when completing LSA for an individual from a nonmajority culture. For example, some children who are African American use African American English (AAE) some of the time. AAE is associated with differences in

Table 3.2 **Rules for Language Sample Analysis and Calculation of Mean Length of Utterance**

1. Identify the first fully intelligible 50 utterances from the child's speech sample. An utterance is marked by a pause, inhalation, and/or falling intonation. Eliminate any utterances that are unintelligible or partially unintelligible from the sample.

2. Place a circle around (or highlight) any bound morphemes including plural *s*, possessive *'s*, third-person singular *s*, past tense *ed*, present progressive *ing* in each utterance.

3. Count each free morpheme (word) and identified bound morphemes in each utterance.

4. Do *not* count the following as morphemes:

   Interjections such as "*you know*" or "*hmm*"

   Words that are used as disfluencies; count only the final production (e.g., *He he he went to the store* = 5 morphemes)

   Words that are used as false starts leading to a revision (e.g., *He went . . . I went to the store* = 5 morphemes)

5. Count the following as one morpheme:

   Compound words (e.g., *snowman, mailbox*).

   Proper names (e.g., *Winnie the Pooh, Snow White*)

   Diminutives (e.g., *birdie, doggie*)

   Reduplications (e.g., *bye-bye, night-night*)

   Irregular past tense verbs (e.g., *went, gone, saw*). The justification is that there is little evidence that children relate to the present form.

   Can't and *don't* (Note: Counting *can't* and *don't* as one morpheme is an exception to the auxiliary rule [#6 below]). The justification is that *can't* and *don't* function as one morpheme for the child.

   Irregular plural forms (e.g., *mice, feet*)

   Catenatives (e.g., *hafta, gonna, wanna*)

6. Count an auxiliary verb as a separate morpheme even when it is in a contracted form (e.g., *He's at the store* = 5 morpheme; *She isn't at the store* = 6 morphemes)

7. Add up the number of morphemes in the entire language sample; divide the number of morphemes in the entire sample by the number of utterances and compute the MLU. Example: 223 morphemes/50 utterances = 4.46 MLU

morphosyntax structure (e.g., *s* plural marker may be omitted; "*I have two book.*") or the auxiliary verb may be omitted ("*He walking.*"). Skilled assessors use variations of LSA so that an individual who uses AAE is not penalized for using AAE features. Learn more in Focus 3.4 about alternative LSA procedures for children who use AAE.

Computing Mean Length of Utterance. SLPs and educators establish a child's mean length of utterance to gauge a child's overall progress in developing mature speech (Rice, Redmond, & Hoffman, 2006). The MLU is completed by dividing the total number of

FOCUS 3.4 *Multicultural Issues*

Multicultural Issues in Language Analysis

- Many African Americans speak African American English (AAE) at least to some degree or some of the time. AAE is associated with differences in morphosyntax structure. For example, the *s* plural marker may be omitted ("*I have two book*") or the auxiliary verb may be omitted ("*He walking*").
- Because AAE linguistic structure varies from General American English, skilled assessors use different language analysis procedures so that children who use AAE are not penalized for using AAE features. Use of more sensitive language analysis procedures avoids a biased diagnosis of language impairment.
- To analyze language samples for students who use AAE, the assessor analyzes simple and complex C-units. A communication unit (C-unit) is an independent clause plus associated modifiers. In simple terms, this means the assessor separates the child utterance at the point where the child uses a coordinating conjunction such as *and*. C-unit analysis also allows the assessor to count words such as *yes* or *uh-uh* when the child responds directly to the adult. (These typically are omitted in MLU analysis.)
- The assessor considers the frequency of production of C-units without complex syntax (simple C-units) as compared to complex C-units and computes a percentage of complex C-units. Examples of C-units with complex structure include simple infinitives ("*They was tryin' to get in*"), noun phrase complements ("*I think this'll work*"), and gerunds ("*They saw splashing*").
- Children developing typically will demonstrate an increase in C-unit length and complexity (Craig & Washington, 2000).
- Learn more about linguistic features of AAE and techniques to more accurately identify nonmajority students with language disorders in Appendix E in this book.

morphemes by the number of utterances in the language sample. This gives the average, or mean, number of morphemes a child uses in his or her communication attempts. As part of a class activity, check the development of MLU across the age ranges for children developing typically and for children with language impairments, at the National Institutes of Health public access journal site: www.ncbi.nlm.nih.gov/pmc/articles/PMC2849178/#!po=1.61290 (Figure 9; Rice et al., 2010).

As you recall from Chapter 2, Brown (1973) outlined stages of syntax development; each stage is associated with a chronological age and morpheme development. So, for example, let us consider a child, Johann, who is 36 months old. Given his chronological age, the assessor expects Johann to produce sentences between 2.5 and 3 words in length (Brown's Stage III). Further, if Johann's morphological development is within normal limits, the assessor expects Johann to produce specific morphological features associated with Brown's Stage III (i.e., irregular past tense verbs [went, saw] and possessives). Johann also should produce grammar forms associated with earlier Brown's stages; in this case, the *ing* verb and plural forms (i.e., bound morphemes associated with Brown's Stage II).

The assessor also knows that a child developing typically will make some morphosyntax errors; some grammar forms will be beyond the child's current level of ability.

For example, a typically developing 36-month-old child may say, "*I cutting my paper.*" In this sentence, the child developing typically omits the auxiliary verb *am* but uses the *ing* verb form. Auxiliary verb errors are expected because auxiliary verbs emerge during Brown's Stage V.

In the case of Johann, the assessor has to determine whether Johann's errors reflect later-developing morphosyntax (Brown's Stages IV–V+) or whether Johann is "behind" compared to a typically developing 3-year-old. In summary, the assessor (a) considers Johann's MLU and morphosyntax skills, (b) considers the MLU and syntax and morphological skills produced by children developing typically, and then (c) compares Johann's actual performance to the predicted performance. This process is the first clinical decision of language sample analysis.

How does the assessor work through this clinical decision-making process? First, the assessor carefully considers Johann's language sample. If Johann's MLU is 2.5 to 3 morphemes per utterance and if Johann uses the morphological features associated with Brown's Stage III, the assessor concludes that Johann's language is within normal limits (given no other outstanding communication problems). Johann's length of utterance and his use of morphological features are appropriate for his chronological age. But what if Johann's MLU is less than expected for his chronological age? Let's consider the clinical decision-making process in more detail by considering three scenarios below. Figure 3.5 visually presents the clinical decisions representing different LSA scenarios.

In Scenario 1, the assessor determines that the child has (a) an MLU consistent with expected chronological age norms and (b) no morphosyntax errors (other than those considered to be beyond the child's developmental level). If the child was referred for assessment due to perceived communication impairments, the assessor completes other criterion-referenced and norm-referenced assessments to confirm or deny deficits in other communication domains (e.g., pragmatics, semantics). It may be that the child is not language delayed; on the other hand, the child may have communication problems that were not "picked up" in the language sample analysis.

In Scenario 2, the assessor notes that the child's MLU is within normal limits but also observes morphosyntax immaturity errors. Consider two utterances, both produced by a child who is 5 years old (i.e., 60 months):

- *Me no go outside mommy.*
- *I want to go outside.*

Both utterances are 5 morphemes in length. In the first case, however, the utterance is immature and ungrammatical. In the second case, the utterance contains an advanced syntax form (i.e., the infinitive verb *to go*). Children with the same MLU level can have very different qualitative differences in their utterance production (Eisenberg et al., 2001). In Scenario 2, the assessor documents the child's average-level MLU but proceeds with a qualitative analysis of language form. I describe the qualitative analysis procedure in the following subsection.

In Scenario 3 (see Figure 3.5), the assessor observes reductions in the child's quantity and quality of language production. For example, in the case of Johann, imagine that his LSA revealed that he speaks in one- to two-word combinations. His MLU is 1.5. He produced the following utterances:

- *"Give it!"*
- *"Me"* (for *"mine"*)
- *"Look doggie!"*

Figure 3.5 Clinical Decision Making for the First Step of Language Sample Analysis

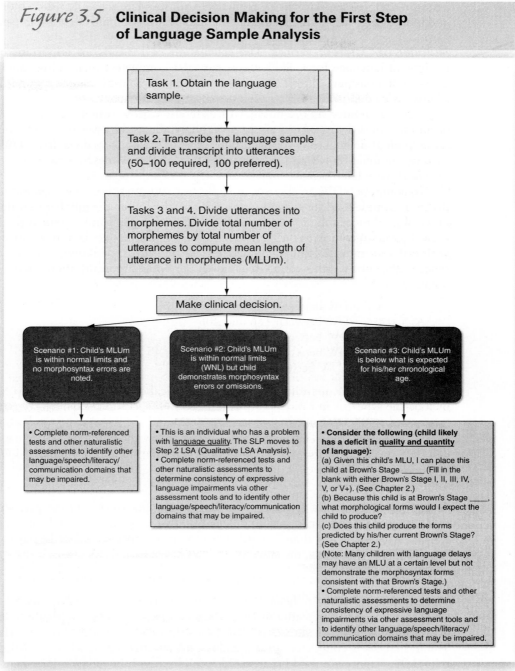

Task 1. Obtain the language sample.

Task 2. Transcribe the language sample and divide transcript into utterances (50–100 required, 100 preferred).

Tasks 3 and 4. Divide utterances into morphemes. Divide total number of morphemes by total number of utterances to compute mean length of utterance in morphemes (MLUm).

Make clinical decision.

Scenario #1: Child's MLUm is within normal limits and no morphosyntax errors are noted.

Scenario #2: Child's MLUm is within normal limits (WNL) but child demonstrates morphosyntax errors or omissions.

Scenario #3: Child's MLUm is below what is expected for his/her chronological age.

• Complete norm-referenced tests and other naturalistic assessments to identify other language/speech/literacy/communication domains that may be impaired.

• This is an individual who has a problem with language quality. The SLP moves to Step 2 LSA (Qualitative LSA Analysis).
• Complete norm-referenced tests and other naturalistic assessments to determine consistency of expressive language impairments via other assessment tools and to identify other language/speech/literacy/communication domains that may be impaired.

• **Consider the following (child likely has a deficit in quality and quantity of language):**
(a) Given this child's MLU, I can place this child at Brown's Stage _____ (Fill in the blank with either Brown's Stage I, II, III, IV, V, or V+). (See Chapter 2.)
(b) Because this child is at Brown's Stage _____, what morphological forms would I expect the child to produce?
(c) Does this child produce the forms predicted by his/her current Brown's Stage? (See Chapter 2.)
(Note: Many children with language delays may have an MLU at a certain level but not demonstrate the morphosyntax forms consistent with that Brown's Stage.)
• Complete norm-referenced tests and other naturalistic assessments to determine consistency of expressive language impairments via other assessment tools and to identify other language/speech/literacy/communication domains that may be impaired.

Source: Reprinted by permission of the publisher from *A First Language: The Early Stages* by Roger Brown, p. 54, Cambridge, Mass: Harvard University Press. Copyright © 1973 by the President and Fellows of Harvard College.

The assessor determines that Johann is (a) below expected levels for MLU and (b) demonstrating immaturity in morphological development. In this example, Johann demonstrates both quantitative (i.e., MLU is below expected levels) and qualitative (i.e., morphosyntax is not age appropriate) differences. In both Scenarios 2 and 3, the assessor completes additional assessments to substantiate the child's difficulties in syntax and morphology and to identify other communication domains that are impaired.

Number of Different Words. The calculation of MLU is an important quantitative analysis of language form. Skilled assessors also complete a quantitative analysis of language content as part of the LSA procedure. Calculation of the **number of different words (NDW) is a quantitative analysis of semantics (language content).**

NDW is defined as the number of different words (sometimes called *tokens*) that occur in a 100-utterance language sample. NDW allows the assessor to determine whether an individual demonstrates appropriate levels of vocabulary diversity. NDW should be used in combination with other measures of vocabulary. (I describe norm-referenced tests for vocabulary later in this chapter.)

To compute NDW, an assessor (a) collects a 100-utterance language sample (typically the same sample used for the MLU calculation), (b) counts the number of different words (a word used more than one time in the language sample is only counted the first time it is used), and (c) compares the student's NDW with normative data. If a root word occurs with different morphological endings (e.g., *walk, walks, walking*), only the first occurrence of the root word is counted. Children developing typically should have the following range of NDW:

- *At 3 years:* NDW between 100 and 164
- *At 5 years:* NDW between 156 and 206
- *At 7 years:* NDW between 173 and 212
- *At 9 years:* NDW between 183 and 235
- *At 11 years:* NDW between 191 and 267

There are other quantitative measures of lexical diversity in addition to NDW. These include the type–token ratio (TTR; that is, the number of different words divided by the total number of words in the language sample) and the number of total words (NTW). When calculating the NTW, every word produced by the child in the language sample is counted—even when the word is produced multiple times. NDW and NTW are better measures of lexical diversity than TTR.

Quantitative Analysis in LSA: Later-Language Learners. In the preceding section, I described MLU as an appropriate quantitative technique for a beginning language learner who uses fewer than 5 words per utterance. Once a student begins to communicate in longer utterances, the assessor uses an alternative technique called T-unit analysis during the LSA process.

Completing a T-unit Analysis. With school-age students, an assessor uses T-unit analysis to segment a student's utterances. A **T-unit** is one main clause, with all the subordinate clauses and nonclausal phrases attached or embedded within the sentence (Paul, 2007). T-unit analysis is completed after a child is 42 months old or when his MLU is greater than 4.00. T-units are used because older children with language impairment often produce run-on sentences linked with coordinating conjunctions.

Consider the following sentence: "*I went to the store, and I bought some bread, and I bought some candy, and I bought some pop.*" The individual's MLU equals 20 words; however, you can see that the sentence form is very simple, and it represents a series of four simple sentences: *//I went to the store// (and) //I bought some bread// (and) //I bought* *some candy// (and) //I bought some pop//.* An MLU analysis would not be useful because the individual's output is beyond Brown's stages in terms of sentence length. An MLU analysis would not reliably identify language impairment. The assessor must determine whether the individual's sentence complexity is acceptable compared to that of his or her peers and whether the sentence complexity is adequate for reading and writing.

T-unit analysis and LSA are important components of written language assessment for older students. Teachers and SLPs use LSA to analyze the writing samples of older students who struggle with reading and writing. I provide more information on reading and writing assessment and intervention in Chapter 10. I provide more details about T-unit analysis in Focus 3.5 in this chapter and a step-by-step tutorial explaining how to complete a T-unit analysis in Appendix B.

Qualitative Language Analysis.   As described above, during a quantitative analysis, an assessor answers the question "Are the child's utterances an appropriate length?" To answer this question, the assessor compares the child's production with that of an age-matched peer (e.g., a child of the same chronological age).

During the qualitative analysis, the assessor answers the question "Now that I have evaluated the child's length of utterance, what qualitative differences do I see in the child's language output?" Individuals with language impairment typically exhibit both quantitative and qualitative language variations. I call the quantitative *and* qualitative analysis the "two-step process" of LSA. The two-step LSA process is visually demonstrated in Figure 3.6.

During the second step of LSA, the assessor compares the individual's language output with a language–age match. A **language–age match** is a chronologically younger individual with an equivalent MLU. So, for example, when evaluating a child with an MLU of 1.0 word per utterance, I compare his or her language output with the communication patterns of a child at Brown's Stage I.

FOCUS 3.5   *Learning More*

A T-unit is one main clause, including all the subordinate clauses and nonclausal phrases. When a child uses long, run-on sentences consisting of many independent clauses connected with conjunctions *and, but,* or *so,* dividing the discourse into T-units avoids an inflated MLU (i.e., an MLU that is high, potentially indicating that the child had sophisticated verbal output when in actuality his or her output was a series of linked simple sentences). Consider the following:

I went to the store and my mom had given me some money so I went and bought

some bread for her and I come back and gave her the bread and she said "OK, thanks, now you can go to the ball game."

The sentence above is one utterance. Consider the difference when the output is divided into T-units:

- *I went to the store*
- *(and) my mom had given me some money*
- *(so) I went and bought some bread for her*
- *(and) I come back and gave her the bread*
- *(and) she said "Ok, thanks, now you can go to the ball game.*

Figure 3.6 **The Two-Step Process: Qualitative and Quantitative Language Sample Analysis**

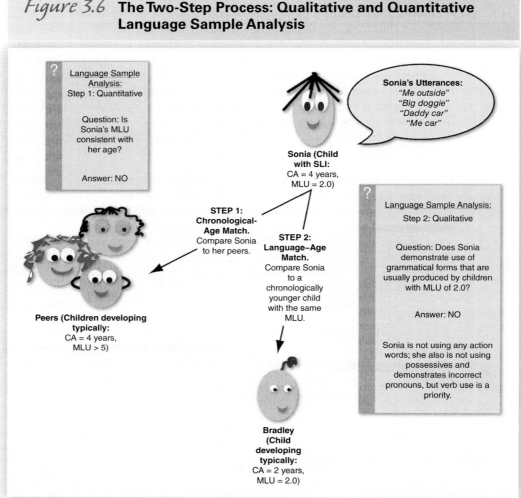

Qualitative analysis is typically completed at both the micro- and macroanalysis levels. **Microanalysis** considers each utterance as it stands alone. Microananalysis for the beginning language learner includes an analysis of the child's pragmatic abilities, semantic abilities, and morphosyntax skills at the utterance-by-utterance level. I provide a sample language analysis form in Table 3.3 to illustrate how an assessor documents microanalysis data for the beginning language learner. Microanalysis for later-language learners considers the individual's use of complex sentences at the utterance level.

Macroanalysis considers an individual's ability to interact during a conversation; it considers his or her discourse skills. It moves beyond the utterance level to consider the individual's ability to initiate a topic, repair communication breakdowns, and use a back-and-forth conversational style. I discuss in the section below both micro- and macroanalysis qualitative procedures used in the second step of LSA.

Table 3.3 **Utterance-Level Worksheet for Beginning Language Learners with MLU between 1 and 3**

Child's Name: S. B.	Chronological Age: 3:8	*Language Sample Analysis (LSA)* **Step # 1** *(Quantitative Analysis):* S. B.'s MLU *is* 3.0; given his age, he *should* be at an MLU +4 (Brown's Stage V considering his chronological age of 3 years, 8 months). However, his MLU is like that of a younger child.							
Examiner: J. K.	Date of sample:	*LSA* **Step #2** *(Qualitative Analysis):* Because S. B.'s current MLU is 3.0, he should be producing morphemes consistent with Brown's Stage IV (i.e., morphemes such as articles, regular past tense, 3rd-person regular verbs). However, S. B.'s morpheme use represents Brown's Stages I and II. *Notes:* S. B. demonstrates deficits in quantity (per MLU) and quality of syntax complexity.							
List Utterances Below:	(A) Pragmatic Functions (✓ Check one)							(B) Semantic Roles and Relations (Describe)	(C) Bound Morphemes and Brown's Stage Morpheme Typically Appears	# of morp.
	Requests	*Declarations*	*Answer questions*	*Agree/disagree*	*Social speech*	*Imitation*	*Other*	*Examples:* Agent Action Object Modifier Negation Agent + Action Action + Object Agent + Action Modifier + X Negation + X X + Location	*Examples of bound morphemes:* Present progressive (*ing*) Prepositions (*in, on*) Plural (*s*) Present tense aux. (*can, will*) Possessive (*'s*) Irregular past tense verb Articles (*a, the*) Copula and auxiliary "*BE*" Regular past tense verbs (*ed*) 3rd-person singular verb (*s*)	
No go outside.				✓				Negation + action + location	0/I	3
Kitty drinking milk.		✓						Agent + action + object	Present prog./II	4
Mommy up!	✓							Agent + location	0/I	2

Source: This table was published in *Language Disorders from Infancy to Intervention*, R. Paul and C. F. Norbury, (4th Ed.), p.434, St. Louis, MO: Mosby. Copyright © 2002 by Elsevier.

Microanalyses for the Beginning Language Learner. The assessor evaluates the beginning language learner's pragmatic, semantic, and morphosyntax skills. During the qualitative analysis of pragmatic function, the assessor first considers the six early developing pragmatic categories: requesting, stating/commenting, protesting/denying, responding, socially interacting, and imitating. (See Chapter 2 to review these terms.) The assessor considers overall communication and determines whether or not the child with language impairment demonstrates a range of pragmatic function. If LSA reveals that the child is not able to perform a pragmatic function (e.g., the child does not appear to use the pragmatic function of *request*), the assessor probes this communication skill. A **communication probe** is an interaction designed to elicit a specific child response. For example, to probe for *request,* the assessor may show a child a favorite toy or object and prompt a request. If the probe indicates the child is unable to produce a request, this skill is identified as a possible intervention goal.

Remember that language form, content, and use are never produced in isolation. A child with LI may appropriately produce a pragmatic function but demonstrate morphosyntax errors during the communication act. For example, a child with LI may demonstrate the pragmatic function *request* by saying, "*Outside now?*" The request is produced with rising intonation instead of a grammatically correct sentence, e.g., "*Can I go outside now?*" In this example, the assessor indicates that the child produced a request in the pragmatic category (column A on the LSA form) but documents a morphosyntax error in column C in Table 3.3.

The six pragmatic categories in Table 3.3 (column A) describe pragmatic competency prior to 24 months. Between 24 and 36 months, children demonstrate increasingly sophisticated pragmatic functions, including detailing, predicting, and requesting clarification. After age 3, children learn more sophisticated pragmatic functions, including expressing feelings, giving reasons, and hypothesizing, and begin to maintain and elaborate on conversational topics. The assessor documents the use, or lack of use, of each pragmatic function in relation to the child's chronological age and level of language use.

Once the assessor considers pragmatic function for beginning language learners, he or she considers the semantic skills associated with Communication Subdomains 2 and 3. (See Chapter 2 for a review of communication subdomains.)

At the earliest stage of language development (i.e., Brown's Stage I, up to 24 months), children use word combinations to express a variety of meaning. For example, the utterance "*Daddy car*" could mean a possessive relationship ("*This is Daddy's car*"), a statement ("*Daddy is driving the car*"), or a request ("*Will Daddy take me in the car?*"). Word combinations communicate a child's meaning unfettered by syntax and grammar constraints. As a result, during the second part of LSA (for the beginning language user), the assessor often completes a qualitative semantic analysis. In a semantic analysis, the assessor documents a child's use of semantic combinations such as agent + object, action + object, agent + action, modifier + X, negation + X (X = any word, including a noun, an action word, or even a word such as *more*).

Semantic combinations are building blocks for later-developing sentences. For example, I typically look for children at the two-word level to produce both agent + action ("*doggie eat*") and action + object ("*eat food*") combinations. Without the ability to produce such two-word combinations, children are likely to have difficulty producing the three-word agent + action + object combination "*Doggie eat food.*" The agent + action + object semantic combination represents the noun + verb + noun structure required for more elaborate syntax and grammatical development. Table 2.4 (in Chapter 2) provides a description of all the semantic combinations for children at the early stages of language development.

Given that children with language impairment often have a primary grammatical deficit, analysis of syntax and morphological ability is a critical component of LSA. Grammatical analysis considers a child's use of language form at Communication Subdomain 4.

During grammatical analysis, an assessor (a) describes the child's grammatical errors and (b) calculates the percentage of correct use for grammatical errors. The assessor marks a grammatical form as an error if it is used incorrectly in an **obligatory context,** meaning that the conversation or situation calls for the use of a specific grammatical form. An error is counted if the child attempts to use the form but the grammatical feature is produced incorrectly. Consider the following example in which the percentage of correct use of the present progressive verb *ing* form is computed:

Utterance (from a 50-utterance sample)	Error*	Obligatory?
TEACHER: *What is the boy doing in this picture?*		
8) CHILD: *he <u>run</u>*.	1	Yes
9) CHILD: *I don't know what him <u>do</u>*.	1	Yes
TEACHER: *Tell me what you see happening at the circus.*		
45) CHILD: *That seal want to eat.*	0	No
46) *He <u>throw</u>* ball.*	1	Yes
47) *He <u>riding</u> bike with him hat on.*	0	Yes
48) *That elephant <u>stand</u>* up on him back legs.*	1	Yes
TOTALS	4	5

Number of errors divided by number of obligatory contexts (4 ÷ 5 = .80) = 80% error in present progressive verb production

Note in utterance #45 that an error was not identified in the use of present progressive verb tense. In this utterance, the child produced an error, but the sentence construction called for a third-person regular verb (*wants*) rather than requiring a present progressive verb (*wanting*). The assessor must also consider that some morphosyntax features may represent cultural or linguistic differences and should not be counted as errors (see Focus 3.6).

Microanalysis for the Later-Language Learner. The qualitative morphosyntax analysis for beginning language learners is framed within Brown's Stages II–V+. Once the language learner is beyond 4 words, the assessor begins to consider the use of complex language beyond Brown's stages. As I described above, the assessor segments language output for the older child into T-units.

FOCUS 3.6   *Multicultural Issues*

A morphological feature of African American English (AAE) includes use of subject and verb that differ in either number or person. For example, a speaker who uses AAE might say, "*What do this mean?*"

What implications would AAE use have in the examples given in the text for calculating percentage of obligatory use (e.g., "*He throw ball*" and "*That elephant stand up on him back legs*")?

Typically developing students (with an MLU of more than 5.0) produce sentences with embedded or conjoined clauses 20% of the time (Paul & Norbury, 2012). In contrast, students with LI often produce few complex sentences. As a result, it is important to document an individual's use of complex sentences.

To determine the percentage of complexity, the assessor counts the number of T-units containing complex sentence construction and divides the number of complex T-units by the total number of T-units. If the percentage is below 20%, the assessor completes a more "fine-grained" analysis by looking at specific types of sentence complexity and evaluates whether the student produces early or late complex sentence forms. Early forms of sentence complexity include simple infinitives ("*He likes* to play *baseball.*") and simple *wh* clauses ("Why *did he go?*"). Later forms of sentence complexity include relative clauses ("*That's the dress* that I wore to the party.") and gerunds ("Swimming *is a great sport.*"). I give examples of early and late sentence complexity in Table 3.4.

Table 3.4 Early- and Late-Developing Complex Sentence Types

Early-Developing Complex Sentence Forms (MLU = 3–4) Examples

- Simple infinitive: The word *to* is used. However, the subject is deleted because it is the same as the main sentence. Does not include catenative forms of infinitive (*wanna, gonna*, etc.)
  - *She has to go.*
  - *The dog wants to run.*

- Full propositional complement: Cognitive verbs are used (*think, said, guess, know, wonder, hope*).
  - *She thought the room looked messy.*
  - *Guess how many I have.*

- Simple *wh* clause: Includes a *wh* conjunction: *what, where, when, why, who, how.* Does not include an infinitive *to.*
  - *Why did you say that?*
  - *See how he throws that ball?*

- Simple conjoining: Two clauses joined by a coordinating conjunction (*and, but, so,* etc.) or subordinating (*because, after,* etc.).
  - *The boy likes to eat lunch early so that he avoids the crowd.*
  - *I ate dinner late and I'm tired.*

- Multiple embeddings: Sentences containing more than one embedded clause; may include a catenative.
  - *He's gonna have to go.*

- Embedded and conjoined: Sentence contains both an embedded and a conjoined clause.
  - *He's not really gonna buy it because he didn't wanna spend so much money.*

Late-Developing Complex Sentence Forms (MLU = 4–5) Examples

- Infinitive clause with different subjects.
  - *He realized she wouldn't want to wait any longer.*
  - *The boat sailed next to the boy who wasn't able to swim.*

- Relative clauses: A subordinate clause that acts as an adjective; may or may not include *which* or *that.*
  - *That's the ice cream that I tasted.*
  - *The argument that they had was silly.*

- Gerunds: An *ing* form that is used as a noun.
  - *Reading is my favorite hobby.*
  - *She likes swimming in the outdoor pool.*

- *Wh infinitives:* Use of *to,* along with *wh* conjunctions.

- Unmarked infinitives: *To* is not used; verbs include *make, help, watch,* or *let.*

- *She doesn't know how to do it.*
- *I thought you knew what to say.*
- *Make it go like this.*
- *Let her play it.*

Source: From *Language Disorders from Infancy to Intervention* (4th ed.), p. 434, by R. Paul and C. F. Norbury, 2012, St. Louis, MO: Mosby. Copyright Elsevier (2012). Reproduced with permission.

A child with an MLU between 3.0 and 4.0 (Brown's Stages IV and V) typically produces early sentence complexity; once a child produces an MLU between 4.0 and 5.0 (Brown's Stage V+ and beyond), later-developing complex sentence types emerge.

During intervention, an SLP or educator targets early-developing sentence complexity before targeting later-developing forms. Older children should be able to use complex sentence types during oral and written language production. I describe writing interventions for older students in Chapter 10.

Macroanalyses. The analyses above describe micro-level analyses; micro-level analyses consider the communicator's pragmatic, semantic, and morphosyntax abilities at the utterance level. The assessor must also consider the communicator's abilities beyond the utterance level. Discourse-level analysis is a macroanalysis that considers an individual's language use (Subdomain 5). **Conversational discourse** is defined as the unstructured or unplanned spoken interactions that occur between two individuals.

At the discourse level, the assessor evaluates the child's ability to effectively convey information as a speaker and to adjust and respond to the listener. Consider the following two speakers' descriptions of the same event:

Speaker 1:	Speaker 2:
• The little girl was on the way to school.	• She walked there.
• On the way, she saw a stray dog.	• And she saw it.
• So, she tried to catch it because she didn't want it to get hurt.	• She tried to catch it.
	• She didn't want it to get hurt.

As you can see from this example, at an utterance level, both speakers' utterances are grammatically correct. However, there are significant differences between the two speakers' communication abilities. We can understand the event described by Speaker 1, but we are confused by Speaker 2's version of the event. Macroanalysis reveals communication deficits not identified at the utterance level.

At the discourse level of analysis, the assessor considers a number of factors regarding an individual's conversational skill. For example, a skilled communicator provides sufficient information so the listener understands the speaker's intent. Consider Speaker 2 in the example just provided. If you were talking to Speaker 2, it would be unclear what had happened because the speaker does not provide enough decontextualized information. **Decontexualized information** is information able to be understood without environmental cues.

As another example of the need for decontextualization, imagine that you and I witness a car accident together and I say, "*Look at that! He crashed into her!*" In this instance, you understand exactly what I am saying because we shared the same visual cues and experience.

On the other hand, without a shared experience, the speaker must provide more information to the listener. If I walked up to you on the way to class and said, "*He crashed into her!*" you would be very confused. In the second conversation, in order to be an effective communicator, I must decontextualize the information. I might say, "*I saw a car accident. The driver of one car crashed into a girl who was driving a second car.*" I need to provide clear **referents** (specific nouns) to describe the people and objects (*the driver of one car* and *a girl . . . a second car*) rather than use ambiguous referents such as *that* and *her*. The ability to create clear linkages between new and old information (e.g., "*I saw a* man *driving a car; he crashed into another car*" [here the speaker uses the pronoun *he* to refer back to the "old" noun *a man*]) is called **referencing** (McCabe & Bliss, 2003). The ability to decontextualize language is a very important skill for an effective speaker and writer. I discuss more about an older student's use of decontextualization in Chapter 10. The ability to decontextualize information begins in the late preschool years and continues to develop during the elementary- and middle-school years.

There are a number of other important macro-level discourse skills assessed with children and older students. Important conversational discourse skills include:

- *Topic control:* Topic control is demonstrated when a speaker introduces a new topic. Children should initiate topics in addition to responding to others' topics. Effective speakers can discuss a variety of topics rather than just one or two.
- *Topic maintenance:* Topic maintenance is demonstrated when a conversational turn connects to the previously introduced topic. An effective conversation has linked exchanges in which communication partners share information using topically linked exchanges. Children with LI are less proficient at introducing and maintaining new topics. By the age of 3 years, children developing typically maintain a shared communication topic 50% of the time; by the age of 4, most children consistently maintain a conversation with a communication partner.
- *Conversational repair:* If one partner does not understand the other, or if the speaker senses the listener does not understand the communication, effective discourse partners repair the conversation either by paraphrasing, asking questions, or elaborating. By the age of 3, children developing typically begin to repair a communication breakdown when the listener says "*Huh?*" or "*What?*" The earliest form of conversational repair is repeating the utterance; as children mature, they begin to rephrase their statement to increase listener comprehension.
- *Informativeness:* An effective communicator contributes new information during a conversational turn rather than just repeating the same information. The communication should not be vague or confusing. Children developing typically begin to add information to a conversation at around age 3.
- *Conjunctive cohesion:* Effective speakers use conjunctions to causally and temporally connect information during shared interactions. For example, in the utterance "*I want to go home and take a nap because I didn't sleep last night,*" I link information with the conjunction *because,* highlighting the causal link between the two ideas. Words such as *because, so, before, then,* and *next* make explicit connections between ideas and events. Children typically begin to use conjunctive cohesion between 3 and 4 years of age.

As you can see, there are many clinical issues to be considered at a macroanalysis level. Figure 3.7 provides an example of a decision tree that demonstrates how an assessor evaluates discourse skills. In addition to conversational discourse, individuals with LI often struggle with narrative and classroom-based discourse. I discuss other discourse forms in Chapter 10.

Figure 3.7 **Decision Making at the Discourse Level**

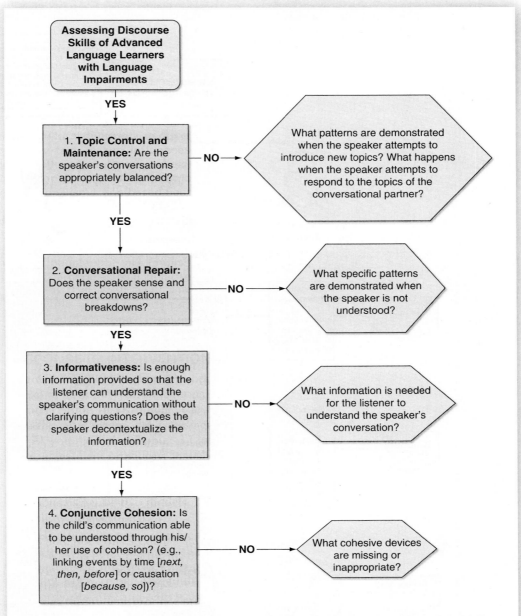

Source: Mccabe, Allyssa; Bliss, Lynn S., *Patterns of Narrative Discourse: A Multicultural, Life Span Approach*, 1st, © 2003. Printed and Electronically reproduced by permission of Pearson Education, Inc., Upper Saddle River, New Jersey.

In sum, it is important to note how the assessment process changes in keeping with a child's communication skills and life experiences. In Figure 3.8, notice how for very young children an SLP uses primarily observational measures and caregiver interviews. During the preschool years, the assessments tend to be play based and the

Figure 3.8 **Assessing Children across the Age Groups**

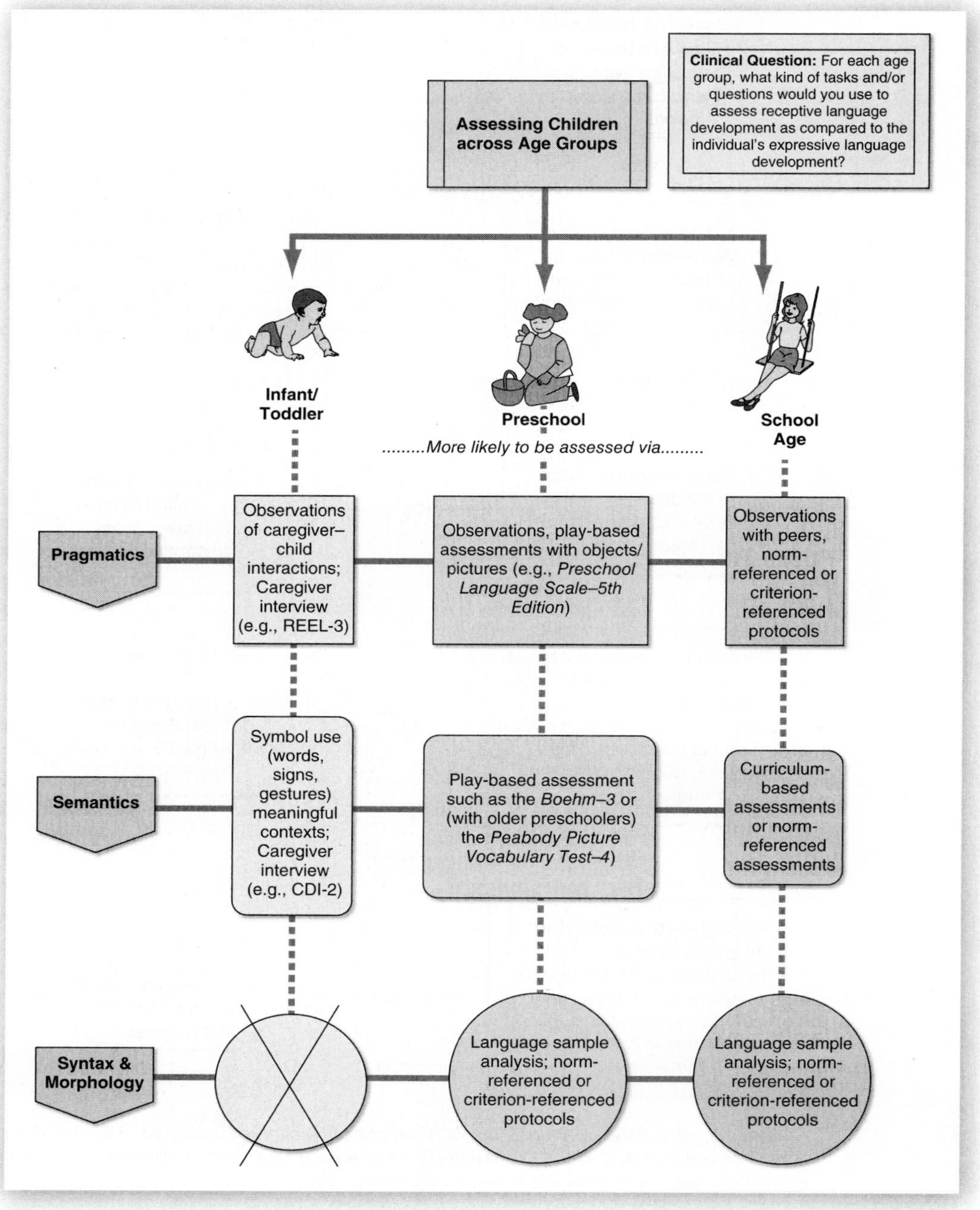

Clinical Question: For each age group, what kind of tasks and/or questions would you use to assess receptive language development as compared to the individual's expressive language development?

Assessing Children across Age Groups

Infant/Toddler — Preschool — School Age

.........More likely to be assessed via.........

Pragmatics
- Infant/Toddler: Observations of caregiver–child interactions; Caregiver interview (e.g., REEL-3)
- Preschool: Observations, play-based assessments with objects/pictures (e.g., *Preschool Language Scale–5th Edition*)
- School Age: Observations with peers, norm-referenced or criterion-referenced protocols

Semantics
- Infant/Toddler: Symbol use (words, signs, gestures) meaningful contexts; Caregiver interview (e.g., CDI-2)
- Preschool: Play-based assessment such as the *Boehm–3* or (with older preschoolers) the *Peabody Picture Vocabulary Test–4*)
- School Age: Curriculum-based assessments or norm-referenced assessments

Syntax & Morphology
- Infant/Toddler: [not assessed]
- Preschool: Language sample analysis; norm-referenced or criterion-referenced protocols
- School Age: Language sample analysis; norm-referenced or criterion-referenced protocols

SLP engages the preschooler in meaningful contexts with pictures, objects, and books. In the school-age years, the SLP includes curriculum-based and more norm-referenced assessments.

Assessment Process

In this section, I describe the process of assessment, including screening, measuring skills and abilities, synthesizing results, counseling families, and writing reports. An overview of the assessment process is visually presented in Figure 3.9.

Figure 3.9 **Overview of the Assessment Process**

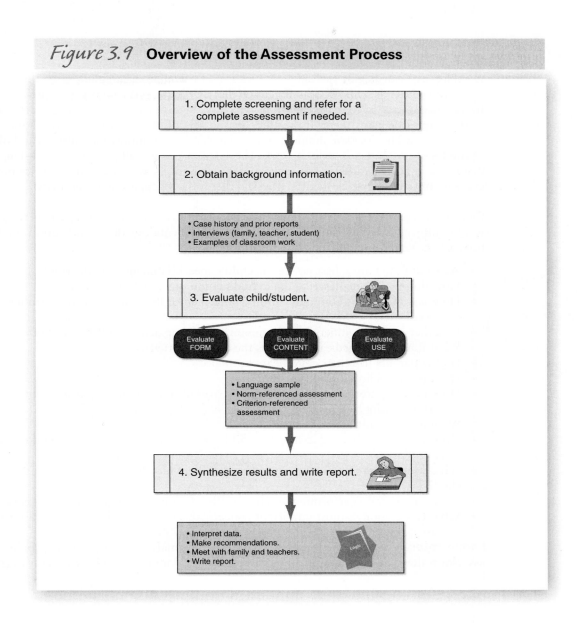

1. Complete screening and refer for a complete assessment if needed.

2. Obtain background information.
- Case history and prior reports
- Interviews (family, teacher, student)
- Examples of classroom work

3. Evaluate child/student.

Evaluate FORM   Evaluate CONTENT   Evaluate USE

- Language sample
- Norm-referenced assessment
- Criterion-referenced assessment

4. Synthesize results and write report.

- Interpret data.
- Make recommendations.
- Meet with family and teachers.
- Write report.

Screening

Screening is the initial assessment process used to identify children or students who require formal evaluation. Failing a screening does not mean an individual has a language delay or disorder. A language delay or disorder is only identified after a full assessment. An assessor uses the screening process to separate children who clearly are developing typical language skills from children who need further assessment. Screening may be accomplished by using a published, norm-referenced test or informal checklist. Sometimes questionnaires are distributed to teachers or parents to identify children needing further evaluation; these also are considered screening measures. Some school districts have mandatory communication screening protocols completed for all children entering school (ASHA, 2000).

DIAGNOSIS AND IDENTIFYING POTENTIAL INTERVENTION TARGETS

A skilled assessor begins the diagnostic process by evaluating a child's environment and considering how the child's communication disorder impacts the family. This process starts by reviewing case history information; typically the family sends this information prior to the diagnostic assessment. If the student is in school, the assessor interviews the classroom teacher. The assessor should observe classroom communication patterns and obtain examples of the student's written work. The assessor reviews all previous speech-language diagnostic reports in addition to reviewing information provided by other service providers (e.g., physicians, psychologists, physical therapists, occupational therapists).

Case History. The assessor begins the case history review by asking parents to supply written information describing their child's developmental, medical, and educational history. The critical questions in a case history include:

- When did the family first notice the child's speech-language impairment?
- How do the parents describe their child's communication at this time?
- How has the child's communication changed since the communication problem was observed?
- Do other family members have communication impairments? What are they?
- What illnesses or medical issues has the child experienced?
- Do the parents feel their child hears normally?
- Has the child's hearing been tested?
- How do the parents describe the child's overall development (physical, motor, self-help skills, eating)?
- What are the child's interests?
- How has the family tried to help the child's communication? What has worked? What has not worked?
- What kinds of therapy or other professional help has the family sought out for their child?
- How is their child performing in school? What (if any) are their educational concerns?
- What is the family's most important concern about their child's communication?

Family Interview. After reviewing the written information that the family provides, the assessor follows up with a family interview. It is important not to ask the parents to repeat all the information they have already provided, because this duplicates the time and effort spent filling out the case history form. However, in order to obtain a clear picture of the child's communication, I summarize the information and then ask the family to give an example or elaborate their answer.

For instance, I might say, "*You indicated that Susan gestures and points to get her needs met at home. Can you give me two examples from the last week of what she 'asked for,' how she indicated what she wanted, and how you responded?*" Or, in order to clarify Susan's hearing ability, I might say, "*Describe for me what Susan does when the phone rings.*" By asking the family to provide examples, I fine-tune my plan for Susan's assessment. For example, if the family indicates that Susan does not look at others when they speak, I take additional time to assess Susan's pragmatic skills in a range of naturalistic interactions. If the parents indicate that Susan's sentences are too simple or too short, I will include several different procedures to assess Susan's morphosyntax skills. Finally, if the family indicates that Susan's written language is unsophisticated and lacks descriptive words, I will plan additional opportunities to assess semantic skills in Susan's oral language and written work.

Remember that family members do not always use the "right" words to describe a child's communication ability. For example, a parent may describe a child's difficulty as a "speech disorder" although technically the deficit is a language disorder. Also, sometimes parents make incorrect assumptions. I interviewed one parent who indicated her child understood many words because when the mother pointed to an item and asked, "*Is that a chair?*" her child would nod *yes*. The mother's description of her child's ability was not substantiated during the assessment; the child did not demonstrate any receptive comprehension of words during the diagnostic session (e.g., she could not point to the correct item when I said, "*Point to the doll.*").

In this example, the mother interpreted the child's nod as an indication of "knowing the word." However, as I'm sure you realize, nodding *yes* does not necessarily indicate word comprehension. It may not even indicate that the child understood the question! To obtain the needed information, I asked the mother for more examples and asked clarifying questions.

When parents lack understanding about their child's communication impairment, the professional provides more in-depth information. However, often all needed information cannot be provided during the initial interview. Instead, the professional knows the family will need more time and counseling to learn more about their child's communication disorder.

Basic Components of the Assessment.   Although this book focuses on language impairment, a professional must consider all aspects of communication during an assessment. Think back to the speech chain model presented in Chapter 1. There, I describe the linkages between the motor system and the linguistic system. The motor system includes the mechanical aspects of hearing and the speech system. The linguistic system is the focus of this book; however, the assessor always remembers that the communication system includes both motor and linguistic components. Many children with LI have impairments in multiple communication components. Therefore, assessors consider all communication components during a diagnostic assessment. Not every area must be assessed with a norm-referenced test, but the assessor formally or informally evaluates all communication components and describes the individual's abilities within the diagnostic report. In addition to the syntax, pragmatic/social, and semantic analyses that are the focus of this book, assessments during a speech-language diagnostic assessment include the following:

- *Hearing screening:* Children who fail a hearing screening need to be referred for a complete audiological assessment. An illustration of a hearing screening is shown in Figure 3.10.
- *Speech-motor assessment:* The assessor evaluates the child's (a) facial symmetry; (b) structure and function of the lips, tongue, jaw, and velopharynx (i.e., the soft palate); and (c) resonance, phonatory, and respiratory systems used for speech.
- *Speech/articulation assessment:* An articulation assessment evaluates the child's motor ability to produce phonemes. The assessor considers the child's sound production in isolation, syllables, words, sentences, and running speech. The norm-referenced Goldman-Fristoe Test of Articulation–Second Edition (Goldman & Fristoe, 2000) is a commonly used articulation test.
- *Phonological assessment and phonological awareness:* Phonological assessment, as discussed briefly in Chapter 2, considers the rules that govern the sound combinations in speech production. To uncover phonological processing disorders, the assessor looks for sound error patterns. Phonological processing disorders are considered a disorder of language form. An example of a test for phonological processing is the Hodson Assessment of Phonological Patterns–Third Edition (Hodson, 2004). Phonological awareness (PA) is a receptive skill. PA refers to the ability to reflect on and manipulate phonemic segments of speech. PA development is highly correlated with early reading skill. (See Chapter 10 for more about PA skills and literacy.)

Figure 3.10 **Student Receives a Hearing Screening as Part of the Assessment Process**

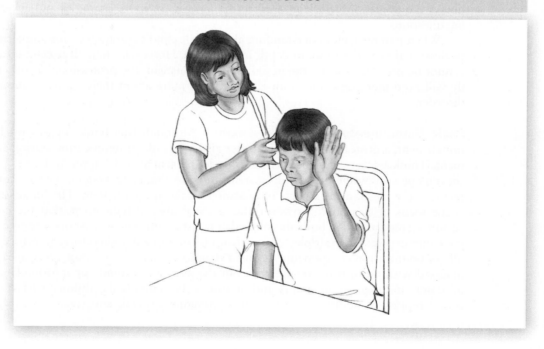

- *Assessment of cognitive ability:* An SLP or educator often documents early cognitive ability by observing child behaviors in play-based tasks (i.e., Piagetian framework for development; see Chapter 2) or by analyzing a child's drawing performance. For older children, the assessment sometimes includes a nonverbal IQ test such as the Test of Nonverbal Intelligence–4 (Brown, Sherbenou, & Johnsen, 2010). (I describe criterion-referenced play-based assessment in Chapter 6.)
- *Analysis of a child's rate and fluency of speech.* A child's fluency is typically evaluated informally during conversation. If a fluency disorder is present, a formal fluency assessment is completed.

Depending on the child's age and developmental level, different components of the assessment are emphasized. For example, a cognitive assessment is less appropriate for an older student when cognitive abilities have already been documented. It is also important to remember that the practitioner may need to include additional or alternative assessments for children who are English language learners (i.e., children for whom English is a second language). Learn more about this issue in Focus 3.7.

Identifying Potential Intervention Communication Targets: Communication Subdomains. During the assessment process, a professional considers the developmental

---

FOCUS 3.7 *Multicultural Issues*

By the 2030s, English language learners (ELLs) will account for approximately 40% of the entire school-aged population in the United States. In some areas in the United States, the number of school-age ELLs already exceeds this projection. For instance, right now in California, approximately 60%–70% of schoolchildren speak a language other than English as their primary language (Roseberry-McKibben & Brice, 2013).

With this changing demographic, there is an urgent need for effective language assessment protocols for children who speak English as their second language (L2). However, it is challenging to identify language and learning disorders in ELLs because their English-language abilities are still developing, and the majority of language tests are normed with monolingual native speakers only. This situation makes it likely that practitioners may overidentify language and learning disorders in the ELL population.

To reduce overidentification, practitioners should use a range of language assessment tools and also obtain information about the child's first-language development from the child's caregivers (Paradis, Schneider, & Duncan, 2013).

Two of the best predictors of language impairment in the ELL population include (a) a parent survey of the child's language development in his or her first language (e.g., Hindi, French, Spanish, Mandarin) and (b) a nonword repetition test.

An example of a parent questionnaire designed to assess a child's language development in his or her first language is The Alberta Language Development Questionnaire (ALDeQ; Paradis, Emmerzael, Sorenson Duncan, 2010). The ALDeQ is a parent questionnaire on early language milestones, current first-language abilities, activity preferences and behavior, and family history. The assessor rates the parent's responses; lower scores reflect what might be expected for children with LI, and higher scores reflect typical development. You can see an example of the ALDeQ and learn more about assessing a child who is an ELL at www.linguistics.ualberta.ca/CHESL_Centre/Questionnaires.aspx.

An example of a nonword repetition test is a subtest included in the Comprehensive Test of Phonological Processing (CTOPP; Wagner, Torgesen, & Rashotte, 1999). The CTOPP nonword repetition subtest measures a child's phonological short-term memory. The child is asked to accurately repeat nonsense words; the nonsense words increase in syllable length and phonological complexity. The child's score reflects the number of words he or she accurately produces.

---

sequence of language and considers the communication subdomains aligned with the individual's age and developmental level. The individual's performance within the five subdomains helps the professional select intervention targets.

Subdomain 1. If a child or an older individual with significant communication impairment is at the initial levels of communication, the assessment focuses on Subdomain 1: early pragmatic development. When focusing on early pragmatics, the assessor considers the individual's communication functions (e.g., asking, naming, requesting, negating) and evaluates whether the individual uses nonlinguistic verbalizations (pointing, gesturing) or meaning-based symbols (words, signs, pictures) to communicate (i.e., the individual's communication means). A summary of Dore's (1975) and Halliday's (1975) pragmatic categories is provided in Table 3.5. The assessor evaluates an individual's pragmatic abilities as compared to the range of pragmatic functions shown in Table 3.5.

Subdomains 2 and 3. Subdomain 2 (vocabulary development) and Subdomain 3 (early word combinations) focus on semantic skills. Parent checklists, such as the MacArthur-Bates Communicative Developmental Inventories (Fenson et al., 2007) can be used to obtain norm-referenced data on children's semantic ability. A short-form version of the MacArthur-Bates–Second Edition is presented in Figure 3.11. In the MacArthur-Bates assessment, parents indicate the vocabulary items produced by their child (between the ages of 8 and 30 months); the number of words produced by an individual child is compared with normative data from other children the same age.

An assessor uses semantic-focused assessment data to determine a child's use of words and word combinations to communicate meaning. The professional combines information from a parent checklist (such as the MacArthur) with information obtained from a conversational language sample.

A few additional basic principles guide the assessment process for a child functioning within Subdomains 2 and 3 (Haynes & Pindzola, 2008):

- Determine whether the child uses a wide range of semantic combinations or only a few. Remember that at Brown's Stage I children should be establishing a variety of semantic categories.
- The child should have the lexicon (i.e., vocabulary) to describe his or her environment and communicate socially to achieve many different outcomes (e.g., greeting, negation, questioning, commenting, imaginative play).

Table 3.5 **Pragmatic Categories for Young Children**

Halliday's* communication function (What is the child trying to accomplish?)	Dore's primitive speech acts (What does the child do?)
Interacting	Labeling—identifies an object
Communication used to maintain contact with others	Answering—responds to a caregiver
	Calling—attempts to gain attention
	Repeating/Imitating
Regulatory	Requesting an action
Communication used to control others	Requesting an answer
	Calling
	Protesting—rejects an action or object
Personal	Greeting—acknowledges a caregiver
Communication used to express emotions	Practicing
	Calling
	Protesting
Heuristic	Labeling
Communication used to explore and categorize	Repeating/Imitating
	Practicing
Instrumental	Requesting an action
Communication used to satisfy wants/needs	Repeating/Imitating
	Calling
	Practicing
Imaginative	Labeling
Communication used during play	Calling
	Practicing
	Repeating/Imitating
Informative	Requesting
Communication used to share knowledge	Labeling
	Practicing

*Halliday (1975) and Dore (1974, 1975) categorized slightly different aspects of early pragmatic function. Halliday's pragmatic skills focus on what the child is trying to accomplish (i.e., What is the child's communication goal?), while Dore's categories focus on the child's communication functions at the one-word stage (i.e., What behaviors do we see the child attempting?). Both category systems are used to characterize early pragmatic skills.

- The child should be able to initiate communication and produce multiword combinations spontaneously (not only in imitation of an adult).
- As the child moves to Brown's Stages II and III, the assessor looks for beginning use of morphosyntax features in multiword combinations (e.g., plurals, past tense verbs).

Some children with language disorders continue to struggle to maintain vocabulary development as they enter school (Brackenbury & Pye, 2005). The reasons for vocabulary delay include difficulty with underlying vocabulary-learning processes such as (a) learning vocabulary through everyday interactions (particularly vocabulary that involves figurative speech), (b) storing the phonological information needed to produce words in short-term memory, (c) storing lexical items in long-term memory, and (d) expressively producing vocabulary. *Figurative speech* refers to nonliteral words or expressions such as metaphors, idioms, and proverbs. For example, when I say, *"My friend flipped his wig!"* you know my

---

Figure 3.11 **MacArthur Short Form: Level II (Form A)**

Vocabulary Checklist: Children understand many more words than they say. We are particularly interested in the words you child SAYS. Please mark the words you have heard your child use. If your child uses a different pronunciation of the word, mark it anyway.

BAA BAA	NECKLACE	PARTY	COLD
MEOW	SHOE	FRIEND	FAST
OUCH	SOCK	MOMMY	HAPPY
OH OH	CHIN	PERSON	HOT
WOOF WOOF	EAR	BYE	LAST
BEAR	HAND	HI	TINY
BIRD	LEG	NO	WET
CAT	BROOM	THANK YOU	AFTER
DUCK	COMB	SHOPPING	DAY
HORSE	MOP	CARRY	TONIGHT
AIRPLANE	PLATE	CHASE	OUR
BOAT	TRASH	DUMP	THEM
CAR	TRAY	FINISH	THIS
BALL	TOWEL	FIT	US
BOOK	BED	HUG	WHERE
GAME	BEDROOM	LIKE	BESIDE
APPLESAUCE	BENCH	LISTEN	DOWN
CANDY	OVEN	PRETEND	UNDER
COKE	STAIRS	RIP	ALL
CRACKER	FLAG	SHAKE	MUCH
JUICE	RAIN	TASTE	COULD
MEAT	STAR	GENTLE	NEED
MILD	SWING	THINK	WOULD
PEAS	SCHOOL	WISH	IF
HAT	SKY	ALL GONE	

Has your child begun to combine words yet, such as "*Nother cookie*" or "*Doggie bite?*"

❑ Not yet   ❑ Sometimes   ❑ Often

Source: Courtesy of Larry Fenson

---

friend was very upset; you do not literally believe that my friend's wig fell off! Nonliteral, figurative language can be challenging vocabulary learning for students with LI. I provide more examples of figurative speech in Table 3.6.

I mentioned above that children with LI have difficulty learning vocabulary because they may not easily learn new words in everyday interactions; this refers to a process called fast mapping. **Fast mapping** is a process in which young children learn a new word with only minimal exposure (Pence, Bojczyk, & Williams, 2007). For instance, young children developing typically hear a word only a few times and then, remarkably, are observed to produce the word spontaneously. Learn more about the research exploring the process of fast mapping in Focus 3.8.

Table 3.6   **Figurative Speech for Older School-Age Students**

Term	Definition	Example
Metaphor	An implied comparison between two unlike things. Metaphors carry meaning from one idea to another.	• *Life is a journey.* • *I'm a night owl; you are an early bird.*
Simile	A figure of speech that draws a comparison between two different words or concepts; usually contains the words *like* or *as*.	• *Her heart soared like an eagle.* • *His headache pounded like a drum.*
Proverb	A well-known saying that expresses a truth or offers advice.	• *Penny wise and pound foolish* • *Practice makes perfect.* • *All's well that ends well.* • *Honesty is the best policy.*
Idiom	An expression that cannot be understood from the combined meanings of the individual words; a colloquial expression.	• *Go the whole nine yards.* • *Come to grips with it.* • *Strikes a chord* • *Out on a limb* • *Not playing with a full deck* • *Taking the bait*

FOCUS 3.8   *Research*

Fast mapping is a process in which young children learn a new word with only minimal exposure (Pence et al., 2007). It is proposed that children, when asked to identify an unfamiliar object, form a tentative hypothesis that leads to a partial construction of word meaning. Over time, with repeated exposure, the meaning of the word is clarified. For example, imagine that a child is helping his mother in the kitchen and she says, "*Give me the whisk.*" Because the child recognizes the spoon, knife, and spatula but does not recognize the fourth item on the counter (the whisk), he hands her the whisk. The child assumes that the novel word is the unfamiliar item. Fast mapping helps explain how children learn so many vocabulary words in such a short time. However, fast mapping is only a step in true vocabulary development; research demonstrates that words must be integrated into a child's lexicon before word meaning is retained (Alt & Plante, 2006).

Children use other linguistic cues to assist in fast mapping; the effects of linguistic features on children's fast-mapping abilities are tested in research studies. To avoid the effect of previous exposure to the words, the examiner often uses nonsense words. For example, imagine that you are testing the effects of a child's knowledge of syntax. You say to the child, "*Show me the blick.*" If the child has syntax knowledge, he is likely to point to an object (i.e., a noun) rather than an action word (i.e., a verb). On the other hand, if you ask, "*Show me 'She is* blicking,'" the child with syntax knowledge is likely to pick an action picture (i.e., a verb).

Children with language impairment (LI) have reduced fast-mapping ability; they need more exposures to a word to complete a fast-mapping task. Research suggests that reduced fast mapping is part of the reason that young children with LI have more difficulty learning new vocabulary items (Alt & Plante, 2006). Researchers continue to investigate how different linguistic information is used to assist (or limit) fast-mapping abilities.

The assessment process of semantic skills assesses a child's receptive and expressive vocabulary. **Receptive vocabulary** refers to the words a child understands, both in spoken and written form, while **expressive vocabulary** refers to the words a child produces. To test receptive vocabulary, the assessor says a word and asks the child to point to a picture representing the word spoken. In an expressive vocabulary test, the assessor shows a picture and asks the child to name the pictured word. Typically, a child comprehends many more words than he is able to produce expressively. A description of some commonly used vocabulary tests is provided in Table 3.7.

Subdomain 4. As a child's sentence length increases, an assessor begins to consider the language features associated with Subdomain 4 (morphosyntax development). In Subdomain 4, an individual developing typically demonstrates the maturing use of adult-like syntax and learns to combine root words with plural and possessive forms. A **root word** is the fundamental or unmarked part of a word (e.g., *look, walk, boy*).

An assessor incorporates a variety of norm-referenced and criterion-referenced tools (such as language sample analysis) into the morphosyntax assessment. Morphosyntax tasks can take several forms:

- Receptive morphosyntax tasks:
  - In order to determine whether a student understands the meaning of a morpheme, the assessor shows several pictures and says, "*Show me the* boys *are running. Now, show me the* boy *is running.*" A student who understands the use of the plural *s* points to a picture of several boys in response to the first sentence and points to a picture of one boy in response to the second sentence.
  - In order to assess the student's understanding of correct sentence structure (i.e., syntax), the assessor tells the student, "*The boy is pushed by the baby.*" The assessor shows several pictures; in one picture, the boy is pushing the baby, and in the other picture, the baby is pushing the boy.
  - The assessor reads a short paragraph and asks the student comprehension questions about the story.
- Expressive morphosyntax tasks:
  - The assessor shows a picture and asks the student to complete the sentence. "*This is David. Whose book is it? It is _____ (his).*" The student demonstrates use of possessive pronouns by completing the sentence with the word *his*.
  - The assessor provides a picture and a word (e.g., *although*). The assessor asks the student to make up a sentence about the picture using the target word.
  - The assessor produces a sentence and asks the student to repeat the sentence. For example, "*Was the boy followed by the girl?*" The assessor notes any errors in morphosyntax during the student's sentence imitation.

Table 3.7 **Examples of Norm-Referenced Vocabulary Tests**

Test	Description	Age norms	Psychometric properties
Expressive One-Word Picture Vocabulary Test–4th Edition (EOWPVT-4; Martin & Brownell, 2010)	Expressive single-word vocabulary. The student is asked to label the word when the examiner points to the picture. Spanish version available.	2.0–80+ years	**RELIABILITY:** The median Cronbach's coefficient alpha was .95. Test–retest coefficient was .98 for the entire sample indicating good reliability. **VALIDITY:** The EOWPVT-4 did well compared to the STAR Reading Test, with a coefficient of .69. When the EOWPVT-4 was compared to the Wechsler Intelligence Scale for Children–Fourth Edition (WISC-4; Full Scale IQ), a coefficient of .35 was obtained; coefficients between .3 and .7 are considered to be "moderate."
Peabody Picture Vocabulary Test–4 (PPVT-4; Dunn & Dunn, 2006)	Receptive, single-word vocabulary; the student points to one named picture when shown four pictures. Spanish version available.	2.6–adult	**RELIABILITY:** Internal consistency alpha: .92 to .98 (median: .95). Split-half: .86 to .97 (median: .94). Alternate-form .88 to .96 (median: .94). Test–retest .91 to .94 (median: .92). **VALIDITY:** The PPVT-3 had an average correlation of .69 with the OWLS Listening Comprehension Scale and .74 with the OWLS Oral Expression Scale. Its correlations with measures of verbal ability are: .91 (WISC-III VIQ), .89 (KAIT Crystallized IQ), and .81 (K-BIT Vocabulary).
Receptive One-Word Picture Vocabulary Test–4th Edition (ROWPVT-4; Martin & Brownell, 2010)	Receptive, single-word vocabulary; the student points to one named picture when shown four pictures. Spanish version available.	2–80 years	**RELIABILITY:** The median Cronbach's coefficient alpha was .97. Test–retest coefficient was .97 for the entire sample, indicating good reliability. **VALIDITY:** The ROWPVT-4 did well compared to the STAR Reading Test, with a coefficient of .69. When ROWPVT-4 was compared to the Wechsler Intelligence Scale for Children–Fourth Edition (WISC-4; Verbal Comprehension Index Subtest), a coefficient of .35 was obtained; coefficients between .3 and .7 are considered to be "moderate."

(continued)

Table 3.7 (*continued*)

Test	Description	Age norms	Psychometric properties
Comprehensive Receptive and Expressive Vocabulary Test–Third Edition (CREVT-3; Wallace & Hammill, 2013)	Receptive and expressive single-word vocabulary. In the expressive subtest, the student is asked to label and define the word.	5.0–89:11 years	**RELIABILITY:** Reliability was assessed by computing coefficient alphas; all subtests were at or above .90 and thus highly acceptable. **VALIDITY:** Validity was assessed by correlating CREVT-3 scores with other vocabulary tests; all correlations were large, in a magnitude ranging from .72 to .87.
The WORD Test–2–Elementary (Bowers, Huisingh, Barrett, LoGiudice, & Orman, 2004)	Semantic concepts. Subtests include associations, synonyms, semantic absurdities, antonyms, definitions, and multiple definitions.	7–11 years	**RELIABILITY:** The lowest test–retest reliability coefficient is .37 in the Flexible Word Use task for the 11 years to 11 years, 5 months age group. The manual explains that several reliability indexes may be low because of the restricted scoring range of the group. The 97.8% of agreement in scoring six protocols among nine SLPs does not provide convincing evidence of high interscorer reliability. **VALIDITY:** A major problem with this test is the lack of validity evidence.

As you review the assessment procedures in the examples above, remember that different test procedures place varying demands on an individual's syntax, morphology, semantic, and phonological abilities. For example, a sentence imitation task taps into an individual's short-term memory; difficulty with an imitative task may be a result of a short-term memory problem rather than a morphosyntax deficit.

The test directions and even the scoring system can alter the student's ability to perform. Specifically, on some tests, approximations of the correct response receive some point value (e.g., a point value of 0 [incorrect], 1 [partially correct], or 2 [completely correct]). On other tests, responses are marked as either correct (e.g., a value of 1) or incorrect (e.g., a value of 0). Assessors should carefully examine individual items to determine the task requirement or even take the test themselves to appreciate task demands.

Subdomain 5. As I discussed earlier in this chapter, an assessor must consider a child's ability to initiate and maintain conversational discourse (Subdomain 5). Advanced pragmatic use also consists of observing a student's use and comprehension of slang, sarcasm, and politeness forms. These subtle language functions become increasingly important in school-age students. A list of pragmatic skills relevant for school-age students is provided in Table 3.8.

Table 3.8 **Pragmatic Skills for School-Age Students**

Social/pragmatic skill	Difficulties that might be demonstrated by a school-age student with pragmatic weaknesses
The student should be able to note the current social situation in which the communication interaction is occurring, including the nonverbal cues.	• Student attempts to enter a conversation where the communication partners are clearly engaged in a private conversation. • Student has difficulty telling when others are teasing or are being sarcastic.
The student should be able to engage in mutually pleasant conversations with others.	• Student talks about a topic that is not interesting to the communication partner. • Student interrupts others. • Student does not link questions or comments to the communication partner's topic. • The student's conversation is disjointed and/or the student does not link his spoken ideas together in ways that promote comprehension.
The student should be able to repair a conversation when others do not understand.	• Student does not note communication partner's nonverbal behaviors that indicate lack of communication. • When the student repairs (attempts to clarify) his message, he repeats himself. The student does not rephrase his communication to increase comprehension. • The student does not adjust his conversation tone (i.e., code switching) when he speaks to varying audiences. For example, the student uses slang or overly casual language when talking to teachers.
The student should follow the implicit rules of a conversational interaction.	• The student stands too close to others when talking. • The student uses inappropriate volume (too loud, too soft). • The student asks too many personal questions. • The student does not raise his or her hand before speaking in a classroom.

SLPs and educators use varying assessment instruments to assess an individual's function in Subdomain 5. It is important to remember that, regardless of the type of assessment used, educators are under increasing pressure to demonstrate the practical benefit of assessment for improving a child's pragmatic communication at home, preschool, or within elementary and secondary classrooms (Zeidner, 2001).

SYNTHESIZING ASSESSMENT RESULTS, COUNSELING FAMILIES, AND WRITING REPORTS

After the assessment protocols are completed, the assessor synthesizes the information that has been gathered. This information includes (a) case history information and information from prior educational or professional tests and reports; (b) interviews with family, teachers, and student (if appropriate); (c) observation of client in conversation with family and peers; (d) criterion-referenced assessment; and (e) norm-referenced assessment. In this process, the SLP or educator answers the following questions:

- Does the child have language impairment?
- What language domains are impaired (form, content, use)?
- Does the child demonstrate consistency of ability across testing procedures?
- What are the child's strengths and weaknesses in communicating?
- What are the most important communication behaviors that limit the child's everyday functioning?

The first challenge is for the assessor to identify information overlap from the tests, interviews, and observations. The SLP or educator seeks to confirm the communication problem across measures or tests.

The second challenge is to summarize the information in a meaningful way so that family members understand the child's communication issues. I have found that using the form–content–use model is a helpful way to communicate information to parents and teachers. I am careful, however, to avoid using jargon and unfamiliar terms. For example, my explanation might go something like this:

> As you described when you came in this morning, Kylee seems behind in her ability to use words and sentences. I completed some different assessments today to check on Kylee's communication. The information you gave me was very helpful. I also want to tell you how much I enjoyed interacting with Kylee today—she really enjoyed playing with the housekeeping center!
>
> First, I completed some assessments of Kylee's ability to communicate her needs. We played together, and I looked at her ability to let me know when she needed a toy, wanted help with something, or wanted to let me know that she didn't like the toy I gave her. I was happy to see that she is very able to communicate what she wants, but as you noted, she doesn't do it with words. Instead, she used pointing and sounds to indicate her ideas. Although she isn't using words to communicate, I was happy to note that she is able to get her needs met nonverbally. This is a very good sign, because sometimes children do not seem to understand that they can communicate with others—even nonverbally—to get their needs met.
>
> Next, I looked at the number of words that Kylee understands and uses. I compared the number of words that she understands to the words she is able to produce verbally. To check her understanding of words, I used an assessment in which I showed Kylee four pictures. After showing her the pictures, I said one of the words and then I asked Kylee to point to the correct word. Kylee's understanding of vocabulary words was somewhat behind what we would expect for her age. In our play interactions, I also saw that she is able to follow very simple one-step instructions, such as "*Show me the book.*" But she has some difficulty with more complex directions, such as "*Put the ball under the table.*" Taken together, the results showed me that Kylee's ability to understand what others say is slightly below what is expected for her age.
>
> Finally, I completed some observations and some formal tests during which I looked at the number of words that Kylee can produce. I would expect at her age that Kylee should have between 50 and 100 words and that she would be beginning to make some word combinations like "*Me go bye-bye*" and "*Baby sleeping.*" But, as you have noticed, Kylee has only one or two words and is not combining words together. Her difficulty in using words to express her ideas demonstrates a moderate level of delay. Do you have any questions about anything I've said so far?

Take a close look at the information I provided to Kylee's parents. In the first paragraph, I summarized the information that her parents provided in the initial interview. Parents are the experts about their child's communication, and I acknowledged this contribution. I also provided feedback on Kylee's behavior during the assessment. I know that parents are typically very anxious about their child's abilities. I used this opportunity to build the ongoing relationship I will need to establish an effective intervention program.

In the second paragraph, I began by describing Kylee's pragmatic skills (i.e., language use). Notice that I did not use the word *pragmatics,* but I described Kylee's ability to use language to request, negate, and question. I also highlighted the importance of pragmatic skills.

In the third paragraph, I described semantics (i.e., language form). I framed this discussion by talking about Kylee's understanding of words (i.e., receptive language). If you read this paragraph carefully, you noticed that I discussed both a norm-referenced test (i.e., the test during which I asked Kylee to point to pictures) and an observational, play-based task in which I asked Kylee to follow directions. This is an example of how I used multiple data sources to understand Kylee's abilities.

Also in the third paragraph, note that during this first explanation of results, I did not provide Kylee's parents with Kylee's standard score on the receptive vocabulary test. I typically give this information to the parents in another discussion; I often discuss test scores when I present the final written report. Many parents are overwhelmed by too much technical information at one time.

In the fourth paragraph, I discussed Kylee's expressive language ability. First, I framed the findings by describing the MLU that Kylee should be using. Then I described Kylee's verbal output in relation to developmental norms. Can you determine (a) the Brown's stage at which Kylee should be from my description and (b) her actual level of performance? If you can do this critical-thinking task, you understand how language sample analysis is used to gauge language development. Finally, at the end of my discussion, I paused and took time to answer questions.

In my discussion of Kylee's results, I used the terms *slightly below* and *moderately delayed.* The use of the terms *mild, moderate,* and *severe* should always be used carefully. However, with this caution in mind, I typically think about a standard score between 1.25 and 1.5 standard deviations as being a mild level of impairment (these are below the 10th percentile) and scores between 1.5 and 2.0 standard deviations as a moderate level of impairment. A standard score at or below 2 standard deviations (2nd percentile of performance) is typically considered a severe impairment. Standard scores are always interpreted in conjunction with observation and criterion-referenced measures.

Clinical Report Writing.   The final challenge in the assessment process is to write the assessment report in a way that clearly summarizes the findings. In Appendix C, I provide a sample of an assessment report and explain the rationale for individual sections and writing style. There is no single right way to write a report except that the report must be accurate, concise, and link the various assessment protocols together in a logical way. However, I ask beginning students to use a report style that is consistent with the form–content–use language model. I do this because often beginning students administer tests but cannot explain what language domains (form, content, use) are being evaluated. This is particularly relevant when interpreting norm-referenced tests (e.g., the CELF-5) where different subtests within the test evaluate different language domains—one subtest evaluating syntax, another evaluating semantics, etc. Whereas a skilled assessor determines what domain is assessed within each subtest, a beginning student sometimes reports test scores without understanding the implications of the subtest score. However, if the report is divided into sections on form, content, and use, the assessor must consider each language domain individually and link information from norm-referenced tests and criterion-referenced assessments.

A skilled assessor also considers the difficulty level of the subtest task. For example, a syntax subtest might ask the child to repeat a sentence (a relatively easy syntax task). Alternatively, in another syntax subtest, the child may be provided with three words and asked to construct a novel sentence (a more difficult syntax task). The assessor looks at an individual's varying ability across subtests and provides an explanation.

Beyond the above-mentioned suggestions, there are general professional writing guidelines used when writing a report. In Table 3.9, I describe writing guidelines and present examples of writing styles to use and avoid.

Table 3.9 **Guidelines for Report Writing**

Guideline	Like this:	Not like this:	Why?
• Use clear, short sentences. • Use specific language rather than ambiguous terms.	Mary has significant difficulty in the classroom following two- and three-step directions.	Following observations, it was revealed[1] that Mary is not functioning up to the norm for her level. She acts confused periodically[2] in the classroom.	[1] An expression such as *it is revealed* adds words but does not add writing clarity. [2] Expressions such as *up to the norm* and *confused periodically* are ambiguous; they cannot be measured.
• Use nontechnical language or explain terms. • Do not use an abbreviation unless it is defined.	The examiner assessed Sonia's ability to point to words when they were named. This is a measure of receptive vocabulary. The Peabody Picture Vocabulary Test–4 (PPVT-4) standard score was within normal limits.	Semantic abilities were assessed using the PPVT-4.	Parents, teachers, and other professionals need to be able to understand the assessment results.
• Avoid colloquial expressions. • Use formal instead of casual word choices.	In a 30-minute period, John left his seat three times. His mother confirmed John's difficulty in attending to tasks at home.	John bounced off the walls[3] during the class; he had difficulty interacting with other kids. His mom[4] said that John is just like this at home.	[3] *Bounced off the walls* is a colloquial expression. [4] Use more formal word choices (e.g., *children, mother*) in written reports.

Table 3.9   (**continued**)

Guideline	Like this:	Not like this:	Why?
• Use active rather than passive sentences.	During an observation of a shared reading, Katrina's mother asked 5–6 questions on each page of the book.	A storybook reading was observed[5] by the examiner. During the observation, the examiner observed that there were numerous examples of direct questioning that were asked by Katrina's mother.[6]	[5] Avoid passive sentence construction such as *a storybook reading was observed.* [6] This sentence is not clearly constructed.
• Avoid qualifiers and noncommittal language. • Describe behavior rather than labeling the individual.	Thomas had difficulty with instructions containing the subordinate conjunctions *before* and *after* (e.g., "*Before you touch the red square, touch the blue triangle.*"). He refused to complete the subtest containing complex commands.	Thomas appeared to have some difficulty with more complex tasks and sometimes[7] struggled to follow directions. He appeared frustrated.[8]	[7] Eliminate noncommittal language. [8] This is a subjective labeling of the student's emotions.

Source: Based on information from "Documenting Clinical Service Delivery: Writing Style and Lexical Selection" by D. L. Wilkerson, 2000, *Contemporary Issues in Communication Science and Disorders, 27,* pp. 6–13.

Summary

- Norm-referenced assessments have statistical properties that allow the assessor to compare the individual's performance to that of his or her chronological peer group. Norm-referenced assessments are typically used to determine whether an individual has language impairment. Criterion-referenced assessments are used to document an individual's ability in a specific domain; the raw data are used to develop intervention plans and document behavior change. Dynamic assessment (DA) is considered a non-static or process-oriented assessment protocol because it evaluates a child's ability to learn; DA is particularly appropriate when assessing a child from a nonmajority ethnic or cultural group. Consider validity and reliability when evaluating an assessment tool. Standard scores are transformed scores that allow an individual's performance to be compared with that of same-age peers on a bell-shaped curve.

- An assessor computes mean length of utterance (MLU) by dividing the total number of morphemes in a speech sample by the number of utterances; this provides an average for utterance length. The assessor can use MLU to quantitatively compare a child's length of utterances with developmental data from Brown's stages. A T-unit analysis is an analysis in which the assessor separates clauses by coordinating conjunctions; it is an analysis used with older school-age children. Microanalysis considers an individual's output utterance by utterance; microanalysis can include analysis of pragmatic function and semantic relationships for beginning language learners and morphosyntax features for later-language learners. Macroanalysis considers an individual's ability to participate in conversation and includes discourse and mazing analyses.

- A professional develops an assessment plan to evaluate the individual's (a) language use (e.g., How does the client communicate? Can he get his needs met? What is conversation like when communicating with this individual?), (b) language content (e.g., What words does the individual know and use? Is the individual's semantic knowledge adequate for school success?), and (c) language form (e.g., What morphosyntax features does the individual understand and use? Do morphosyntax weaknesses negatively impact academic performance?).

- Assessment priorities change depending on the relevant communication subdomain. In Subdomain 1 (early pragmatic), the assessor often uses criterion-referenced assessments and parent surveys to understand the individual's use of pragmatic communication behaviors. When considering Subdomains 2 and 3 (word learning and early word combinations), the assessor uses a semantic focus to document the individual's lexicon and the semantic combinations used when combining words. Norm-referenced, criterion-referenced, dynamic, and observational assessments are all used for individuals at Subdomains 2 and 3. When assessing Subdomain 4 (morphosyntax), an assessor typically uses a combination of language sample analyses, along with norm-referenced, dynamic, and criterion-referenced assessment. When assessing Subdomain 5, the assessor completes a discourse analysis and considers advanced pragmatic skills.

- In addition to evaluating an individual's language abilities, an assessor considers all aspects of the communication system during a speech-language assessment. This includes hearing ability, speech motor ability, cognitive ability, fluency and rate of speech, sound production, awareness of phonemes, and voice quality.

- An assessor evaluates case history data, interviews family members and teachers, evaluates the child or student using a variety of assessment tools, synthesizes test results, and writes a clinical report to complete the assessment process.

Discussion and In-Class Activities

1. Divide into groups with other students in your class. Look over a brief outline of a child with a language disorder given to you by your instructor (e.g., Child 1, who is 8 years old, is having difficulty in school learning to read and write; Child 2 is 5 years old but can only speak with a few word combinations [i.e., child has a severe disability]; Child 3, who is 3 years old, has a slight language delay and is making morphosyntax errors). Together with students in your group, brainstorm activities, observations, interviews, and criterion-referenced assessments that could be used with each case to obtain background information and conduct the assessment. Who should be interviewed before the assessment, and what questions will you ask? What points should be included in the final interview with parents and teachers? What information needs to be obtained during classroom observations?

2. Your instructor will provide a videotape observation of a young child in play with another child or an adult. Use the Language Sample Worksheet (see Appendix D) to document observed behaviors. Did the child you observed demonstrate a sufficient range (given his or her age) of pragmatic function? Could the context or environment be altered to promote a greater variety of pragmatic behaviors? How did the child try to communicate (communication means)? Did he or she use gestures, sounds, words, or word combinations?

3. Your instructor will show you a video of the administration of a norm-referenced test; score at least part of the test using score sheets provided to you. Your instructor may choose to give you score sheets already scored for the target child. After completing the scoring process (with your instructor's guidance), refer to the normative data table from the test manual. Find the page in the manual with standard scores for the target child's chronological age. Use the manual and your test data to (a) compute the raw score, (b) transform the raw score into a standard score, and (c) identify the confidence intervals. Following this exercise, you and your classmates can work together to role-play an interview with a parent in which the assessor explains the student's performance on the norm-referenced test.

4. Your instructor will provide you with a brief example of a child language transcript. Compute the child's MLU and NDW. Answer the following questions: (a) At which of Brown's stages should the child be, given his or her chronological age? (b) Is the child's MLU consistent with this stage? (c) If not, at which of Brown's stages is the child? (d) Is this child within normal limits for sentence length and vocabulary variety?

5. Pick a norm-referenced test (you may be able to choose one from the university speech-language clinic). In an oral or written presentation, provide information about the assessment's (a) reliability data, (b) validity data, (c) purpose (Does it test form, content, and use?), and (d) tasks used to assess different domains.

6. Your instructor will provide you with examples of good, average, and poorly written assessment reports. Edit the reports either individually or in a group with your classmates. Why did you change certain components of each report? Compare your changes with those of the other students. Following your edits, role-play how an SLP might interpret the assessment results to parents.

Chapter 3 Case Study

A student, Michael, is in the fourth grade and is 10 years, 3 months old. He speaks slowly, but his sound production and syntax are correct. He is performing at just below average levels academically. He does not appear distracted but has difficulty following instructions in the classroom.

The assessor administered two norm-referenced tests, the Peabody Picture Vocabulary Test (PPVT-4; a receptive vocabulary test) and several subtests from the Clinical Evaluation of Language Function–5 (CELF-5).

Michael received the following standard scores (SS):

TEST/Subtest	SS (M = 100)	SS (M = 10)
PPVT-4	87	
CELF-5		
Concepts		8
Following Directions		7
Word Classes		9
Semantic Relationships		7
RECEPTIVE CELF-5 SCORE	84	
Formulated Sentences		13
Recalling Sentences		8
Sentence Assembly		5
EXPRESSIVE LANGUAGE SCORE	92	

Overall, Michael's normative assessment data indicated that his receptive-expressive language and vocabulary knowledge were generally within normal limits, but he demonstrated significant levels of difficulty with sentence assembly. The assessor noted that Michael had difficulty organizing the sentences into more than one sentence type (a requirement of this sentence-assembly subtest).

The assessor evaluated some of Michael's written work. Michael's written work was grammatically accurate, but he used simple rather than complex sentence constructions. His story writing was "flat," lacking descriptive language or temporal or clausal connections.

Questions for Discussion

1. Explain why Michael could score reasonably well on most of the CELF-5 and PPVT-4 but have the described difficulties in the classroom.
2. Describe a criterion-referenced task that you might use to further evaluate Michael's abilities.
3. Find a copy of the PPVT-4 and the CELF-5; look at the different tasks that are used to assess each language domain. Which tasks are easier? Which are more difficult?
4. Role-play an explanation to Michael's parents and teacher regarding Michael's assessment. Explain the results of his standardized scores.

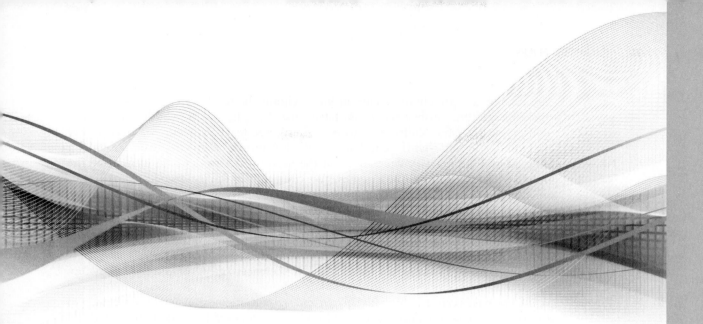

4 Decision Making in Assessment and Intervention

Chapter Overview Questions

1. What are the three critical-thinking parameters? Give two examples of critical-thinking questions that reflect each parameter.
2. How does a practitioner use decision trees to increase understanding of clinical decision making? Draw a simple decision tree.
3. How is the response to intervention (RTI) model different from a more traditional model of assessment? Give three examples of critical-thinking questions that reflect the RTI model.
4. What changes in public policy have influenced decision making for students with language impairment?
5. What are some examples of questions used to elicit information from a family during a routines-based interview?
6. How does IDEA affect progress monitoring? What role does IDEA play in implementation of the RTI model?

As a speech-language pathologist (SLP) or special educator, you will be making daily decisions that directly affect the lives of children and families. Read the following case examples and consider the decisions you might be called on to make in the following situations:

1. Tanzia is 7 and is significantly impaired. She communicates in simple sentences, and her verbal productions are often off-topic. Last year, her teacher worked on increasing Tanzia's sentence length and complexity. This year, Tanzia has been assigned to you.

2. Mrs. Shultz is a preschool teacher in your school; she teaches in an inclusive class-room. Six children in her classroom have special needs, and six children are developing typically. Mrs. Shultz used to be a first-grade teacher. When you observe her classroom, you find that the children spend a lot of time completing worksheets at a table. Mrs. Shultz is very worried about the need for her students to identify all the alphabet letters and write their names. You want to help the children learn these concepts but also want to promote a more active learning style.

3. Jahara is 16 and has an intellectual disability. In the past year, her intervention has focused on improving her syntax (e.g., correct use of pronouns) and working on correct articulation of the /r/ and /l/ sounds. You are meeting with Jahara and her family and need to develop her intervention goals for the upcoming school year.

4. Thomas is 8 and is struggling in school. His sentences often contain morphosyntax errors, including errors with verb forms and subordinating conjunctions (i.e., *because, so, if*). He makes errors in both his spoken and written language. You will be working to develop a progress-monitoring protocol for his Individualized Education Program (IEP).

This chapter will highlight strategies you can use to make important clinical decisions in situations like the case examples described above.

A Model of Decision Making

The world you will be entering as a professional is very different from the professional world I entered over 30 years ago. When I began my training in the 1970s, undergraduate education focused on teaching vocabulary terms and the facts and figures connected with language disorders. We did not have the Internet, and teachers focused on providing terminology and basic knowledge fundamental to the field.

As students in the new millennium, you have grown up accessing facts at the click of a mouse. The quantity of easily available information changes how young professionals should be trained. Now, rather than presenting only the facts, training must focus on helping students synthesize and evaluate available information. Young professionals must learn how to use theory and data to make clinical decisions. This chapter focuses on that important challenge: learning to become an effective clinical decision maker, someone who has moved beyond simply knowing the basic facts. An effective clinical decision maker:

- Knows how to choose among a wealth of information and is able to select credible information.
- Is able to understand and explain to parents and teachers—who also have access to a great deal of information—(a) the theories that underlie specific approaches and (b) the pros and cons associated with various intervention approaches.
- Understands how to weigh research evidence to choose approaches that demonstrate strong efficacy, evidence, and efficiency. **Efficacy** is measured by studies that determine the extent to which a specific intervention, procedure, or service produces a beneficial result under ideal conditions (e.g., in a very controlled clinical study when it is administered by highly trained interventionists). **Effectiveness** is determined in studies that examine the extent to which a specific intervention results in a positive outcome when it is used in routine practice (e.g., in a school setting administered by regular SLPs). **Efficiency** is a priority when funding sources are limited; a decision maker

must consider the most efficient means to rehabilitate an individual's communication disorder (Stout & Hayes, 2004).

- Understands the *why* and *how* associated with various intervention approaches. A skilled decision maker understands when to choose one approach over another, sets specific and targeted goals supported by research evidence, and documents change in an individual's communication behaviors.
- Is sensitive to a multicultural environment, because increasingly SLPs and educators are providing services for children and families with a variety of life experiences and cultural practices.
- Develops a professional approach that welcomes innovation and change. A skilled decision maker recognizes that continual professional training is required to keep abreast of what works, as demonstrated by high-quality research.

This chapter is designed to help you begin to develop important decision-making skills. I set you on the course to becoming a skilled decision maker by (a) presenting a series of three critical-thinking parameters, (b) linking the critical-thinking parameters to questions you can use to implement high-level thinking skills, and (c) connecting the critical-thinking parameters to four components of clinical practice (i.e., assessment, intervention, the environment, and progress monitoring/dismissal). Throughout this chapter, I give examples and illustrate decision-making processes by providing case examples.

I have divided the important critical-thinking skills into three parameters: (1) accuracy and scope of information, (2) evaluating the evidence, and (3) change and adaptability. These three parameters characterize important elements of thought demonstrated in higher-order decision making. See Figure 4.1 for a graphic presentation of the three parameters.

In the following section, I briefly describe each of the three critical-thinking parameters. These parameters are adapted from the work of Paul and Elder (2008).

Figure 4.1 **Graphic Presentation of Critical-Thinking Parameters**

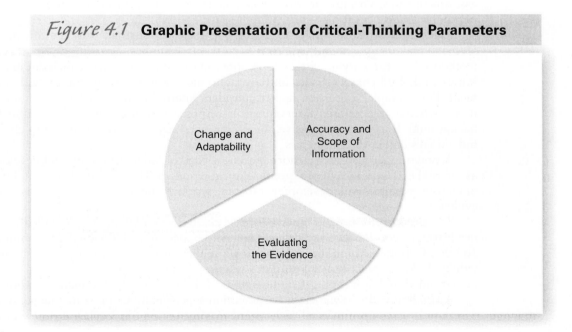

CRITICAL-THINKING PARAMETERS

The first critical-thinking parameter is *accuracy and scope of information*. The need for accuracy prompts a decision maker to gather supporting evidence to identify the communication problem and make conclusions. A communication problem cannot be remediated until it is objectively described. A decision maker uses both objective and subjective data to accurately document a communication disorder; **objective data** are based on observable phenomena (e.g., ratings scales, behavioral/classroom observations, test scores). **Subjective data** represent an individual's opinion. A family's belief about a child's communication disorder is subjective; however, this information must be included as part of the decision-making process. Accuracy also is an essential feature of intervention; a practitioner makes recommendations based on a child's data, carefully documents intervention outcomes in high-quality reports, and accurately documents a child's progress.

The data must be accurate, but a decision maker also must take care to gather enough pertinent information to reach a meaningful conclusion. In Chapter 3, I discussed issues of reliability and validity. Accuracy is most similar to reliability: The decision maker wants to accurately capture and describe the individual's communication behavior. But, as you recall, validity is even more important than reliability! In order for clinical conclusions to be valid, a decision maker must gather sufficient scope of information to document an individual's communication skills in real-life settings. For example, a decision maker may consider the scope of information by asking a family, "Can you give me an example or illustration of that behavior?" or "Could you elaborate on that point?" during the assessment interview. Scope of information also provides the rationale for completing classroom observations and working closely with classroom teachers.

The second critical-thinking parameter is *evaluating the evidence*. This second parameter underlies the need for practitioners to know and understand how to use scientific evidence to identify high-quality assessment tools and intervention programs. In Chapter 3, I presented information about adequate correlation levels to document reliability levels in assessment tools. This information helps you consider the evidence supporting the use of particular assessment tools.

Practitioners also evaluate evidence when they choose an intervention program. Decision makers use external evidence (e.g., research studies) as well as internal evidence to choose between varying intervention approaches. Internal evidence includes individual family and child characteristics and a practitioner's knowledge of theory and development. For example, a decision maker considers internal evidence when he or she determines whether a proposed intervention is responsive to a client's cultural and family background. If it is not responsive, the practitioner acquires more evidence to clarify the individual's unique circumstances.

A practitioner also uses a thorough knowledge of language theory and development as internal evidence to support specific clinical practices. Throughout this book, I provide numerous examples and developmental frameworks to build your ability to use internal evidence.

The third decision-making parameter is *change and adaptability*. A skilled practitioner learns to consistently note and document change in an individual's communication abilities. Communication interventions must make a real difference in the life of an individual. A skilled practitioner also notes whether an intervention is motivating for a particular individual; if it is not, the intervention should be modified to increase motivation.

Adaptability also requires that a practitioner personally be open to change. A skilled practitioner stays open minded with regard to intervention approaches and new evidence.

It is easy to fall into "intervention habits" and use the same or similar approaches for different children with dissimilar communication challenges. A professional should beware of entering a "clinical comfort zone"; it is easy to use a familiar approach. Skilled professionals continually seek out new information to determine whether another approach may be more helpful.

In summary, a skilled decision maker uses critical-thinking skills to (a) gather relevant and sufficient information to aid the decision-making process, (b) compare decisions via internal and external evidence, (c) consider multicultural influences on communication behavior, (d) observe and document change in communication behavior, and (e) flexibly adapt interventions to promote effective outcomes.

QUESTIONING AS A TOOL FOR CRITICAL THINKING

We are all familiar—through Court TV or television dramas—with the proceedings of the courtroom. The prosecuting attorney faces the witness and asks a number of focused questions. The assumption is that questioning reveals information that allows the jury or judge to reach a verdict. The process of asking and answering questions is central to this process. Focused questioning allows facts to be less distorted, clarifies confusing issues, and guides thoughtful reasoning (Browne & Keeley, 2007; Nelson, 2011; Paul & Elder, 2008; Phillips & Duke, 2001).

As a developing critical thinker, you must learn to ask and answer critical-thinking questions. At first, you will need to deliberately ask yourself questions and write down your answers. As you become a skilled decision maker, the question asking and answering process will become automatic and internalized. Asking and answering questions will guide you to become reflective and increase thinking clarity, and it will help you achieve important critical-thinking skills.

Examples of the critical-thinking questions you will learn to use are provided in Table 4.1. You should notice that the questions are aligned along the three critical-thinking

Table 4.1   **Critical-Thinking Parameters, Questions, and Aspects of Clinical Practice**

Critical-thinking parameters	Critical-thinking questions	Assessment, intervention, environment, or progress monitoring
Accuracy and scope of information	1. What information have I learned from screening the student? Is a more in-depth assessment warranted?	Assessment
	2. What details have emerged regarding the student's language disorder that help me understand the issues?	Assessment, intervention, environment
	3. What multicultural issues may be occurring? How might they potentially be impacting this language disorder?	Assessment, intervention, environment, progress monitoring

(continued)

Table 4.1 (**continued**)

	4. What specific language domains are impacted?	Assessment, intervention, environment
	5. Can I clearly explain the relevant issues facing this individual?	Assessment, intervention, environment, progress monitoring
	6. Have I considered this student's language disorder from all relevant points of view (e.g., family, teacher, employer, student)?	Assessment, intervention, environment, progress monitoring
	7. What sources have I used to collect data? How have I cross-verified the information (e.g., norm-referenced tests, criterion-referenced protocols, environmental scans)?	Assessment, intervention, environment, progress monitoring
Evaluating the evidence	1. What research evidence exists to support my assessment protocol and intervention approach?	Assessment, intervention
	2. Does all the information I have about this individual make sense together?	Assessment, intervention, environment
	3. How have I used student outcome data to foster my intervention decision making?	Intervention, progress monitoring
	4. How does my data-monitoring system track student progress?	Progress monitoring
Change and adaptability	1. What alternative perspectives may be useful to help me consider this student's intervention program?	Assessment, intervention, environment, progress monitoring
	2. Will the intervention be motivating to the student? If not, how can I change it?	Assessment, intervention, environment
	3. How will the selected intervention target behaviors make a real difference in the student's life?	Intervention, environment
	4. Am I providing intervention in an environment (i.e., family routines, classroom) that is likely to promote change?	Intervention, environment
	5. Am I providing the intervention that is best for the client, or does my intervention reflect what is convenient for my schedule and me?	Intervention, environment
	6. Have I continued to learn and grow as a professional? What have I learned to do differently or better in the past year?	Assessment, intervention, environment, progress monitoring

parameters (accuracy and scope of information, evaluating the evidence, change and adaptability). Although you might not ask yourself every question with every student, you should consider each of the three parameters during the clinical decision-making process. This list does not include all the possible questions that could be asked; it is only a beginning to help you get started.

Not only are the questions in Table 4.1 aligned with the three critical-thinking parameters (the column on the left in Table 4.1), I have also aligned questions in relation to important aspects of clinical practice: assessment, intervention, environment, and progress monitoring. The rest of this chapter is organized around these four important aspects of clinical practice.

DECISION TREES AS A TOOL FOR CRITICAL THINKING

A **decision tree** is a graphic that shows the alternatives in the decision-making process. I incorporate a number of decision trees throughout this book to efficiently help you become a skilled decision maker. A decision tree allows you to see the thought process that underlies the decision-making process. A very simple example of a decision tree is illustrated in Figure 4.2: It is an illustration of my thought process at age 18 when I was deciding on a major as an undergraduate student. I considered different occupations and

Figure 4.2   **Example of a Decision Tree**

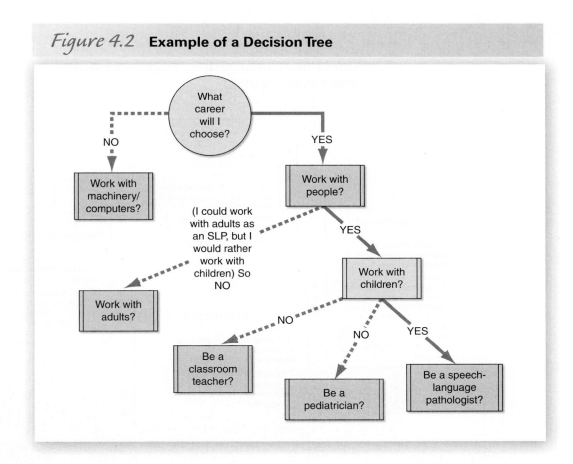

chose speech-language pathology. The decision tree illustrates how I chose among the various alternatives.

I include decision trees and graphic illustrations of critical-thinking processes throughout this book; this is to help you understand underlying decision-making processes. Take time to consider the decision trees included in this book. Use the decision trees to address the provided case examples. Just as one needs practice to become a skilled athlete, you must practice decision-making skills to become proficient.

When an SLP student or student teacher is assigned his or her first clinical experience, the student often looks at the supervisor in horror and says, "But what should I DO?" Although the student has learned a great deal of information prior to the first clinical assignment, he or she often fails to master critical-thinking skills. Do not let this happen to you! Start now to develop the critical-thinking skills you will use throughout your professional career.

In the sections below, I describe critical-thinking skills as they relate to four aspects of clinical practice: assessment, intervention, environment, and progress monitoring. I explain how critical-thinking questions are used to fine-tune the decision-making process. In Figure 4.3 I illustrate critical-thinking questions and how they relate to the four aspects of clinical and educational practice.

Figure 4.3 **Critical-Thinking Questions as They Relate to Assessment, Intervention, Environment, and Progress Monitoring**

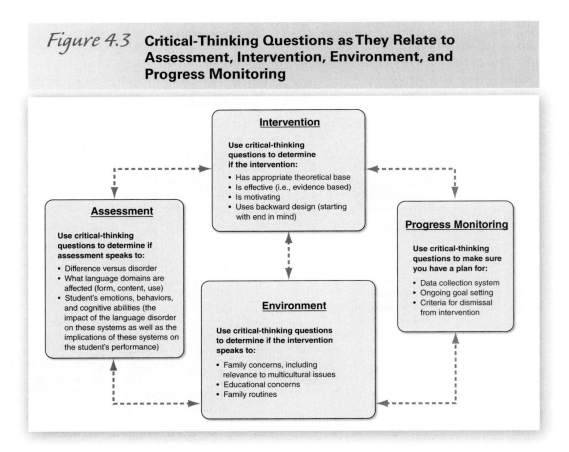

Intervention

Use critical-thinking questions to determine if the intervention:

• Has appropriate theoretical base
• Is effective (i.e., evidence based)
• Is motivating
• Uses backward design (starting with end in mind)

Assessment

Use critical-thinking questions to determine if assessment speaks to:

• Difference versus disorder
• What language domains are affected (form, content, use)
• Student's emotions, behaviors, and cognitive abilities (the impact of the language disorder on these systems as well as the implications of these systems on the student's performance)

Environment

Use critical-thinking questions to determine if the intervention speaks to:

• Family concerns, including relevance to multicultural issues
• Educational concerns
• Family routines

Progress Monitoring

Use critical-thinking questions to make sure you have a plan for:

• Data collection system
• Ongoing goal setting
• Criteria for dismissal from intervention

Decision Making: Assessment

As you recall from Chapter 3, assessment is used to (a) describe a child's communicative functioning, (b) determine what domains or communication functions should be targeted during intervention, and (c) determine a child's eligibility for special educational or rehabilitative service. In the clinical decision model, the practitioner begins this process by asking some of the following questions:

- What aspects of language should be evaluated for this student (e.g., form, content, use)?
- What kinds and varieties of clinical measures are used to describe the student's language disorder (e.g., norm-referenced and criterion-referenced tools)?
- What referrals should be made for this student?

These are some of the questions to consider during the assessment process. In the section below I highlight additional points with regard to the critical-thinking parameter of *accuracy and scope of information*.

The need for *accuracy* significantly impacts the assessment process. You learned a great deal about assessment in Chapter 3. Now, expand your ability to use this knowledge by looking at Table 4.2, and consider how you might use questions to guide your assessment with (a) a toddler who is not interacting socially with his communication partners, (b) a preschool child who is not speaking in word combinations, and (c) an older school-age student who is having difficulty following the teacher's instructions.

Table 4.2 **Critical-Thinking Questions Related to Aspects of Communication or Related Skills**

Prelinguistic

- Does the child or student have the basic principles of communication (i.e., imitation, joint attention) underlying social interactions (first evidenced at a nonverbal level)?

Cognitive

- Does the child or student demonstrate the cognitive skills (i.e., means–end, object permanence, cause and effect) that impact language development?

Pragmatic (early skills)

- Does the child or student have early communication behaviors (e.g., turn taking, range of pragmatic acts [requesting, commenting, protesting]) needed for social interaction (verbal or nonverbal)?

Lexical

- Is the beginning language learner putting words into two- and three-word combinations using a variety of semantic combinations (i.e., agent + action, action + object, agent + object)?
- Are there vocabulary items or concepts that would significantly improve communication or make a clear impact in the child's academic setting or workplace? Does the student have the needed vocabulary to be successful academically?

(*continued*)

Table 4.2 (**continued**)

Morphosyntax

- Are there morphosyntax features that, if targeted, would improve social communication and/or academic achievement? Does the student have appropriate levels of syntax complexity for his or her age or grade?

Pragmatic (discourse)

- Does the student have good ability to introduce topics, maintain a topic, switch topics appropriately, and ask questions in ways that promote social interaction?
- Can the student make conversational repairs?

Literacy

- Are early literacy skills being targeted in ways that engage young children in active learning?
- Are there reading and writing skills for the older student that, if facilitated, would improve communication, academic skills, work skills, or quality of life?
- Are there learning strategies that an older student can learn that will help him or her be more successful in the classroom?
- Can the student tell and/or write a narrative? Is the student motivated to work on narrative production?

Assessment also requires the practitioner to consider the *scope of information*; remember this when considering whether the child's language behaviors reflect a language difference vs. a language disorder. In order to determine if you are observing a true language disorder, you need to ask:

- Does this student score significantly lower than average on standardized testing and/ or naturalistic testing, *and* is the student perceived by his or her significant communication partners as having a communication disorder?

If you can answer yes to both parts of the question, you are likely to have identified a language disorder instead of a language difference (Paul & Norbury, 2012). Use the Internet address provided in Focus 4.1 to learn more about language differences, multicultural language, and the importance of multicultural awareness. I highlight additional information with regard to multicultural issues throughout this book. It is a very important aspect of your clinical training.

Scope of information also implies that you have considered the breadth of behaviors that may be affected by a student's disability. Ask yourself about the student's cognitive and perceptual skills, coping behaviors, social interactions, and academic skills. Consider whether any related domains are affected by the communication impairment and, if so, whether your proposed intervention will accommodate the student's associated deficits. If they won't, take the time to complete more observations and conduct more interviews with the student, teachers, or family members during the assessment process. What do the stakeholders feel are the student's most significant communication issues? To determine whether you have met this critical-thinking threshold, you can ask yourself, "Has my assessment evaluated the student's most critical communication challenges, as perceived by those closest to him or her?"

FOCUS 4.1   *Multicultural Issues*

The American Speech-Language Hearing Association (ASHA) considers it of utmost importance that students training to be SLPs learn all they can about the issues related to cultural diversity in the United States. Consider the following information from ASHA's multicultural board (ASHA, 2004, p. 1):

> The ethnic, cultural, and linguistic makeup of this country has been changing steadily over the past few decades. Cultural diversity can result from many factors and influences including ethnicity, religious beliefs, sexual orientation, socioeconomic levels, regionalisms, age-based peer groups, educational background, and mental/physical disability. With cultural diversity comes linguistic diversity, including an increase in the number of people who are English Language Learners, as well as those

who speak non-mainstream dialects of English. In the United States, the percentage of racial/ethnic minorities increased to over 30% of the total population. The makeup of our school populations continues to diversify so that in 2010, children of immigrants represented 22% of the school-age population.

You can access more information about the multicultural knowledge and skill requirements outlined by the American Speech-Language Hearing Association at www.asha.org/practice/multicultural/.

_____

Source: Based on information from American Speech-Language-Hearing Association. (2004). *Knowledge and skills needed by speech-language pathologists and audiologists to provide culturally and linguistically appropriate services* [Knowledge and Skills]. Retrieved from www.asha.org/policy/KS2004-00215/.

RESPONSE TO INTERVENTION

You will be making assessment decisions in a constantly evolving professional world. As an example, in 2004 an educational model was proposed, the response (or responsiveness) to intervention (RTI) model. The RTI model begins with a different set of assumptions than the more traditional assessment model described in Chapter 3.

As you recall, in Chapter 3 I introduced the concept of static vs. dynamic assessment. Static assessment provides a snapshot of an individual's abilities at a particular moment in time. Dynamic assessment, on the other hand, identifies an individual's learning potential. The RTI model is a form of dynamic assessment. Consider the differences between clinical questions using the two models. In a traditional model of assessment, a practitioner poses the following questions:

- Where does this student's standard score on a norm-referenced test fall as compared to what is expected for his or her age?
- What is the child's mean length of utterance as compared to children who are the same chronological age?
- Does the student produce utterances with sufficient levels of complexity?
- How are this student's everyday communication abilities compared to those of other students his or her age?

In contrast, in the RTI model, a practitioner begins with a different set of critical questions:

- Has this student had previous exposure to the concepts or skills required for a particular task?
- What evidence-based (i.e., scientifically proven) instructional methods have been implemented in the classroom?
- How will I continuously monitor the student's communication or academic development?

With the RTI model–framed clinical questions, a practitioner considers that a child's poor performance on a language/literacy task may be due to the student's (a) lack of experience with the task or (b) lack of evidence-based instruction (i.e., instruction was not based on scientific research).

For example, many preschoolers have few opportunities to practice rhyming words (e.g., "What word rhymes with *hat*?"). In a preschool-level screening test, a child without sufficient rhyming experience may perform very poorly when asked to rhyme. In the RTI model, the practitioner makes certain that every child has many learning opportunities to rhyme before assuming that there is a "rhyming deficit."

The need to focus on rhyming ability in young children is based on scientific research. Consequently, classroom-based opportunities for rhyming must be provided to all children during their preschool years. In the RTI model, exposure to key language and literacy targets within the general education classroom is called Tier 1 intervention. Tier 1 intervention is typically provided by a general education teacher and involves the use of instructional methods with good efficacy, effectiveness, and efficiency. The assumption is that a child should not be identified as being impaired until he or she has had many opportunities to learn important language/literacy skills at the classroom level.

The RTI model applies to preschool children (as in the rhyming example above) and also to older, school-age students. In elementary school, practitioners do not wait until a student is diagnosed as learning disabled before they initiate scientifically based educational interventions. With the RTI model, all students receive high-quality evidence-based educational instruction in the classroom. Reading instruction has been a significant focus in the RTI model. Scientifically based reading instruction for school-age students includes a focus on phonological awareness skills, reading comprehension, and reading fluency. I describe the important components of scientifically based reading research in more detail in Chapter 10.

In summary, the RTI model is based on the principles that (a) there are specific instructional practices (identified in scientific research) linked to academic success that should guide instruction for all children, (b) it is easier and better to prevent academic failure than to wait until a child experiences academic failure, (c) all children should receive Tier 1 instruction at the classroom level, and (d) most children will learn with high-quality Tier 1 instruction.

However, some children—even with high-quality classroom instruction—will fall behind. A second important component of the RTI model is that children who do not develop at the Tier 1 level are provided more intensive instruction at the Tier 2 level. Tier 2 instruction is typically provided several times a week in small groups; an SLP, a teacher, a teacher assistant, or a tutor provides the instruction (Ehren, et al., 2006; Haager, Klingner, & Vaughn, 2007).

In the RTI model, children's skill development is used as an indicator for more intense levels of instruction. Therefore, a child failing to progress with high-quality classroom instruction alone will be moved to Tier 2, where he or she will receive more explicit and intense exposure to the targeted skill. Explicit instruction is more adult directed and provides more opportunities for focused skill repetition. For example, a Tier 2 intervention for preschoolers is likely to focus on a particular skill, such as alphabet letter recognition. During a Tier 2 small-group intervention, the adult may read a storybook and provide multiple opportunities for children to look for, point to, and name letters during the shared book reading.

Some children may continue to struggle, even with Tier 2 small-group intervention. A student who does not show adequate skill development in Tier 2 is referred for Tier 3 instruction (i.e., highly specialized and focused intervention). Children referred for Tier 3 instruction often include students with more severe levels of disability (i.e., children with intellectual disabilities, children with significant language disabilities). An example of a Tier 3 approach for an older school-age student may include training the student to use specific strategies prior to reading to improve his or her comprehension. The student may be trained to list specific key words to look for during the reading process. At the Tier 3 level, the practitioner helps the student implement the comprehension strategy during classroom reading assignments and monitors the student's successful use of the new strategy. Figure 4.4 shows the relationship between Tiers 1, 2, and 3. It is important to note that

Figure 4.4   **Response to Intervention (RTI) Model and Critical-Thinking Questions**

Tier 3 Intervention
(Student is provided with scientifically based instruction and specialized interventions intensively at an individual level or in a small group.)

Critical-Thinking Question (Accuracy): *What data document the student's progress at each level?*

Students move between levels as appropriate.

Tier 2 Intervention
(Student is provided with scientifically based instruction regularly in a small group.)

Critical-Thinking Questions (Scope of Information): *Are there additional educational supports and/or modifications that would allow the student to maintain his or her progress at the Tier I level?*

Students whose skill levels do not develop move to Tier 2. Students who catch up move back to Tier I.

Critical-Thinking Question (Evaluating Evidence): *Is the classroom Instuction scientifically based?*

Tier 1 Intervention
(Student is provided with scientifically based instruction in the classroom.)

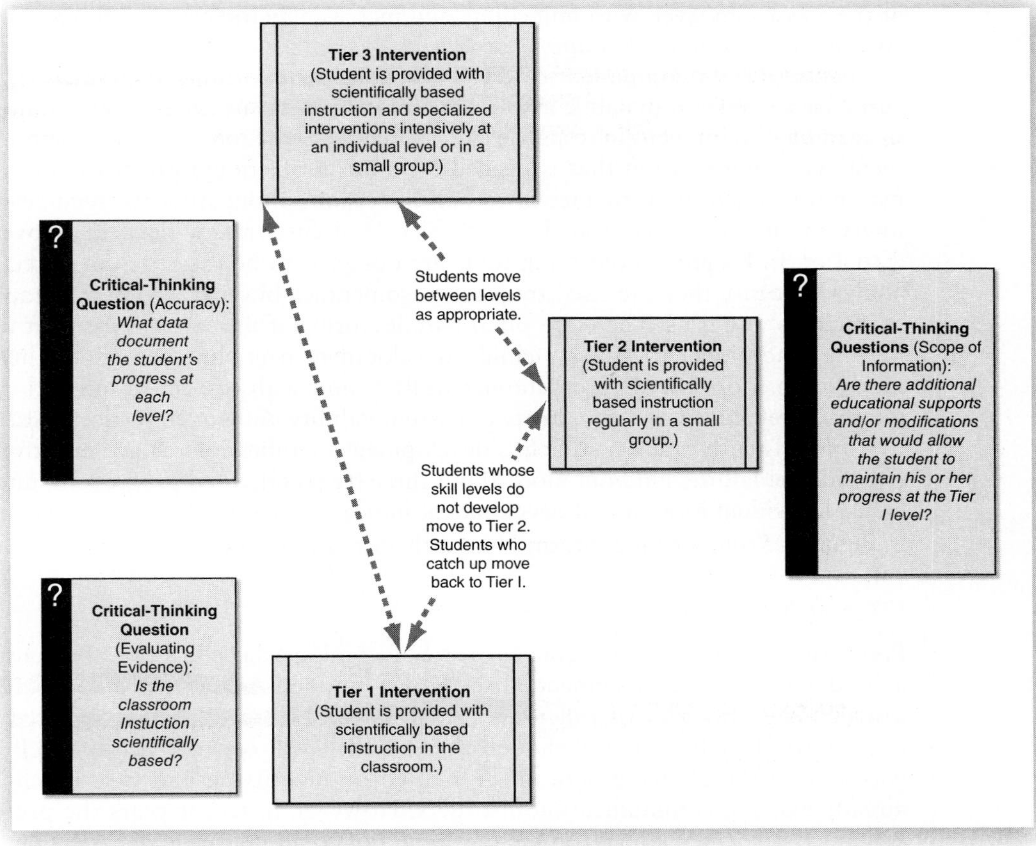

the RTI model is compatible with important U.S. educational policies—specifically the Individuals with Disabilities Education Act (IDEA) and a component of IDEA called the free, appropriate public education (FAPE) requirement. I discuss the relationship between RTI and U.S. educational policy later in this chapter.

To reiterate the fundamental principle of RTI, a student's response to instruction is used as the criteria for placement in Tier 1, 2, or 3. If a student improves after Tier 2 or Tier 3 intervention, he or she moves back down to the Tier 1 level. This approach varies from a discrepancy criterion model. Prior to implementation of the RTI model, the discrepancy criterion model was used to qualify children as having a learning disability. The discrepancy model required that a child demonstrate a significant difference between IQ (i.e., overall cognitive ability) and school achievement in order to qualify for educational services. Use of the discrepancy model often resulted in delaying intervention until the student's achievement had fallen significantly below that of his or her peers.

Educationally, there are clear limitations for the discrepancy criterion model. Once a child has fallen behind in school, it is difficult to help the child catch up. The common pattern of reading failure typifies this problem. A child who struggles to read reads less often and often dislikes reading. With less practice, the struggling reader has less exposure to new vocabulary, causing the poor reader to fall further behind. Skilled readers, in contrast, enjoy reading, tackle increasingly difficult texts, and become more and more proficient. This has also been called the "Matthew effect" because—as in the biblical reference—"the rich get richer and the poor get poorer" (Stanovich, 1986). To counteract the downward spiral of reading disability, the RTI model advocates high-quality instruction for children at the classroom level, with immediate and increasingly intensive levels of instruction for students who do not catch up.

An important component of RTI is progress monitoring. Progress-monitoring measures are considered dynamic assessments because they measure student communication or reading development in response to systematic instruction. Progress-monitoring assessments yield information that is needed to tailor instructional practices appropriately to maximize student performance or to make decisions about students' readiness to exit an intervention (e.g., move from Tier 2 to Tier 1) or enter a new tier (e.g., move from Tier 2 to Tier 3). Progress-monitoring tools are designed to be easy to administer, score, and analyze because they are used frequently (sometimes biweekly) to permit rapid analysis of students' progress. There are often parallel forms of the same assessment tool, allowing the practitioner to assess a child's development over time. A high-quality progress-monitoring tool should be psychometrically sound with respect to internal consistency, interrater reliability, and construct/concurrent validity (Gillam & Justice, 2010). The ability to consistently track a student's development qualifies RTI as a preventive approach to academic failure. Find out more about three frequently used progress-monitoring tools called individual growth and development indicators (IGDIs) by reading the information in Figure 4.5 and viewing information at the listed websites.

PREVENTION

Prevention is an important concept for SLPs and special educators. Prevention also is a fundamental concept embedded in the RTI model. A **preventive approach** provides instruction or modifies an individual's environment before a deficit is observed. A preventive approach reduces the likelihood that a deficit will occur. When the SLP profession was new, in the 1940s, practitioners focused on identifying and treating children with already-existing communication disorders. However, in recent years the profession has expanded to include a focus on the prevention of communication disorders and academic

Figure 4.5 **Examples of Progress-Monitoring Assessments: Individual Growth and Development Indicators (IGDIs)**

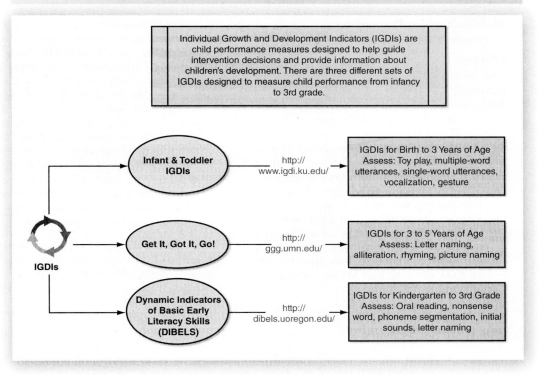

failure. There are a number of important skills related to prevention. To prevent communication disorder, SLPs and special educators should:

- Use prevention terminology appropriately (see Focus 4.2 for definitions).
- Understand conditions that place individuals at risk for various communication disorders.
- Understand factors, either biological or environmental, that cause communication disabilities.
- Understand practices and educational strategies that enhance children's communication abilities.
- Identify and intervene as early as possible to prevent serious communication disabilities.

In this book, you begin to learn about prevention approaches by reading about (a) the conditions that place students at risk for language disorders, (b) risk factors for language impairments, (c) effective practices for preventing communication disorders, and (d) intervention approaches appropriate for very young children. Your knowledge in these areas will continue to develop throughout your professional career. As an SLP or special educator, you will ask yourself critical-thinking questions to determine whether you (or your school or organization) are implementing an effective prevention program. Critical-thinking questions may include the following:

- What screening programs exist in my community that can identify children at earlier ages?

FOCUS 4.2 *Learning More*

Terminology for Prevention of Communication Disorders

Effective prevention of language disorders requires the appropriate use of prevention terminology. Below I provide prevention definitions and explain how these terms are applied throughout this text:

- *At risk:* The potential to develop a disorder based on specific biological, environmental, or behavioral factors. In Chapters 7 and 10, I will discuss risk factors associated with hearing loss and autism.
- *Primary prevention:* The elimination or inhibition of the onset and development of a communication disorder by altering susceptibility or reducing exposure for susceptible persons. Use of Tier 1 instruction

in the response to intervention (RTI) model is an example of primary prevention.
- *Secondary prevention:* The early detection and treatment of communication disorders. Early detection and treatment may lead to the elimination of a disorder or the retardation of the disorder's progress, thereby preventing further complications. Screening is an example of secondary prevention.
- *Tertiary prevention:* The reduction of a disability by attempting to restore effective functioning. I will present a number of intervention approaches in this text as examples of tertiary prevention.

For more information about prevention in speech-language pathology, see www.asha.org/policy/PS1988-00228/.

- What information is provided to community members or school personnel to help parents and teachers recognize language disorders at an early age?
- What kinds of early intervention programs are available in my community for very young children and their families?

CASE EXAMPLE: DECISION MAKING DURING ASSESSMENT

Review Case Example 1 at the beginning of this chapter. Tanzia is 7 years old and has a significant impairment that prevents her from interacting socially with her peers. She avoids interactions, does not initiate communication with adults or children, and plays by herself. Tanzia often demonstrates repetitive activities (e.g., spinning a top). She speaks in simple two- to three-word sentences, but her sentences often do not relate to the ongoing activity. Before completing an assessment, you answer this critical-thinking question:

- What domains of communication (i.e., form, content, use) are most impaired for Tanzia?

Before you read further, reflect on what you have already learned and try to think of the answer.

After thinking about Tanzia's communication problems, I hope you considered the communication subdomains and remembered that Subdomain 1 (social interaction) is the foundational skill underlying advanced language learning. It is likely that you determined that Tanzia has difficulty with this underlying social interaction skill because she has problems in requesting, responding, turn taking, and eye contact.

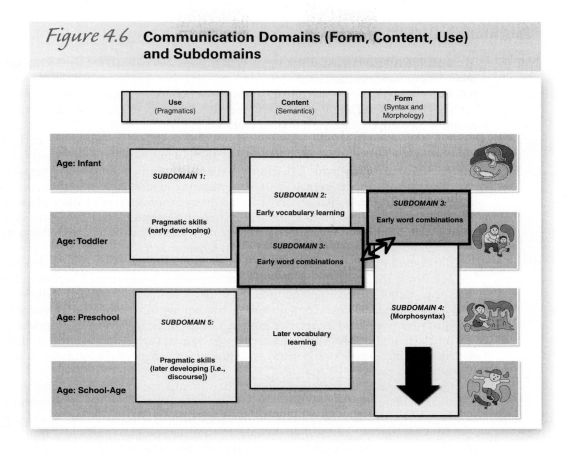

Figure 4.6 **Communication Domains (Form, Content, Use) and Subdomains**

Now, let's continue with this critical-thinking exercise. Answer a second question:

- What assessments should I use to understand Tanzia's communication challenges?

Finally, answer this question:

- Am I more likely to use norm-referenced or criterion-referenced assessments as part of the assessment protocol?

At this point in your professional training, I do not expect you to name specific tests. Instead, I want you to describe several tests or procedures appropriate for a student such as Tanzia. Refer to Figure 4.6 to review the communication subdomains, which should help you respond to this case example.

Decision Making: Intervention

In this section on decision making and intervention, I outline the general goals of intervention with respect to various age groups; I then describe how critical-thinking questions help a skilled practitioner relate language theory to language intervention. In the second and third subsections, I describe how public policies and issues of motivation influence decision making.

GOALS OF INTERVENTION: INFANTS, TODDLERS, PRESCHOOLERS, AND SCHOOL-AGE STUDENTS

The goals of speech-language intervention change with respect to the age of the individual with communication impairments (ASHA, 2004a). For infants and toddlers who are at risk for communication impairment, a practitioner concentrates on increasing the caregivers' sensitivity to the infant's needs and teaches caregivers to facilitate preverbal communication (i.e., eye contact, turn taking, imitation).

Early intervention also includes teaching caregivers to facilitate early speech (i.e., babbling, word approximations) and the communication skills associated with Communication Subdomains 2 (early words) and 3 (word combinations). Social interaction, play, and emergent literacy skills (e.g., engaging in joint action routines, interactions using toys and books) also are included as intervention targets at the earliest ages. In Figure 4.7, I show how an SLP could use clinical questions and a decision tree to plan intervention for a preschooler with language delay. As you can see, the decision tree uses the communication subdomains presented in Chapter 2.

Intervention for preschoolers continues to focus on social interaction, play, and early literacy. Now, the practitioner also targets increasing sophisticated receptive language skills (e.g., building attention and listening skills, developing vocabulary, following directions, understanding sentences and stories, responding to communicative intent of peers and adult partners) and expressive language skills (e.g., using age-appropriate phonology and articulation skills, using a variety of words, formulating simple and complex sentences, telling simple oral narratives, expressing a variety of communicative functions, engaging with peers).

During the school-age years, intervention includes a focus on the student's educational curriculum, future vocational needs, and peer interaction. The practitioner considers the student's knowledge and use of language for listening, speaking, reading, writing, and thinking. Interventions often include an emphasis on phonology and print symbols, complex syntax structures, advanced vocabulary, discourse structures for comprehending and organizing spoken and written texts, pragmatic skills for communicating appropriately in varied situations, and metacognitive and self-regulatory strategies for handling complex language, literacy, and academic demands (ASHA, 2004a).

In summary, the goals of communication intervention at any age include (a) facilitating communication development, (b) changing or eliminating an individual's underlying communication problem, (c) changing specific aspects of the individual's communication function by teaching specific skills, or (d) teaching compensatory techniques to improve the individual's communication functioning. Throughout an intervention, a skilled practitioner asks this critical-thinking question:

- Is this individual's intervention focusing on goals that reflect abilities consistent with age and communicative needs?

CRITICAL-THINKING QUESTIONS DURING INTERVENTION: CONSIDERING UNDERLYING LANGUAGE THEORY

One important question regarding intervention is motivated by the critical-thinking parameter *evaluating the evidence.* As I described at the beginning of this chapter, evaluating assessment and intervention approaches requires both external and internal evidence. In Chapter 5, I discuss how to evaluate external evidence. Weighing the scientific

Figure 4.7   **Critical-Thinking Questions and Decision Tree For Preschool Intervention**

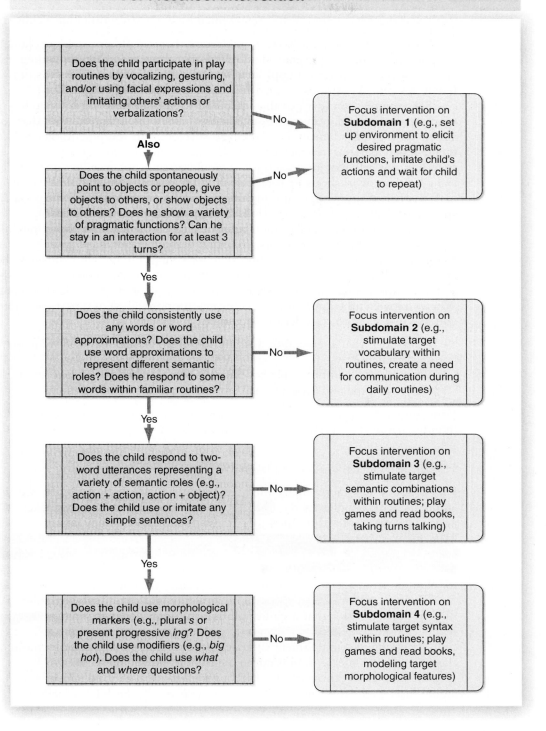

evidence supporting (or not supporting) a particular approach is an essential component of evidence-based practice. To begin this process, let's consider how a practitioner evaluates an intervention's internal evidence using a critical-thinking question such as this one:

- What theoretical approach is represented by the intervention I have chosen?

Different professionals have very different theoretical approaches to language intervention. In Chapter 2, I discussed a number of language theories, including behaviorism and the social interactionist approach. Different intervention approaches draw from different theoretical positions.

For example, consider possible intervention choices for a student who has difficulties with vocabulary and grammar. If an SLP or a special educator believes that social interaction theory is fundamental to language development, the practitioner is likely to use theme-based materials to engage the student in meaningful conversations during intervention. It is unlikely that the practitioner would attempt to remediate the targeted syntax skills by using worksheets or rote drills. On the other hand, a practitioner who believes in behaviorist theory might use highly controlled interactions and focus on reinforcing specific student responses with a skills-based approach (Ukraintez, 2005).

There are differences of opinion regarding appropriate interventions for children with different communication disorders. For example, some experts propose that interventions based on behaviorism are most appropriate for young children with autism. Other experts argue that children with autism should participate in interventions based on social interactionist theory. Some practitioners use a combination of methods (Solomon et al., 2007). When you weigh the appropriateness (or inappropriateness) of a particular intervention, you will first want to consider the following questions:

- How does the intervention I am proposing fit with my beliefs about language development?
- What kinds of information have I provided to parents and teachers to help them understand the underlying principles that frame this intervention?

Your ability to answer these critical-thinking questions will demonstrate the critical-thinking parameter of *evaluating the evidence*.

PUBLIC POLICY (IDEA) AND DECISION MAKING

Public policy has increasingly impacted educational interventions in recent years. A landmark federal policy is the **Individuals with Disabilities Education Act (IDEA)**; this policy was reauthorized in 2004'; the latest revision took effect in October 2006. IDEA 2004 ensures that all eligible children with disabilities have a right to a free, appropriate public education (FAPE) in the least restrictive environment (LRE) and that the rights of children and parents are protected. IDEA mandates that schools provide special education for children from age 3 through age 21 and ensures the effectiveness of these services.

The term *least restrictive environment* is a fundamental concept under IDEA 2004. LRE policy mandates that a child with special educational needs must receive services within the general education classroom to the greatest degree possible. That is to say, a child with language impairment should receive services outside the classroom only when classroom-based intervention is not in the child's best interests.

The implementation of the LRE and FAPE are very compatible with the RTI model discussed earlier in this chapter. As you recall, the RTI model's Tier 1 requires research-based interventions provided to all students in the classroom, while Tier 2 provides more intensive and specialized services to students who are not performing as well as their peers academically. The RTI model is designed to be a system that keeps children in the general education classroom but also provides interventions as appropriate. As a result, by implementing the RTI model, schools are compliant with the FAPE requirement mandated by IDEA.

Students with disabilities in the following areas are eligible for services under IDEA: hearing loss, deafness, speech or language impairments, intellectual disability, visual impairments, blindness, serious emotional disturbance, orthopedic impairments, autism, traumatic brain injury, other health impairments, specific learning disabilities, deaf-blindness, and multiple disabilities.

Part C of IDEA focuses on services for infants and toddlers (birth to age 3) with disabilities; it is a federal grant program that helps states provide early intervention services for children and families. In order for a state to participate in the program, it must ensure that early intervention will be available to every eligible child and his or her family. Children served under Part C of IDEA have developmental delay in domains including cognitive development, physical development (e.g., vision and hearing), communication development, social or emotional development, and adaptive development (i.e., difficulty performing activities needed for daily living).

For school-age children, IDEA regulations specify that academic failure is not a requirement for receiving special education and related services (i.e., the student does not have to demonstrate a discrepancy between IQ and achievement). Assessment should be broad based and consider educational performance across school environments (i.e., classroom discussions, peer interactions, extracurricular).

Identification of a disability that impairs a student's academic performance results in the development of an **Individualized Education Program (IEP)**. An IEP is a plan outlining special education and related services specifically designed to meet the unique educational needs of a student with a disability. Every child who receives special education and related services under IDEA must have an IEP. The IEP has two general purposes: (1) to set reasonable learning goals for the child and (2) to state the services that the school will provide for the child. Parents, general education teachers, school administration, and members of the special education team (including the SLP) all participate and agree to the final plan during the IEP process.

Critical-thinking questions considered during the IEP process include:

- To the maximum extent possible, how does this IEP guarantee that the student with a disability will be educated with children who are nondisabled?
- For students who cannot be educated solely in the general education classroom, is there a continuum of alternative placements (i.e., from less restrictive [as in receiving supplementary services part of the day] to more restrictive [as in a self-contained classroom for children with disabilities])?

Two final concepts are motivated by IDEA and the critical-thinking questions listed above: inclusion and differential instruction. The first term, *inclusion,* requires children to be educated in the LRE. Inclusion means that children with disabilities are educated in the same context as nondisabled peers. Inclusion is different from **mainstreaming**, in which students with disabilities spend a portion of their school day in the general education program and a portion in a separate special education program. The term *inclusion* is the preferred term; professionals avoid the use of the older term, *mainstreaming* (Idol, 2006).

Research demonstrates that children in inclusive preschool classrooms have improved developmental abilities, auditory comprehension, expressive language, and social skills compared to their language-delayed peers in segregated classes (Rafferty, Piscitelli, & Boettcher, 2003). Inclusive education also benefits older school-age students. Idol (2006) studied elementary and secondary schools and reported that inclusion benefited students with special educational needs. Further, data demonstrated that inclusion did not negatively impact educational outcomes for students developing typically—which is a concern voiced by critics of IDEA.

The second term is *differentiated instruction*. When children are in inclusive classrooms, teachers must use **differentiated instruction** to determine what children will learn, how they will learn it, and how students can express what they have learned (Tomlinson, 2003). Differentiated instruction may include altering the content of what is taught, altering how the content is taught, or altering a student's curriculum goal (i.e., reducing task demands). Differentiated instruction increases the likelihood that each student will learn as much as possible, as efficiently as possible. For example, when altering content, a practitioner may decide to reduce the number of pages a student is required to read to complete an assignment. If the practitioner decides to alter how the student is instructed, the student may be provided simultaneous auditory and written instruction instead of auditory-only instruction.

Critical-thinking questions motivated by the principle of differentiated instruction include:

- Will this student benefit if he or she is taught self-management skills (i.e., checking work, planning prior to beginning the task) to facilitate the curriculum goal?
- Will this student benefit by being trained to use reflective questions prior to and during the curriculum task?
- Would simplifying the task (e.g., reducing the number of spelling words for a spelling assignment) be an appropriate curriculum modification?
- Should this student focus on a foundational communication goal during a higher-level classroom activity (e.g., the student [who has a significant language impairment] practices initiating conversation during a small-group science activity)?

A skilled SLP or special educator helps teachers develop a range of differentiated instructional strategies. By using differentiated instruction, children with special educational needs remain in inclusive classrooms but receive the specialized intervention required by their IEPs.

STUDENT MOTIVATION AND DECISION MAKING

When you are a skilled practitioner working with a student with communication impairment, you are likely to ask this question:

- Is this intervention motivating for the student?

A student's level of motivation profoundly impacts academic achievement (McTigue, Beckman, & Kaderavek, 2007). Students who are motivated to learn will spend more time on a task and will seek out opportunities to practice the targeted skill (Lepola, Salonen, & Vauras, 2000). Moreover, students who exhibit high task motivation internalize the targeted skills, resulting in more permanent behavior change (Edmunds & Bauserman, 2006). The issue of student motivation is prompted by the critical-thinking parameter *change and adaptability.* If a student is not motivated during intervention, the practitioner must flexibly adapt the intervention to improve motivation and improve the student's opportunity for a good outcome.

Increasingly, trends in special education emphasize choosing interventions to impact an individual's daily activities and classroom achievement (Whitmire, 2002). This movement has stemmed from IDEA requirements, along with current research demonstrating the relationships between language skills and academic ability (Catts & Kahmi, 2005). Student motivation is enhanced when the practitioner emphasizes the positive effects of the intervention in everyday events. For example, imagine that you are working with a high-functioning student with social communication impairment who has difficulty with peer interactions. As a skilled practitioner, you explain and give examples to the student to demonstrate how improved discourse skills will positively affect peer relationships. Your goal is to enhance the student's understanding of how the targeted skills will be used in daily life to increase motivation and use of the intervention strategies.

BACKWARD DESIGN

Considering the parameter *change and adaptation* motivates a practitioner to focus on communication behaviors most likely to impact an individual's everyday interactions. One way to achieve this goal is to begin intervention with the end in mind (Ehren, 2007). This approach is called backward design. **Backward design advocates that the practitioner first consider the desired results for a particular student.** Then, after clearly outlining the ultimate goal, the practitioner identifies interventions needed to equip students to achieve the goal. Using backward design prompts several critical-thinking questions, such as:

- What does the student need to understand?
- What does the student need to do that he or she cannot do now?
- What interventions and approaches will promote understanding, interest, and competency in the targeted area?

The issue of backward design is relevant whether the individual is a preschooler, a school-age child, or an older student preparing for a career. A skilled SLP or special educator continually considers the individual's environment by asking the overarching question "Will this intervention make a real difference in the individual's daily life?"

CASE EXAMPLE: DECISION MAKING IN INTERVENTION

Consider the case of Mrs. Shultz, the preschool teacher (Case Example 2 at the beginning of this chapter). You are concerned about what you see in the classroom because you are thinking about the critical-thinking parameter *evaluating the evidence.* You are aware that having preschoolers sit for extended periods doing worksheets is not a recommended educational practice. You know the importance of early literacy skill building and need to answer the following question:

- What language theory should guide early language/literacy intervention for preschool children?

Your knowledge of language theory prompts you to reflect on social interactionist theory; social interactionist theory suggests that young children learn best when they are actively engaged with others. Because of your training, you know that young children need to explore and "think, do, and talk" to learn early literacy skills.

Reflect on how you might share your critical-thinking questions with Mrs. Shultz. Do you have any suggestions for changing how preschoolers could learn alphabet letters or name-writing within a preschool classroom with a more active learning approach? (You will learn more about how to foster early literacy skills in Chapter 10.) Use the sample questions in Table 4.2 to guide your critical thinking. An example of a preschool literacy activity incorporated within an engaging art activity is illustrated in Figure 4.8.

Decision Making: Environment

Undoubtedly, a child's environment makes a difference in language development. A child's exposure to high-quality language at home results in significantly higher child language output and vocabulary development. In a preschool environment, rich and frequent high-level teacher language results in improved academic gains for children (Wasik, Bond, & Hindman, 2006). Peers also influence language development: Preschoolers in classrooms with higher peer language levels demonstrate improved receptive and expressive language development (Mashburn et al., 2009). During the school years, opportunities for peer socialization and interaction with a caring, supportive adult promote positive language outcomes for students with language impairment (Gillam et al., 2008). Finally, children who come from culturally or linguistically different homes are likely to have differences in language use. A skilled practitioner considers the impact of environment and considers *scope of information.* Questions include:

- What perspectives do the child and/or the child's family have about the child's communication impairment?
- Am I considering all communication environments and environmental influences on language development?

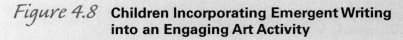

Figure 4.8 **Children Incorporating Emergent Writing into an Engaging Art Activity**

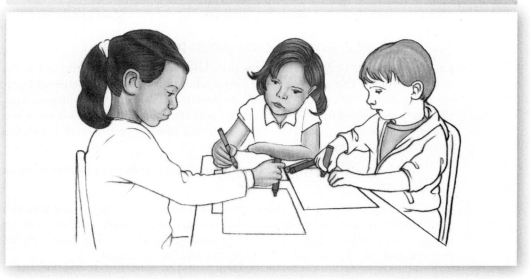

- How do family discourse patterns between adults and children (and children with other children) differ from what I might expect? Have I considered discourse patterns as they may vary for individuals from a minority culture?

In the following subsections, I highlight two issues to help you more carefully consider communication environments: routines-based interviewing and classroom contexts for language learning.

ROUTINES-BASED INTERVIEWING

It is important to remember that children are part of a multilayered system. When a practitioner considers the complex interactions of a family system, she is basing her thinking on the **ecological approach** (Bronfenbrenner, 1979; Schalock, Luckasson, & Shogren, 2007) and related approaches such as family systems theory. Family systems may be very nurturing or may be dysfunctional. Some teachers may be highly sensitive to the needs of a particular child. In contrast, other teachers may need a great deal of support to provide individualized instruction. When using an ecological approach, and in order to demonstrate the critical-thinking parameter *accuracy and scope of information,* skilled practitioners often use a routines-based interview (McWilliam & Clingenpeel, 2003).

A practitioner uses **routines-based interviewing (RBI)** to pose questions to family members to (a) assess a child's developmental and communication status, (b) gain information about day-to-day life, and (c) tune in to a family's feelings about their child. The goal is to gather a sense of the family's most important concerns in order to prioritize intervention goals. The word **routine** is used to describe times of day and/or familiar activities such as eating, bathing, bedtime, hanging out, going to the store, and traveling in the car.

This is an introductory question to initiate RBI:

- What does a typical day look like for your family?

This question is used to determine those routines that are most important for the family. The interviewer also asks:

- What activities does your family enjoy for fun?
- What does your family do on holidays?
- What do you do on weekends?

After identifying four to six of the most important routines, the interviewer asks the following questions about each of the important routines:

- What does everyone do during this routine?
- What does your child do?
- Is the child highly engaged (e.g., eager, high attention) or poorly engaged (e.g., "wandering," low attention) during the routine? (See Focus 4.3 for more information on engagement.)
- What does the child do independently as part of this routine?
- How does the child communicate during this routine?
- How satisfied are you with your child's interaction and participation during this routine?

Gathering routines-based information helps a practitioner target meaningful outcomes that build on a family's strengths. For example, imagine that you have Tabitha on

FOCUS 4.3   *Clinical Skill Building*

Special educators have developed a hierarchy to code preschool children's level of engagement during classroom routines (e.g., circle time, center activity, mealtimes). The following scale has been adapted (McWilliam, Scarborough, & Kim, 2003):

Child Level of Engagement

1 *Low engagement:* (a) The child demonstrates undifferentiated behavior; he or she interacts with the environment without differentiating behavior (i.e., performs low-level actions in a repetitive manner). (b) The child demonstrates non-engaged behavior such as staring blankly, wandering aimlessly, crying, whining, committing aggressive or destructive acts, breaking rules (i.e., throwing or kicking toys).

2 *Moderate-to-low engagement:* The child demonstrates attention to the activity by looking at an object or people; attention must be sustained for at least 3 seconds.

The child evidences engagement at this level when he or she is observed to demonstrate a serious facial expression and a quieting of motor activity.

3 *Moderate-to-high engagement:* (a) The child intentionally manipulates objects to create, make, or build something. He or she puts together objects in some type of spatial form (not just handling an object or banging blocks together). (b) The child demonstrates differentiated behavior that includes active interaction with the environment (e.g., typical play) and demonstrates adaptation to environmental demands and expectations

4 *High engagement:* (a) The child demonstrates problem solving and persistence following a failed first attempt. (b) The child uses language, pretend play, drawings, etc., that allow him or her to reflect on the past, talk about the future, and construct new forms of expression through combinations of different symbols and signs.

your caseload. Tabitha is 14 and is hearing impaired; she wears hearing aids and communicates verbally, although her language is delayed. She is struggling in school, and her reading skills are below average. After interviewing the family, you find that family members typically spend time together after dinner. You ask if reading chapter books (e.g., the Harry Potter series) together with Tabitha would be an enjoyable shared family event. The parents are enthusiastic about taking turns reading aloud. At first, Tabitha is reluctant, but eventually she is willing to read aloud with her parents' support. Eventually, she rereads the books independently because she is familiar with the vocabulary. In this example, you used RBI to integrate a language/literacy goal into a family's daily schedule.

Routines-based questions are also used to target the most important opportunities for intervention during child care. Frequently occurring child care routines include entering the classroom at the beginning of the day, free play, center time, mealtime, nap time, outdoor play, transitions (e.g., moving from one activity to another), and going to the bathroom. The practitioner asks the child care provider routines-based questions (e.g., "What does the child do when it is time to change activities?") and uses classroom observations to clarify the child's participation and engagement during the child care routines (McWilliam et al., 2003). Using RBI focuses a practitioner on the parameter *accuracy and scope of information.*

During RBI, a practitioner also considers the critical-thinking parameter *change and adaptability*. This parameter reminds the practitioner to consider issues of child motivation; motivation in young children is sometimes called **engagement**, and this refers to a child's duration and complexity of play and quality of interaction with others.

When young children exhibit positive engagement in classroom routines and activities (i.e., when they are highly focused, cooperative, or self-directed), students learn more. Further, classrooms where more children are engaged more of the time promote positive academic achievement (Powell et al., 2008). Consequently, skilled SLPs and educators evaluate child engagement levels to monitor classroom environments and facilitate change if engagement is not high.

Child engagement levels vary from high to low and are typically ranked on a four-point rating scale. A hierarchy of the levels of engagement and the scoring system used to rate child engagement levels is detailed in Focus 4.3. A child can be highly engaged in some activities (e.g., free play) but demonstrate low engagement during more structured activities. A practitioner uses engagement ratings to help a teacher modify instructional practices to increase a child's engagement across the school day. Combining family and child care provider information, in addition to using direct observation of child levels of engagement, demonstrates a practitioner's commitment to critical-thinking parameters.

CLASSROOM CONTEXTS FOR REMEDIATION

Considering *scope of information* motivates a practitioner to consider the location of school-based interventions. In **pullout models** of service delivery, a special educator or an SLP works with an individual or a small group of children in an area outside the classroom (McGinty & Justice, 2006). In contrast, when a practitioner provides intervention using a **classroom-based approach** to service delivery, he or she works with a student in the classroom. In a classroom-based approach, the curriculum materials or ongoing classroom activities typically are the stimulus for communication. Language intervention is embedded within the child's familiar activities and incorporates the child's teachers and peers.

Pullout intervention and classroom-based intervention represent two different service delivery models. A **service delivery model** refers to an intervention protocol aimed at achieving a particular educational goal. A service delivery model includes the personnel, materials, specific intervention procedure, schedule for provision of services, settings in which intervention services will be delivered, and direct or indirect roles of the practitioner as he or she provides language intervention to students with language impairments.

Despite IDEA's focus on classroom-based interventions as the optimal model of service delivery, most practitioners continue to provide school-based services using a pullout model of therapy. At present, only one-third of SLPs provide interventions with general education classrooms (ASHA, 2012).

There are several reasons for the limited use of classroom-based approaches with school-age students. First, many school-based SLPs have high caseloads; a high caseload reduces planning time and limits the time needed to complete paperwork and collaborate with teachers (Chiang & Rylance, 2000). Second, many SLPs currently working in schools were not trained to use curriculum-based assessment and intervention. Despite the challenges, ASHA continues to advocate the use of classroom-based intervention approaches with school-age students (ASHA, 2002).

Young children also benefit from a classroom-based model of service delivery. Inclusive, classroom-based service delivery is advantageous for young children with language disorders because the practitioner can focus on enhancing the preschooler's communication within classroom routines. During conversational routines, the child practices his new communication behaviors with his typically developing peers.

Direct vs. Indirect Classroom-Based Intervention. The classroom-based service delivery model can be implemented in several ways; the approaches are typically categorized into indirect and direct approaches (McGinty & Justice, 2007). In the **indirect service classroom-based approach**, an SLP or a special educator serves as a consultant to the general education teacher. The practitioner provides expert guidance so that the teacher can adjust instructional methods to meet a child's special needs. In the **direct service classroom-based approach**, a practitioner (a) collaborates with the teacher using a team-teaching method or (b) the teacher and the SLP take turns providing specific lessons to the entire class. Often practitioners use a combination of direct and indirect methods as part of the classroom-based approach.

Skilled practitioners ask themselves critical-thinking questions to evaluate their level of classroom-based service delivery approaches. These questions include:

- Am I serving as a "coach" to the teacher?
- If not, how can I increase my support to facilitate differentiated instruction for the child with language impairment?

The implementation of classroom-based approaches requires that the practitioner coach other adults (Dinnebeil, Pretti-Frontczak, & McInerney, 2008). Coaching helps the classroom teacher acquire intervention skills to help children meet IEP goals and objectives.

When a practitioner coaches another adult, he or she (a) models specific strategies that can be used in the classroom to increase communication, (b) demonstrates how the approach can be implemented in the classroom, (c) observes the teacher using the strategy, and (d) provides feedback and reinforcement to the teacher in his or her implementation of the targeted strategy. The goal of high-quality classroom intervention is to help teachers embed differentiated instruction throughout the school day, in keeping with the child's level of ability. For example, the classroom teacher is trained to prompt question asking during snack time or naming during outdoor play. An embedded intervention for an older student might include reminding a student to use a series of prompts (posted on the student's desk) to organize a writing assignment.

Embedded learning opportunities take place as part of children's contextualized interactions as they occur in the classroom. In an embedded approach, the adult is seen as a facilitator of a child's communication (Justice & Kaderavek, 2004). When teachers—supported by an SLP or a special educator—provide instruction across classroom activities and routines, children have learning opportunities that match everyday communication demands. This match facilitates generalization. **Generalization** refers to the ability of an individual to take a learned skill and apply it in a novel situation. Embedded instruction also ensures that instruction is provided when children are highly involved in an interesting activity; this increases children's engagement and motivation.

The concepts of embedded learning and classroom-based instruction lead the practitioner to consider the positive effects of distributed practice. **Distributed practice** refers to providing children with opportunities to practice a skill frequently throughout the day. Distributed practice contrasts with **massed practice,** where skill training is massed into less-frequent and longer sessions. Experts suggest that distributed practice promotes learning (Cepeda et al., 2006).

When SLPs think about the optimal service delivery model, they also consider dosage by asking, "How much intervention is required to achieve the required outcome?" *Dosage* refers to the amount and frequency of intervention (i.e., How many weeks are required? How long should the session last? How many exposures to the target stimuli?). More is not always better! For example, it has been demonstrated that young children receive the maximum benefit from some early literacy interventions with less than 20 hours of instruction. I will be discussing the issue of dosage in Chapter 5.

CASE EXAMPLE: DECISION MAKING AND THE ENVIRONMENT

In Case Example 3, you are meeting Jahara and her family for a family interview. You remember to consider issues related to *accuracy and scope of information* (i.e., having enough information to help make decisions) and *change and adaptability* (i.e., making a real difference in an individual's life). You decide to use the principle of backward design to focus on the family's perceptions for Jahara's ultimate communication goals. You also want to carefully consider Jahara's communication environments. You ask the family the following question:

- What are your hopes and wishes for Jahara in the next 5 to 10 years?

You discover that Jahara will be entering a vocational training program, and she hopes to work in a hospital. She will be trained to work in the hospital laundry. This is likely to be her long-term employment setting. With more questioning and assessment, you find that Jahara communicates in simple sentences, but unfamiliar listeners understand her about 50% of the time (i.e., her speech is poorly articulated and she often mumbles). Jahara is motivated and excited to begin her job training.

Now, after learning this information, ask yourself some critical-thinking questions. Look back at Table 4.1 for possible questions. What language domains do you feel should be targeted in intervention? How do Jahara's future work environment and motivation to succeed affect her intervention program? Use this opportunity to improve your critical decision-making skills.

Decision Making: Progress Monitoring and Dismissal

A skilled practitioner maintains data to continuously monitor the changes in a child's language abilities. Data document specific child outcomes and also reflect the type and frequency of intervention. Both IDEA policy and the response to intervention model require frequent progress monitoring and the use of child response data to make educational decisions (Ehren et al., 2006). Progress monitoring reflects the critical-thinking parameters *evaluating the evidence* and *accuracy and scope of information.*

Deciding when a child or student should be dismissed from treatment is one of the most important decisions in the clinical process. ASHA and IDEA both provide guidelines for dismissal. I discuss these guidelines later in the chapter.

PROGRESS MONITORING

Progress monitoring provides data about a student's communication progress during intervention and guides decisions and programmatic changes (ASHA, 2006a). In the RTI model, an SLP or a special educator uses progress monitoring to document a student's status in response to evidence-based instruction within the classroom (i.e., the Tier 1 level of intervention). The practitioner considers the following question at Tier 1:

- What progress-monitoring system is in place to document the student's change as a result of classroom evidence-based instruction?

If the student does not progress, or if he or she falls behind expected levels of performance, the progress-monitoring system triggers movement to Tier 2 or 3, where the student receives more frequent, intense, and specialized intervention.

If a student is placed on an IEP, progress monitoring continues to play an important role. IDEA 2004 requires that parents receive regular reports on a student's progress toward annual goals. Progress is measured by comparing changes in a student's speech-language skills to established performance baselines, including curriculum-based language assessments and classroom observations (ASHA, 2004c).

Additional critical-thinking questions that the practitioner may ask include:

- Do I have a progress-monitoring system that allows me to document the student's progress across time?
- Have I shared the progress data with the student (if appropriate) and the student's teachers and parents?
- Is the progress-monitoring system efficient and effective?

Several methods of data collection are appropriate for progress-monitoring systems; they are discussed next.

Data Collection. Data collection procedures (a) allow a practitioner to track a student's progress from one session to another, (b) document the effectiveness of the intervention approach, and (c) maximize the effectiveness of the intervention (Paul & Cascella, 2006). The practitioner uses record forms and documentation procedures consistent with the underlying theory guiding the intervention. For example, data keeping in an intervention based on a behavioral approach is likely to reflect a student's correct or incorrect attempt when performing a targeted skill. Counting the number of correct attempts reflects quantitative data. **Quantitative data** are numbers expressing quantity, amount, or range of a targeted behavior.

In contrast, a social interaction or systems-based intervention is likely to result in the practitioner using qualitative data to document progress. **Qualitative data** are words or labels describing observed attributes or properties. Qualitative data can be organized into categories and assigned a number. However, with qualitative data, the numbers do not have value by themselves; rather, they represent descriptive attributes. A rubric is a data system commonly used for qualitative behavior documentation. A **rubric** is a set of criteria and standards used to assess an individual's performance on a specific task. In Table 4.3 you can see an example of a rubric used to document a student's ability to tell a

Table 4.3 **Rubric for Evaluating Storytelling**

Category	4	3	2	1
			Rating	
Characters	The main characters are named and clearly described (through words and/or actions). The audience knows and can describe what the characters look like and how they typically behave.	The main characters are named and described (through words and/or actions). The audience has a fairly good idea of what the characters look like.	The main characters are named. The audience knows very little about the main characters.	It is hard to tell who the main characters are.
Pacing	The story is told slowly where the storyteller wants to create suspense and told quickly when there is a lot of action.	The storyteller usually paces the story well, but one or two parts seem to drag or to be rushed.	The storyteller tries to pace the story, but the story seems to drag or be rushed in several places.	The storyteller tells everything at one pace and does not change the pace to match the story.
Knows the story	The storyteller knows the story well and has obviously practiced telling the story several times. The storyteller does not need notes and speaks with confidence.	The storyteller knows the story pretty well and has practiced telling the story once or twice. He or she may need notes once or twice but is relatively confident.	The storyteller knows some of the story but did not appear to have practiced. He or she may need notes three or four times and appears ill at ease.	The storyteller could not tell the story without using notes.
Audience contact	The storyteller looks at and tells the story to all members of the audience.	The storyteller looks at and tells the story to a few people in the audience.	The storyteller looks at and tells the story to one or two people in the audience.	The storyteller does not look at or try to involve the audience.

Source: RubiStar, 2000–2009. Copyright ALTEC at the University of Kansas. Development of this educational resource was supported, in part, by the U.S. Department of Education award #R302A000015 to ALTEC (Advanced Learning Technologies in Education Consortia) at the University of Kansas. Reprinted with permission.

story. In this example, the practitioner rates the storyteller on a series of four components of good storytelling (e.g., introducing characters, familiarity with the story, pacing, and audience contact). The storyteller is rated on each component with a rating varying from 4 (very good demonstration of the skill) down to a level of 1 (very poor demonstration of the skill). Chapter 5 provides more details on data-keeping systems.

DISMISSAL FROM THERAPY

A practitioner uses critical-thinking skills to determine when an individual should be dismissed from language intervention. Careful progress monitoring allows dismissal from therapy to be tied to student outcomes and achievement. Experts suggest that the SLP or special educator use the following factors to determine a school-age student's continued eligibility for intervention (Steppling, Quattlebaum, & Brady, 2007):

- Student's age
- Rate of student progress as documented by progress monitoring
- Student's motivation

The practitioner also considers ASHA standards when making decisions about dismissal from intervention. ASHA standards indicate that dismissal is appropriate when (a) an individual's communication disorder no longer negatively affects health status or social, emotional, or vocational performance; (b) there is no longer any measurable progress; (c) the individual's goal and objectives have been met; or (d) the individual has obtained the desired level of enhanced communication (ASHA, 2004a). A decision tree illustrating the dismissal decision-making process is presented in Figure 4.9.

Once a student is dismissed from direct therapy, indirect support in the student's classroom may be a viable option. IDEA also has criteria governing dismissal from speech-language school-based services. Under IDEA, dismissal occurs when a student's speech-language impairment no longer negatively affects educational performance.

CASE EXAMPLE: DECISION MAKING IN PROGRESS MONITORING

In Case Example 4, at the beginning of this chapter, you were asked to develop a progress-monitoring tool to document Thomas's morphosyntax skills. Thomas demonstrates frequent errors with verb forms and subordinating conjunctions. You consider issues related to *accuracy* (i.e., keeping accurate data) and *change and adaptability* (i.e., documenting real-life changes) and ask the following critical-thinking questions:

- What method of progress monitoring will best document changes in Thomas's morphosyntax?
- How can I gather data to help Thomas, Thomas's parents, and his teacher see changes in morphosyntax during everyday speaking and writing tasks?

In order to document change in verb forms, you decide to incorporate both quantitative and qualitative data-keeping systems. To keep quantitative data, you decide to have Thomas describe an event for 2 minutes and count the number of correct and incorrect verb forms. As a qualitative procedure, you create a rubric to evaluate changes in the quality of Thomas's written work.

Figure 4.9   **Dismissal Decision Tree**

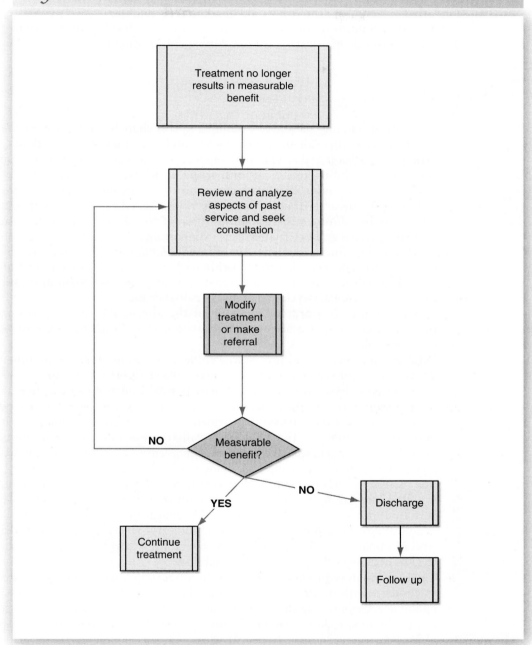

As a clinical skill-building exercise, develop a rubric to capture qualitative differences in Thomas's use of verb forms during his writing assignments. After you develop a rubric for verb use, write out how you would quantitatively and qualitatively evaluate Thomas's use of subordinating conjunctions. Your ability to develop appropriate progress-monitoring tools demonstrates your developing critical-thinking skills.

Summary

- The critical-thinking parameters outlined in this chapter are (a) accuracy and scope of information, (b) evaluating the evidence, and (c) change and adaptability. *Accuracy* prompts a decision maker to gather supporting evidence to identify the communication problem and make conclusions; *scope of information* creates critical-thinking questions to motivate careful documentation of an individual's communication reflecting the breadth of communication skills needed in multiple settings and considers cultural differences. *Evaluating the evidence* demands that the practitioners evaluate internal and external evidence supporting assessment tools and intervention protocols. The final parameter, *change and adaptability,* demands critical-thinking questions to make sure that the practitioner looks for real change in real-life settings for individuals with communication impairments, assesses student motivation, and is open to professional development and personal change.
- A decision tree is a graphic example of the alternatives in the decision-making process. A decision tree helps a practitioner see the thought process that underlies decision-making.
- Different approaches and procedures influence decision making. An important new approach is called the response to intervention (RTI) model. In the RTI model, intervention is based on scientific, research-based evidence using a tiered approach. Intervention is organized with three tiers of intervention. Tier 1 (classroom-based intervention on a daily basis) is provided to all children. For children who do not improve in response to Tier 1, Tier 2 (small-group or individualized intervention) is provided on a regular, weekly basis. Tier 3 intervention, consisting of intense, individualized intervention, is provided for children who do not progress with Tier 2 intervention. RTI is a preventive approach in that it provides scientifically based intervention for all children at the Tier 1 level to reduce the occurrence of later academic problems; it is an approach that is aligned with U.S. educational policy. In the RTI model, a child's ability to respond to intervention indicates whether a child has a significant level of impairment. In traditional assessment, test scores and observational data are used to document the presence of a disability.
- The Individuals with Disabilities Education Act (IDEA) is a law that ensures services to children with disabilities throughout the nation. IDEA governs how states and public agencies provide early intervention, special education, and related services to eligible infants, toddlers, children, and youth with disabilities. IDEA has prompted SLPs and special educators to provide classroom-based intervention in inclusive classrooms and train teachers to provide differentiated instruction to students with special educational needs.
- When making decisions about a student's environment, an SLP can use routines-based interviewing (RBI) to pose questions to family members. RBI is used to

(a) assess a child's developmental and communication status, (b) gain information about day-to-day life and family routines, and (c) tune in to a family's feelings about their child. A family routine includes familiar activities such as eating, bathing, bedtime, hanging out, going to the store, and traveling in the car.

- Progress monitoring results in data about a student's communication progress during intervention and guides decisions and programmatic changes. Progress monitoring helps an SLP develop goals, monitor progress, and formulate dismissal criteria. Progress monitoring is needed in the RTI model to move students between the three tiers of intervention; it is a requirement under IDEA policy.

Discussion and In-Class Activities

1. Alone or in a small group, develop critical-thinking questions to guide assessment and intervention for an individual at Communication Subdomains 1, 2, 3, 4, and 5; each small group will be assigned a different subdomain. As an elaboration to this activity, write critical-thinking questions for an individual with language challenges in your assigned subdomain who is (a) a preschooler and (b) an older school-age student. Note how the questions change in relation to the child's age and environmental expectations (i.e., classroom, vocational, peer).

2. Use the Internet and research information on the response to intervention model. Two good sites are:
   - www.rti4success.org
   - www.asha.org/slp/schools/prof-consult/RtoI.htm

   Prepare a brief report of additional information on RTI beyond what is presented in this chapter.

3. Use the Internet and research information on IDEA. Two good sites are:
   - http://idea.ed.gov
   - www.asha.org/advocacy/federal/idea/default.htm

   Prepare a brief report of additional information on IDEA beyond what is presented in this chapter.

4. Read more about embedded learning in preschool classrooms and develop embedded learning activities to engage young learners in early literacy learning. The following are some good sources:
   - Justice, L. M., & Kaderavek, J. N. (2004a). Embedded-explicit emergent literacy intervention I: Background and description of approach. *Language, Speech, and Hearing Services in Schools, 35,* 201–211.
   - Kaderavek, J. N., & Justice, L. M. (2004b). Embedded-explicit emergent literacy intervention II: Goal selection and implementation in the early childhood classroom. *Language, Speech, and Hearing Services in Schools, 35,* 212–228.

5. Develop a rubric to document (a) a preschooler's topic initiation and maintenance in the preschool classroom, (b) the quality of an oral presentation in front of the class for a fourth-grade student, or (c) social interaction with peers for an older school-age student. An Internet resource is http://rubistar.4teachers.org/index.php.

Chapter 4 Case Studies

1. Sandeep's parents brought their son into the clinic and said, "We've only ever had one real worry about Sandeep and that was just before his first birthday. Sandeep had always had a lot of colds and chest infections, but this time it developed into pneumonia and a collapsed lung. That was bad. Apart from that, he has always seemed quite happy, but quiet. We noticed he was not saying very many words but were not overly worried until we realized his younger brother had more words and was putting them together. We ignored it for a time and then went to our doctor for help. He suggested we see you."

Sandeep is now 2 years, 8 months. During the assessment, he was a very quiet, shy child who was reluctant to separate from his mother. No words or vocalizations were heard in the clinic, and he was not cooperative during the formal assessment. Sandeep's mother and father immigrated to the United States from India.

Questions for Discussion

1. An SLP uses clinical decision-making skills to formulate questions. With your classmates, discuss the quality and characteristics of the questions listed below. (a) What critical-thinking parameters guide each of the questions? (b) What aspects of clinical practice are covered by these questions? (c) What additional questions might you ask? (d) How would you modify these questions if Sandeep were older or from a majority culture?

Questions to ask Sandeep's parents:

1. What are Sandeep's favorite activities/toys? How does he request these items? What does he do when he wants something but it is not in sight or is out of reach? How does he indicate that he is hungry or tired?
2. What words does he understand? How do you know he understands these words (e.g., what does Sandeep do or say that indicates he knows these words)?
3. Describe a family activity or routine (e.g., dinnertime, bedtime, bathing, weekend outings). What do you do during this routine? What does Sandeep do during this routine? In what routine(s) do you feel Sandeep is highly successful? Are there any routines that are problematic for Sandeep? Why? What would you like to see Sandeep do differently during a problematic family routine?
4. Describe how Sandeep plays by himself. What does he do to entertain himself? How long can he play by himself or with his younger brother?
5. If you could change or improve one thing for Sandeep right now, what would it be?
6. Would you describe Sandeep as spending most of his or her time interacting with just the two of you, interacting with you and siblings, or interacting with you and other adult friends or family members?
7. When do you and Sandeep do most of your talking—while driving in the car, at the dinner table, at night when getting ready for bed, or at other times of the day?

Questions to ask yourself when you are observing Sandeep and his parents in a play interaction:

1. What kinds of symbolic play behavior does Sandeep evidence?
2. Does he point at objects or show objects to his family members?

3. What evidence indicates that Sandeep is comprehending language?

4. Does Sandeep imitate what his parents or brother are doing? Does he imitate sounds that they make? If so, does he vocalize vowels, consonants, or consonant + vowel syllables?

5. What kinds of turn-taking behaviors are evident? Does Sandeep engage easily with his parents and younger brother? What kinds of activities does he seem most interested in? How long does he sustain each interaction?

6. How does Sandeep request items or show his parents that he doesn't like something?

7. Does Sandeep make eye contact and show social behaviors (e.g., waving) when he comes to the clinic or upon leaving?

8. What does Sandeep do when his back is turned and his parents call his name or make a verbal request?

Source: The Communication Trust (2013). *A collection of case studies highlighting effective practice in speech, language and communication.*

2. Cameron is 4 years old and has autism. His parents ask you if they should enroll him in an intensive behavioral communication intervention. Cameron would be receiving one-on-one intervention learning (at the initial level) to point to pictures and follow one-step commands. He will receive 3 to 4 hours of intervention per day. Describe some of the points you want to consider when you talk to them. Base your discussion on internal evidence. In other words, give them background on the different theoretical approaches that can be used with children with autism (i.e., behavioral vs. social interaction theory).

   a. List some critical-thinking questions that help you clarify this situation.

   b. Research information about interventions for children with autism at www .autismspeaks.org.

   c. Role-play a conversation in which you explain to Cameron's parents the theories that underlie each approach.

3. Alana is 3 years old and is in a preschool classroom. She has a language delay and communicates with one-word utterances. Describe some classroom routines that might be appropriate opportunities to facilitate Alana's verbal communication.

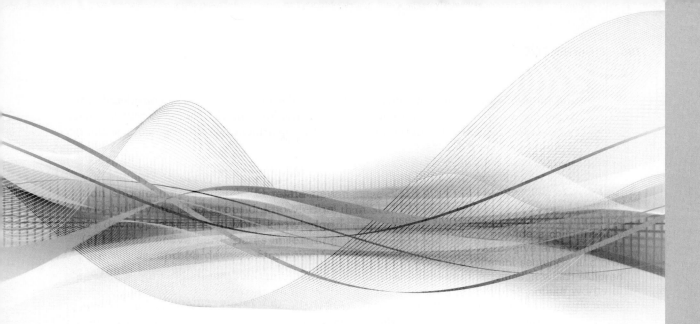

5 *Principles of Intervention*

Chapter Overview Questions

1. What does an interventionist consider when choosing stimuli to use in intervention? What techniques elicit responses? What factors influence reinforcement?
2. Describe five different language facilitation techniques. How are they related to social interactionist theory? How are they used in language intervention sessions?
3. How does an interventionist use the assertiveness–responsiveness scheme and

the continuum of naturalness for intervention planning?
4. What are the basic components of an intervention goal?
5. What are two different techniques for maintaining intervention data?
6. What intervention techniques are important when considering a student's competencies in language form, content, and use? Give examples.

In this this chapter, and throughout this book, my goal is to provide you with a toolbox of theoretical principles, developmental guidelines, and underlying state-of-the-art practices to guide your clinical work as a speech-language pathologist (SLP) or as an educator. This chapter focuses on tools and techniques you will use during language intervention. It begins by reviewing important components of intervention planning, providing information about specific intervention techniques and describing the links between techniques and underlying theories. This chapter also provides information to be considered when designing an intervention approach. I also discuss how an SLP uses different language intervention strategies based on an individual's impairment, within pragmatic, semantic, or morphosyntax domains.

Structuring and Planning Intervention

INTERVENTION TECHNIQUES AND THEIR RELATIONSHIP TO LANGUAGE THEORY

Recall from Chapter 1 that within the guidelines of evidence-based practice (EBP), a skilled professional considers both external and internal evidence in selecting an appropriate intervention plan. Internal evidence focuses on the theory or rationale that underlies a proposed intervention (Ratner, 2006). Review Chapter 4 for clinical questions related to evaluating internal evidence. In the following subsection, I highlight connections between frequently used intervention techniques and theoretical perspectives.

Intervention Techniques: Influences from Behaviorist Theory. In Chapter 2, I discussed several concepts, including the following ones based on behaviorist theory: reinforcement, behavioral extinction, punishment, and chaining. In the section below, I highlight additional intervention concepts related to behavioral theory. Specifically, I discuss information to guide (a) selection of stimuli used to elicit target behaviors, (b) techniques to elicit communication, and (c) reinforcement used during interventions.

Choosing Stimuli for Intervention. In keeping with the behavioral model, a professional carefully considers and defines aspects of an intervention to elicit the target behavior. Stimuli are either nonlinguistic or linguistic. Examples of nonlinguistic stimuli include showing a picture to elicit naming, making eye contact, and touching the child to prompt a pointing response. Linguistic events include calling the child's name, asking a *wh*-question, and initiating a conversation.

Choosing the right stimulus type and context is an important component of an effective intervention. For example, young children learn most easily when they are engaged in an activity (McWilliam & Casey, 2007). Consequently, it makes sense to use objects rather than pictures when teaching words to very young children or children with significant levels of delay. Object use also allows the object name (e.g., *ball*) to be paired with actions (e.g., *throw, catch, roll*). When a child is learning to use verbs and prepositions (e.g., *in, on, under*), the ongoing activity makes word meaning more transparent (Gentner, 2006).

Interventionists often use pictures to elicit language when they work with older children. Usually by age 2, children developing typically can learn new vocabulary by looking at pictures and transferring newly learned vocabulary to the real world (Ganea, Bloom-Pickard, & DeLoache, 2008). For children at early levels of language learning, realistic photographs promote more word learning than do illustrations (Ganea et al., 2008). Shared storybook reading is a frequently used and effective stimulus for language intervention; a book's illustrations connect children to the written text. Importantly, incorporating storybook reading into interventions not only facilitates a child's vocabulary, morphological, and syntax abilities but also fosters children's emergent literacy skills (Kaderavek & Justice, 2002).

SLPs and educators increasingly use computers and communication applications (i.e., apps) to deliver stimuli during language interventions. However, skilled professionals carefully consider EBP when choosing an app, because research indicates that adult-delivered intervention using imitation, modeling, and elicited production is more effective than a computer-delivered approach for students with morphosyntax deficits (Cirrin & Gillam, 2008). In another example, Bishop, Adams, and Rosen (2006) reported that computerized intervention treatments using slowed speech or modified speech input did not produce better results than regular school services.

Although computers do not replace adult-provided intervention, professionals can use computers and software apps effectively in specific contexts. Computer games and apps provide an engaging topic of conversation for many school-age students. Some software programs allow the user to create and illustrate stories, create greeting cards, or use problem-solving strategies (e.g., SimCity). Software programs can in such cases serve as a context for discourse between a practitioner and an individual with language impairment (Cress & Green, 2006). The onscreen stimuli function much like the board games or arts-and-crafts activities used traditionally in language interventions. As an in-class activity, go online and examine features of the language software programs listed in Table 5.1. Discuss how you might use the software in different ways to meet the needs of individual students.

Computers also provide practice opportunities for school-age students who struggle to develop topics for papers, organize writing assignments, or edit and revise written work. In this case, adults train students to use brainstorming software (such as Inspiration) to improve prewriting skills and word processing programs to facilitate editing and writing revisions.

Eliciting Responses. SLPs and educators use a variety of intervention techniques to elicit children's responses. I discuss the following terms and concepts: prompting, shaping, and modifying contexts.

Table 5.1 **Language-Oriented Software Programs**

Software program*	Website	Materials available that can be reviewed online
Webber Interactive WH Questions (Super Duper Publications)	www.superduperinc.com	Online demo available
Processing Auditory Directions (Academic Communication Associates)	www.acadcom.com	Sample pages
Acorn's Tree House Vocabulary and Language Skills (Janelle Publications)	www.janellepublications.com	
No Glamour Grammar; No Glamour Language & Reasoning; No Glamour Sentence Structure (LinguiSystems)	www.linguisystems.com	Online demo available

*The author and publisher do not necessarily endorse these software programs. However, they are typical of the kinds of software programs that SLPs use.

Prompts are instructions or stimuli used to ensure that a child responds correctly. Generally, an adult uses combinations of multiple prompts at early stages of learning and then reduces the number of prompts as the child develops skill. For example, imagine that you are an interventionist responsible for the communication program for Isaac, a 3-year-old minimally verbal child. Isaac uses some gestures and a few words to communicate in his preschool class. After "morning circle," the children typically request to move to a preferred activity (e.g., art table, dramatic play, sand table, book center). Along with Isaac's preschool teacher, you develop a sequence of prompts to facilitate Isaac's verbal productions. First, the teacher shows Isaac a series of pictures that visually demonstrate activity choices (pictures = prompt #1); the teacher then asks, "What do you want to do today, Isaac?" (teacher request = prompt #2). If Isaac does not respond, the teacher touches Isaac's arm and says, "Show me what you want to do today" (tactile = prompt # 3). If needed, the teacher uses a hand-over-hand method (physical support = prompt #4) to help Isaac point to his favorite activity—the sand table. The teacher then says, "Isaac, say 'sand table'" (imitation = prompt #5). Gradually, Isaac learns to respond to the teacher's question "What do you want to do today?" without the use of additional prompts.

Shaping also is used to teach increasingly complex behaviors. Consider the following example: An interventionist works with a nonverbal child to pair motor actions with verbalizations. Specifically, the professional decides to train the word *in* paired with an action (e.g., dropping blocks into a coffee can). At the beginning of the shaping procedure, the adult models and rewards the client as he imitates the motor act of dropping a block into the can. As this behavior emerges, the adult pairs a sound, *uh!*, along with dropping the blocks. Then, the adult shapes the child's behavior by providing reinforcement only when a sound and an action are produced together. Eventually, the adult uses the word *in* as she drops the block. Once again, she uses shaping; she now reinforces the child only when an approximation of the word *in* is paired with the motor action. Eventually the word and action are transferred to other similar motor activities (e.g., putting trash into a trash can, loading laundry into a basket).

Rewarding Communication Responses. As I discussed in Chapter 2, reinforcement increases the probability that a target behavior will occur. There are many decisions to consider regarding how to implement reinforcement during intervention. Professionals choose the most appropriate reinforcement for an individual and modify the reinforcement schedule to facilitate generalization of new behaviors.

When considering reinforcement, professionals prefer to use social reinforcement rather than primary reinforcement (e.g., food). Social reinforcement is preferred because it is always available and because responsiveness to social cues is programmed into our species and serves as a powerful tool for changing behavior within a social context (Baum, 2005). Just as adults view a smiling baby as highly reinforcing and a crying baby as highly aversive, children have a predisposition to respond to the positive and negative social responses of others. Social reinforcement includes smiling, nonverbal responses, "high fives," and positive sounds and verbalizations (e.g., *Oh! Yea! Good job!*; Baum, 2005). When food is used as reinforcement (e.g., for a child with very significant disabilities), the goal is to use it only at the initial stages of intervention, to pair food with social reinforcement, and to fade food reinforcement as quickly as possible.

Several intervention techniques are important when an interventionist considers how to generalize a new behavior into other communication contexts. **Fading** is a technique in which adult prompting is reduced, with the goal of the spontaneous occurrence of child behaviors in daily interactions. Generally at initial stages of intervention, target behaviors are elicited with strong modeling, cuing, and prompting. Eventually, the intensity of the elicitation behaviors is faded. Fading is a part of intervention at all levels, from the initial stages of teaching a behavior through the final stages of generalization. In fact, an interventionist's overall goal is to "fade out of the picture." The real goal of language intervention is to help a child produce the appropriate communication behavior with complete independence.

Part of fading from the picture is fostering a child's ability to produce the target behavior with less externally provided reinforcement. At first the adult provides frequent reinforcement and feedback; ultimately the goal of intervention is for new behaviors to be used and reinforced via everyday social interactions (Fernald, 2008). At the initial stages of intervention, the adult often uses **continuous reinforcement,** in which every correct response is followed by an event to increase the probability that the response will be repeated. Once the behavior is established, the adult reinforces the target behavior intermittently. In **intermittent reinforcement,** sometimes called **partial reinforcement,** only some correct responses are followed by the reinforcing event.

Intervention Techniques: Influences from Vygotsky and Social Interactionist Theory. Vygotskian theory (1978, 1987) maintains that initially a learner completes a task with the support of a more skilled participant, but with repeated opportunities, the learner internalizes underlying concepts and learns to perform the task independently. The social interactionist perspective motivates the practitioner to promote children's communication attempts within positive and socially relevant interactions. The practitioner builds on a child's communication bids by using modeling and by indicating that the child's efforts are important and accepted (Prizant, Wetherby, & Rydell, 2000).

Below I describe techniques used to facilitate children's language learning during adult–child interactions as they occur within SLP-provided intervention. Parents and teachers also use these language facilitation techniques when they interact with language learners.

Language Facilitation Techniques. A child with language impairment (LI) is less likely to engage in conversation than are children developing typically (Westby, 2008). Children with LI have reduced vocabulary and are less skilled at producing word combinations to verbalize their experiences. Once they begin to use word combinations, children with LI typically have unsophisticated morphology and syntax. In order to facilitate children's communication output, adults use a variety of strategies to encourage children to say more (i.e., increase the frequency of talk, vocabulary richness, and sentence length) and to elaborate their output (i.e., increase morphosyntax complexity). Techniques discussed below include self-talk, parallel talk, modeling, expansions, extensions, buildup/breakdown, and sentence recasts. Figure 5.1 demonstrates a teacher using modeling techniques.

Self-talk is language in which the adult describes what he is thinking, feeling, or seeing. Self-talk statements typically begin with *I.* For example, while playing with a dollhouse, an adult might say, "I'm putting the baby to sleep. Night-night, baby. I'm rocking the baby. Rock, rock!" The adult uses words to link the ongoing experience with interesting words, phrases, and sentences. Self-talk is a particularly helpful technique for children who are reluctant to talk; it is most effective when the adult observes what the child is doing and then performs similar actions with similar materials.

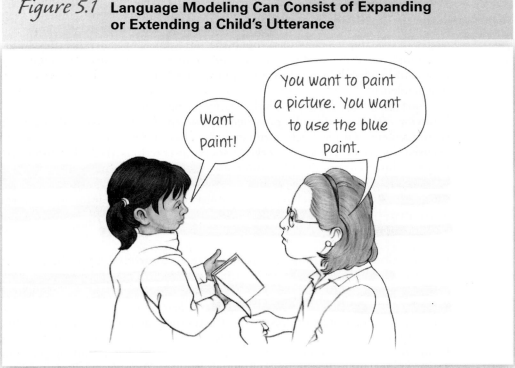

Figure 5.1   **Language Modeling Can Consist of Expanding or Extending a Child's Utterance**

Parallel talk differs from self-talk in that the adult uses language to describe what the child is thinking, feeling, and doing. As in self-talk, the adult does not require the child to respond; instead, the adult provides "play-by-play" descriptive language connected to the child's actions.

Both self-talk and parallel talk are consistent with language modeling. **Modeling** is a technique in which an adult talks and a child listens. Modeling is an opportunity for the child to deduce linguistic structures because the communication partner provides multiple examples of the language target.

During self-talk and parallel talk, the adult typically uses simplified language; sentences have less vocabulary variation, are shorter, have less complex syntax, and are semantically redundant. For example, the adult uses redundancy when he says, "I see a doggie. The doggie is big! He is barking! The big doggie is barking at the cat!" This simplification draws on Vygotsky's principle of operating in a child's zone of proximal development (van Kleeck et al., 2010).

Children are most likely to talk when they are highly engaged (McWilliam, Scarborough, & Kim, 2003). Parallel talk is likely to be effective because the adult's communication is based on the child's interests, level of engagement in the ongoing activity, and focus of attention. In early stages of language development, children also are more likely to talk about their own actions than to talk about what others are doing. Consequently, parallel talk stimulates a child's independent utterances. Adults subsequently build on children's independent utterances through elaboration and expansion. (Elaboration and expansion are defined below.)

There is controversy regarding the level of simplification adults should use in their utterances to young children and children with language delays (van Kleeck et al., 2010). For example, with a child who is very language delayed or very young, an adult might say "doggie walk" instead of "The dog is walking." This sentence construction pattern is similar to children's early word combinations, sometimes called telegraphic speech. **Telegraphic speech** typically includes only content words, such as nouns, verbs, and a few adjectives/adverbs, with few or no function words (e.g., auxiliary verbs, articles, conjunctions, and prepositions) or morphemes (e.g., present progressive *ing*, plural *s*, past tense *ed*). Function words and morphemes are not needed to communicate the meaning of a sentence. Examples of telegraphic speech include word combinations such as *Mommy fix* and *put table*. The adult uses telegraphic speech in the following example (Hancock & Kaiser, 2006):

Child: (points to cookie)
Adult: "Say, 'want cookie.' "
Child: "Cookie."
Adult: "Want cookie."

As a counterexample, consider the following interaction, where the adult uses short utterances but includes function words and consequently avoids telegraphic speech (van Kleeck et al., 2010):

Child: "Truck."
Adult: "Say, 'push the truck.' "
Child: "Push truck."
Adult: "I'll push the truck. Now you push the truck!"

Many experts suggest that telegraphic speech should never be used; in contrast, some language specialists argue that telegraphic speech is appropriate for children with a mean length of utterance less than 2.0 and appropriate within language interaction programs (Kaiser & Trent, 2007). However, all experts agree that adults should avoid using decidedly nongrammatical sentences, such as asking a child, "What doing?" (in contrast to using the correct form, "What are you doing?") and agree that adults should not use telegraphic speech in everyday conversations with children.

A child is not required to talk during self-talk and parallel talk; however, the adult's use of self-talk and parallel talk encourages the child's spontaneous communication. The adult subsequently builds on the child's spontaneous communication by using **language expansions** and **language extensions**. In an expansion, the adult repeats the child's verbalization but adds morphemes or words to make the sentence an acceptable adult sentence (Vigil, Hodges, & Klee, 2005). An example of an expansion follows:

Child: "Daddy go outside?"
Adult: "Yes, Daddy went outside!"

An extension is very similar to an expansion, but during an extension, the adult adds additional information related to the ongoing event. For example:

Child: "Baby night-night"
Adult: "The baby is going night-night. The baby is tired. Night-night, baby."

To summarize, an expansion is an elaboration of a child utterance in which the adult fills in missing grammar; an adult produces an extension when he or she adds grammatical forms as well as semantic information.

Researchers have documented the use of expansions between parents and children developing typically; parents expand about 30% of the utterances of their 18-month-old to 3-year-old children. Children developing typically imitate 10 to 24% of the parents' expansions (Goldstein, 1984).

A technique called buildup/breakdown is another powerful language facilitating technique. The **buildup/breakdown technique** was proposed in the early 1960s. It is designed to deconstruct a sentence into its separate components (e.g., noun phrase, verb phrase, prepositional phrase, adverb and adjective clauses). Buildups and breakdowns are observed in conversations between parents and young children. Parents say a sentence, repeat smaller segments of the sentence, and then finally repeat the entire sentence. Buildups and breakdowns are associated with positive language growth in young children developing typically. Here is an example of a buildup/breakdown. In this example, the adult and child are playing with building blocks:

Child: "House."

Adult: "I'm building a tall house with my blocks. A tall house! Building a tall house. I'm building. I'm building a tall house. I'm building a tall house with my blocks."

Child: "Build house."

A final language facilitation method, **sentence recasts**, is a technique often used in morphosyntax-focused intervention. Sentence recasts are similar to expansions except that in sentence recasts the language facilitator changes the modality of the sentence structure (e.g., changes the sentence from a statement to a question). Consider the following feedback during an intervention session. The intervention goal is to facilitate auxiliary verbs (e.g., *is* and *are*) within a noun phrase + verb phrase sentence. The interventionist chooses this goal because the child omits auxiliary verbs; he says, "The dog barking outside" instead of "The dog is barking outside." The child also does not use auxiliary verbs when asking questions; he says, "Dog barking?" instead of using an interrogative reversal, "Is the dog barking?"). The adult and child are playing with a farm set.

Adult: "The pig *is eating* his dinner. *Is* the pig *eating* his dinner? Yes, the pig *is eating* his food!" (SLP makes eating noises.)

Child: "Pig is eating!"

Adult: "Yes, the pig is eating! I liked how you used the special *is* word. You said, 'The pig *is* eating!'"

In this example, the adult produced the auxiliary verb during a statement ("*The pig is eating*") and also produced the sentence as an interrogative reversal ("*Is the pig eating?*"). It is hypothesized that alternating sentence modalities puts the targeted syntax feature at the forefront and increases the student's awareness of the language target. It should be noted, however, that experts caution that the use of the inverted auxiliary (e.g., "Are you going to the store?") during language intervention is a challenging linguistic task for children with LI, and SLPs might want to delay this intervention technique until the child shows some ability to produce auxiliary verbs (Fey & Loeb, 2002).

Expansions, extensions, buildup/breakdown, and sentence recasts are all highly contingent on a child's behavior. **Contingency** refers to how closely a language facilitator's communication relates to a child's output. Language facilitation techniques start with the child's communication and then modify the child's output to correspond to the adult language form. The frequency of contingent language during adult–child interactions positively predicts child language development (Hoff, 2006).

Assertive–Responsive Communication Scheme. Fey (1986) proposed a scheme in alignment with the social interaction approach; he proposed that an interventionist should observe an individual's **conversational assertiveness** and **conversational responsiveness** within a social context. An assertive communicator initiates a conversational turn. A responsive communicator responds to others' communication attempts. An effective communicator is both assertive and responsive. However, individuals vary along a continuum of assertiveness and responsiveness during conversations; the assertiveness–responsiveness scheme profiles an individual according to levels of social participation. A visual representation of the scheme is shown in Figure 5.2. Consider the following example as an illustration of the scheme.

Imagine that you are at a party, and you introduce yourself to the people around you. First, you begin a conversation with a woman who is extremely talkative. You have difficulty fitting in a comment. When you do make a statement, she ignores your comment. She continues to talk about her own ideas and thoughts, without fostering the expected back-and-forth flow of conversation. In the assertiveness–responsiveness scheme, this individual is classified as highly assertive and minimally responsive (+ assertive, − responsive).

You seek out another conversation partner. Your second conversation is completely different. Now you are talking to a man who answers your questions but does not elaborate on his ideas and does not bring up new topics. You feel frustrated because you are doing all the conversational "work," and your communication partner is passive during the interaction. In the assertiveness–responsiveness scheme, this individual is classified as an unassertive but responsive communicator (− assertive, + responsive).

The examples above are exaggerations; however, I imagine you have experienced a version of the events I have described. In contrast to the two examples above, an effective communicator achieves a balance between assertiveness (i.e., is able to initiate a topic as needed, makes statements or comments) and responsiveness (i.e., responds to what other people say). An individual who is + assertive and + responsive generates the expected back-and-forth conversational pattern.

As Figure 5.2 demonstrates, there are four communication types in the scheme. Beyond the three types discussed above (+ assertive, − responsive; − assertive, + responsive; + assertive, + responsive), there is a − assertive, − responsive classification. In this case, the individual does not initiate or respond to others' communication. This communication type describes an individual with a severe disability.

The assertiveness–responsiveness scheme is helpful when the interventionist considers the aspects of communication to be targeted within an individual's intervention program. Remember, an effective communicator (+ assertive, + responsive) produces a range of assertive communication acts and also responds well to others' conversational attempts. Assertive conversational acts include asking for information from others, requesting actions or objects, making comments and statements, joking, and teasing.

Other communication behaviors are classified as responsive communication. Responsive communication acts include responding to others' requests for action or

Figure 5.2 **Fey's Assertiveness—Responsiveness Scheme**

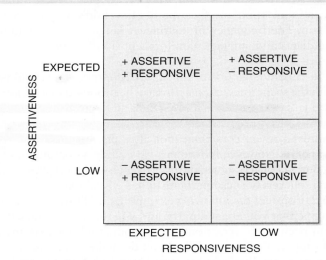

Source: Fey, Marc E., *Language Intervention with Young Children*, 1st, © 1986. Printed and Electronically reproduced by permission of Pearson Education, Inc., Upper Saddle River, New Jersey.

objects and acknowledging others' comments. A list of assertive and responsive communication acts is shown in Table 5.2.

An SLP or educator provides intervention for children who vary along the continuum of assertive and responsive communication. For example, as a language facilitator, you might work with an individual who is highly verbal but has difficulty responding contingently to others' conversational attempts. In this case, the communication profile is classified as + assertive, − responsive.

The intervention focuses on improving the individual's communication responsiveness. An example of a goal for a + assertive, − responsive student is *Elissa will respond contingently to a conversational partner's comments at least three times within a 3-minute conversation*. Elissa's intervention program includes (a) practicing responsive communication behaviors using prompts (prompts include a written set of directions to serve as a reminder of the conversational rules and an adult hand gesture to signal the responsive act; prompts are faded), (b) videotaping and analyzing videotapes of conversations (Elissa participates in analyzing her conversational skills), and (c) practicing the responsive communications skills with peers in the classroom setting.

In contrast to the example demonstrated with Elissa, you may work with a student who is − assertive, + responsive. Imagine that in this case the student, Daniel, is having difficulty in the classroom because he fails to initiate comments to peers, does not request objects or actions when needed, and fails to ask for clarification when he is confused. You and the student's teacher design the following goal: *Daniel will use assertive communication acts at least three times during classroom small-group science activities*. Daniel practices completing assertive communication with you during role-playing simulations.

Table 5.2   **Examples of Assertive and Responsive Communication Acts**

Assertive Acts

- Requests for information
  - *"Why you going?"*
  - *"Where my Mommy?"*
  - *"You want you Mommy?"*
  - *"Wanna go outside?"*
  - *"It's nice, isn't it?"*
- Requests for action
  - *"Gimme that!"*
  - *"Push the chair in."*
  - *"You say it."*
- Requests for clarification
  - *"What?"*
  - *"No?"*
  - *"Excuse me?"*
- Requests for attention
  - *"Look at this!"*
  - *"See this?"*
  - *"Mommy!"*
- Comments, statements, and disagreement
  - *"This is the biggest one."*
  - *"They hanged up."*
  - *"That's my dog, Jackie."*
  - *"Do it this way."*
  - *"You have to push it."*
  - *"That's not mine."*
  - *"No."*
  - *"I'm not telling you."*
- Discourse-level assertive conversational acts
  - Initiating a new topic
  - Extending a topic (adding new information)

Responsive Acts

- Responses to requests for information
- Responses to requests for action
- Responses to requests for clarification
- Responses to requests for attention
- Responses to comments and statements and disagreement
  - *"Sure."*
  - *"I know."*
  - *"Yeah."*
  - *"Right."*
- Discourse-level responsive conversational acts
  - Maintaining topic (does not add information)

Source: Fey, Marc E., Language Intervention with Young Children, 1st, © 1986. Printed and Electronically reproduced by permission of Pearson Education, Inc., Upper Saddle River, New Jersey.

Prior to each small-group science activity, Daniel and his teacher write out three assertive communication acts (i.e., comments, statements, or requests). The first several times Daniel tries his assertive acts, you visit the classroom and help with the science activity. You cue and support Daniel's use of assertive communication acts; gradually Daniel's teacher provides the needed level of support. Eventually, Daniel practices embedding assertive conversational acts into other classroom activities.

Note that in the above examples, I did not mention the students' diagnoses. One of the compelling features of the assertiveness–responsiveness scheme is that it is not organized around an individual's diagnostic label (e.g., autism, intellectual disability, hearing impairment). Instead, the assertiveness–responsiveness scheme focuses on an individual's quality of participation during social discourse. An interventionist uses this scheme to make sure there is a focus on how the individual interacts with others in daily life. The assertiveness–responsiveness scheme is a valuable tool for your intervention toolbox as it can be used to plan intervention approaches for children with varying disabilities.

Intervention Techniques: Influences from Cognitive Theory. As you learned in Chapter 2, cognitive theories include the concepts proposed by Piaget. Cognitive constructivist theories focus on individuals' mental processes, including perception, memory, and problem solving. The influence of cognitive constructivist theories on language intervention is profound, ranging from facilitating early learning strategies to enhancing sophisticated processes associated with high-level cognition.

Imitation and Practice. The most fundamental cognitive processes are facilitated through imitation and practice. **Imitation** occurs when one communication partner copies another's actions or sounds. Imitation often is used as a first step in teaching a specific language target. Providing a gesture, sound, word, phrase, or sentence for imitation gives a child more opportunities to talk and more opportunities for pragmatic, phonological, semantic, and morphosyntax practice. Adults also reciprocate by imitating children's behaviors and communication attempts. Young children increase vocalization and communication attempts when adults imitate child utterances or motor acts (e.g., waving "bye-bye" back to a child). Imitation can be used to foster back-and-forth conversational turns within interactions (MacDonald, 2004).

Children must practice language to become proficient communicators. **Practice is** defined as the repetition of a task to gain proficiency; practice fosters cognitive development. To understand the importance of practice in language learning, think of the skills needed to become a skilled dancer.

Learning to dance is a good analogy for language learning (Moerk, 2004). Dance is based on basic stepping patterns that are likely to be innate. Dance occurs in all world cultures, in different forms, and is a learned social skill. To become a skilled dancer, an individual learns different dance components from different sources; individual components of dance must be separated and then recombined into new combinations. Much of this learning is internalized unconsciously. Dance is primarily taught through modeling and imitation, but it can also be taught didactically (e.g., through formalized and explicit instruction). The individual internalizes concepts to become proficient. Practice is essential.

As a language facilitator, you will facilitate multiple opportunities for individuals to practice their communication skills, just as a dancer must practice dance steps. During intervention, skilled practitioners monitor the frequency of adult talk in relation to the amount of child talk. A practitioner waits for a child to respond. Children with communication disorders often need more time to compose their ideas and more opportunities for practice.

Direct questions (questions requiring only a brief answer) are avoided. Instead, modeling procedures and open-ended comments (e.g., "What's happening now?") are preferable because they provide increased opportunity for practice. To facilitate even more practice, practitioners work closely with teachers and family members so children can practice communicating more often. When intervention goals are highlighted throughout the day, the individual has more opportunities for practice.

Metacognition. Practitioners foster high-level cognitive skills when they facilitate a student's metacognition and metalinguistic skills. **Metacognition** refers to the conscious recognition and application of abstract concepts. The student learns to "think about thinking." **Metalinguistics** refers to a student's ability to focus on and talk about language. A student uses metacognitive tasks to (a) consider how to approach a learning task, (b) monitor comprehension during reading, or (c) evaluate progress on an academic task. A number of intervention strategies build meta-awareness (Margolis & McCabe, 2006). To facilitate metaskills, a language facilitator can:

- *Describe* the learning strategy so the student internalizes the skill. For example, if the practitioner is teaching strategies to improve reading comprehension, he or she first explicitly describes the underlying process (e.g., "I will outline at least five important paragraphs in each science chapter and ask myself questions about it, so I can understand the material.")
- *Model* the strategy for the student. In this example, the practitioner shows the student how he or she selects the important items from the text.
- *Rehearse* the strategy with the student both verbally and in guided practice. The practitioner breaks the task into separate steps; together the practitioner and student take sections of the step and practice the task.
- *Discuss* how the student can use the strategy in a variety of situations. The practitioner plans time for the student to use the strategy during class.
- *Teach the student to monitor* his or her use of the strategy. In the example above, the practitioner and student make a check sheet with basic *wh-* questions (e.g., "What is the primary point of the text?" "What facts support the primary point?"). The student learns to use the check sheet to monitor his or her comprehension.
- *Teach struggling learners to reinforce* themselves when they correctly use the strategy. In this example, the practitioner and student have fun looking in a mirror and saying "I am doing great; I used questions today after I read my science assignment!"
- "*Provide task-specific feedback* (e.g., "You made an excellent topic sentence for each section of your outline."). Specific feedback, in contrast to general feedback (e.g., "Good job!"), promotes meta-awareness.

There is an increasing emphasis on enhancing metaskills as students move past the early primary school years into middle school. The assumption is that early learning focuses on skill acquisition, but older students should focus on applying effective strategies to guide thinking and language use (Law et al., 2008). An SLP's focus on building metaskills differentiates the SLP's intervention approach from that of an academic tutor. An academic tutor assists a student with the goal of producing a better product (e.g., helping the student complete homework). In contrast, an SLP facilitates a student's metaskills, focusing on the *process* needed to produce a good product so the student learns to independently use appropriate strategies during academic tasks.

STRUCTURING INTERVENTION: THE CONTINUUM OF NATURALNESS

In the sections above, I discussed how varying intervention approaches are aligned with different language theories. For example, focusing on the stimuli and reinforcement schedule during intervention draws from behaviorist theory, while incorporating language facilitation techniques such as self-talk and parallel talk reflects a social interactionist theoretical base. The choice of different techniques also impacts the naturalness or unnaturalness of language intervention. Some language intervention is highly natural in that the social turn taking during the intervention session is very much like a child's everyday interactions. A practitioner waits for a child to communicate and uses contingent response to foster more language output. In contrast, when an SLP asks a student to name many pictures or imitate a sequence of utterances, the interaction is less like what a child experiences in his everyday life. This variation represents the concept underlying the **continuum of naturalness** (Fey, 1986). Intervention activities are placed along the continuum of naturalness to the degree that they are more or less like everyday communication. The activities, location, and social context are variables that contribute to an intervention's naturalness or unnaturalness; Figure 5.3 illustrates how these variables contribute to an interaction's naturalness rating. In the section below, I discuss how the activities, the location, and the social variables contribute to an intervention being classified as unnatural (structured), natural (unstructured), or at the midpoint, using Fey's continuum.

Continuum of Naturalness: Highly Structured Intervention. The activities that are used during the intervention contribute to the naturalness rating. An example of a structured language activity is **drill**, an activity often completed in response to pictures. Drill

Figure 5.3 **Continuum of Naturalness**

		drill	organized games	daily activities
1.	Activity	0	+1	+2
2.	Physical Context	clinic 0	school +1	home +2
3.	Social Context	clinician 0	teacher +1	parents +2
4.	Overall Naturalness	low 0	+3	high +6

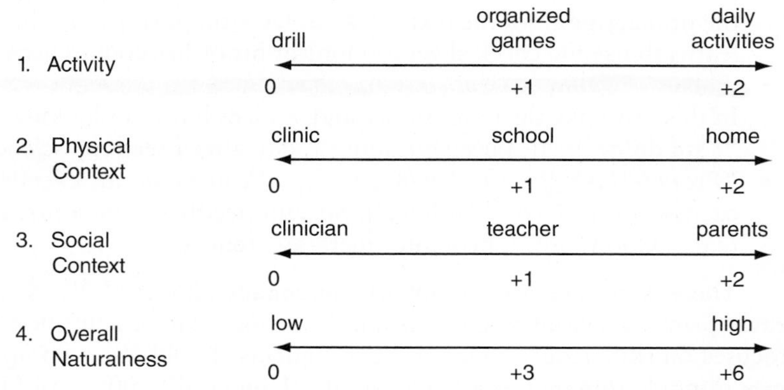

Source: Fey, Marc E., Language Intervention with Young Children, 1st, © 1986. Printed and Electronically reproduced by permission of Pearson Education, Inc., Upper Saddle River, New Jersey.

activities typically elicit a high number of child responses produced in response to adult questions. Drill play is somewhat more natural but still highly structured. In **drill play**, an element of a play routine is used to increase motivation. Examples include having the child "mail" a picture into a pretend mailbox after he or she names the picture, asking the child to produce a language target in response to a selected object (e.g., child selects miniature items from a toy box), and playing a game in which multiple child productions are elicited.

Location and social variables also contribute to an intervention being classified as less natural. The location of a less-natural interaction occurs outside the child's classroom or without family participation. This approach sometimes is called *pullout therapy*.

The social variation characteristic of highly structured or unnatural intervention is one-on-one and adult directed. Extended one-on-one, skill-based interactions generally do not occur in a child's everyday life. Adult-directed intervention contrasts with child-directed intervention (discussed below). The dichotomy of adult-directed vs. child-directed intervention describes who is "in charge" and leads the interaction.

In **adult-directed intervention**, the adult leads the interaction by (a) choosing the stimulus items; (b) regulating how the child will respond; (c) prompting particular responses through pointing, modeling, or the use of questions; and (d) providing direct feedback on the child's performance (e.g., "Good talking!"). One of the common features of the adult-directed approach is the three-part question sequence consisting of (1) the adult's request to produce specific information, (2) the child's response, and (3) the adult's evaluative feedback. Adult-directed approaches tend to use many of the intervention strategies from behavioral-based intervention discussed previously in this chapter. I provide a treatment sequence illustrative of an adult-directed approach in Focus 5.1.

FOCUS 5.1   *Learning More*

An adult-directed intervention sequence has a typical question–statement–feedback format. Here is an example:

> **Adult:** *"Joshua, I have different kinds of balls in this box. I am going to pull one out and throw it to you. Each time, catch it and then tell me about the ball. Remember to use your descriptive words!"*
> **Adult:** *"What kind of ball is this?"*
> **Joshua:** *"It is a red ball."*
> **Adult:** *"Yes, it is red. Is it big or little?"*
> **Joshua:** *"It is big."*
> **Adult:** *"Try to put all your descriptive words together to make a big sentence."*
> **Joshua:** *"This is a big, red ball."*
> **Adult:** *"Good. You told me about the size and the color. You could have also told me about how it feels. Like this: 'This is a soft, bouncy ball.'"*
> **Joshua:** *"This ball is soft and bouncy."*
> **Adult:** *"Good try! Try it this way: 'This is a soft, bouncy ball.'"*
> **Joshua:** *"This is a soft, bouncy ball."*
> **Adult:** *"Good! That time you used your descriptive words before the word ball. You said, 'This is a soft, bouncy ball.' Let's try this next one. What about this ball?"*

Continuum of Naturalness: Natural Intervention. On the opposite end of the continuum of naturalness is highly natural interaction. An example of a highly natural language intervention occurs when the practitioner creates opportunities for a child to communicate in the classroom or interacts with a child with toys, following the child's lead. The locations of natural interactions tend to be a student's typical communication environments—the classroom or home. The social variables include working with the student with his or her peers or with family members. The classroom-based model of intervention discussed in Chapter 4 reflects a more natural intervention approach.

In contrast to the adult-directed format discussed previously, highly natural approaches tend to represent **child-directed intervention.** Here, the adult follows the child's lead, responds contingently to the child's responses, and waits for the child to respond before initiating another conversational sequence. Social interaction is viewed as the reinforcing event in contrast to explicit reinforcement. Rather than taking on the leader role, in child-directed intervention the adult modifies the situation's interactional and interpersonal characteristics to enhance the child's communication functioning. The approach reflects the modeling and balanced turn-taking strategies influenced by social interactionist theory.

Continuum of Naturalness: Midpoint Intervention. Some language approaches, referred to as **hybrid intervention,** represent a midpoint on the continuum of naturalness. Hybrid approaches are more natural than drill and drill play but are not completely child-directed. For a midpoint intervention, an interventionist may work with a child one-on-one in the classroom environment (i.e., at a separate table inside the classroom) or in a pullout intervention. Social variables may include communication just with the adult or with a small group of peers or siblings. In either case, the SLP works to make the interactions pragmatically meaningful and to reflect real-life communication patterns.

In a hybrid approach, the practitioner focuses on a small subset of language behaviors and focuses a great deal of attention on identified targets during the intervention session. However, rather than use the direct question sequence often seen in the adult-directed approach, the adult manipulates the context to prompt the child to spontaneously use the targeted linguistic features. Often hybrid interventions use toys and play routines to create opportunities for practice. During a play routine, a practitioner uses specific modeling and responsive strategies to emphasize targeted features. An example of a technique consistent with the hybrid approach is sentence recasting. As discussed earlier in this chapter, during sentence recasting, the practitioner varies sentence structure in modeled sentences (i.e., interrogative vs. declarative sentences) to increase the child's attention to the language target.

Focused stimulation is an intervention technique that is considered to be a hybrid therapy. In **focused stimulation,** a child is exposed to multiple examples of a linguistic target in a meaningful communication context. The practitioner does not require an imitative response but rather elicits spontaneous communication. Focused stimulation can be used to facilitate features within form, content, or use language domains (Weismer & Robertson, 2006).

Empirical evidence supports the clinical use of focused stimulation for children who have language impairments, toddlers who are language delayed, and individuals with intellectual disability. Level I research studies have demonstrated that focused stimulation intervention results in significant gains in toddlers' total number of words, number of different words, and mean length of utterance (Weismer & Robertson, 2006) and that stimulation techniques fostered growth in school-age children's use of grammar forms (Leonard et al., 2006). There is an interesting finding reported in the Leonard et al. study: The authors hypothesized that children may have improved more if SLPs had exposed the children to a higher frequency of grammar targets; the SLPs produced about 12 stimulations per 15-minute period. This finding underscores the importance of considering issues related to dosage. **Dosage refers to the frequency, intensity, and duration of services required to achieve optimal intervention outcomes.** Learn more about the issue of dosage as it relates to language intervention in Focus 5.2.

FOCUS 5.2   *Learning More*

As you know, EBP involves providing evidence-based interventions and choosing the interventions with the strongest outcomes. However, very little attention has been given to the issue of intervention intensity. An SPL not only selects an intervention but also makes decisions regarding dosage. Dosage includes the rate of teaching episodes provided per minute or hour, the number of hours of intervention per specified time period (e.g., a day, a week), and the total amount of intervention, in weeks, months, or year. The SLP must determine how much is enough (Ukrainetz, 2009).

To understand this issue, I describe six aspects of dosage (Warren, Fey, & Yoder, 2007) and pose a question an SLP might ask related to each:

- *Dose:* This refers to the number of times teaching occurs per session (e.g., 100 trials, 40 expansion recasts). The SLP might ask, "Did I provide the right number of exposures to the target during the session to maximize student outcomes?"
- *Dose form:* This refers to the type of task or activity in which the intervention target is delivered (e.g., drill, play, storytelling). The SLP might ask, "What kind of activity will promote the most significant improvement?"
- *Length of a session in time:* This refers to the length of one session (e.g., 50 minutes). The SLP might ask, "Is a longer session better, or can I achieve the same outcome with a shorter session but more intense exposures to the target?"

- *Number of sessions per unit of time:* This refers to how often the intervention should take place over a period of a week, a month, or a school year (e.g., twice per week). The SLP might ask, "Would it be better to think about my caseload as cycles, working with a group of students intensively for 4 weeks (four times per week) and then rotating to a second group that I see intensively, and then cycling the groups throughout the school year?"
- *Total intervention duration:* This refers to how much total time is needed to achieve maximum improvement (e.g., 12 weeks, 30 weeks). The SLP might ask, "If I work with kindergarteners for 12 sessions over a period of 6 weeks on phonological awareness (PA) skills, is that enough dosage to ensure that the majority of students have the PA skills they need to become good readers?"
- *Cumulative intervention intensity:* This is the relationship that occurs when all the features of dosage are considered. It can be thought of as a mathematical formula (e.g., dose : dose frequency : total intervention, or 100 trials : 3 times per week : 30 weeks = 9000 trials overall). The SLP might ask, "How often does my student require intervention, and how much, to achieve a positive outcome?"

A great deal of research is currently under way to answer these questions. The interdependent and complex factors of service delivery make it challenging to complete research investigations.

Future studies examining service delivery should systematically examine discrete aspects of service delivery to children using well-designed and highly controlled methodologies. Dosage will be an area of research that you will want to follow in your career as a speech-language pathologist (Schooling, Venediktov, & Leech, 2010).

Developing a playlike, engaging context is an important component of focused stimulation. For example, imagine that a practitioner wants to teach a child to use auxiliary forms. The practitioner selects the modal auxiliary form *can* because modal verbs typically emerge earlier than *be* auxiliary verbs. In this interaction, the child and adult manipulate superhero action figures:

Adult: *"Can Superman fly? Yes, he can fly! Superman can fly. How about Aquaman? Can he fly?"*

Child: *"Aquaman no fly. Aquaman swim."*

Adult: *"Oh, I see. Aquaman can swim. Superman can fly."*

Adult: *"I wonder if Hulk can fly? What do you think?"*

Child: *"Hulk can fly!"*

Adult: *"Wow, I didn't know Hulk can fly! Show me again, how Hulk can fly!"*

Classic characteristics of focused stimulation are demonstrated in the previous example. The activity is carefully constructed so that repeated exposure to the targeted form is modeled and produced. Play routines consist of dramatic play enactments (e.g., setting up a grocery store, getting ready for school) or manipulating toy figures and objects. Examples of play routines to elicit different form, function, and use targets are provided in Table 5.3.

As discussed in the previous example, the practitioner does not demand that the child imitate a response but creates a context in which child productions are elicited. As the child's skill level improves, the practitioner decreases the number of focused models and increases opportunities for child responses.

The notion of adult- vs. child-directed therapy, and the use of hybrid approaches, is a helpful concept for intervention planning. It is important to remember, however, that an intervention does not have to be entirely one approach or another. Typically, practitioners use a combination of approaches within a therapy session. For example, a child might participate in an adult-directed warm-up activity at the beginning of each therapy session, followed by a child-directed or hybrid approach during the rest of the therapy session. The duration and intensity of different approaches is varied in relation to the child's abilities, motivation level, and the intervention goal.

As a final note on this topic, one caution when considering Fey's continuum is the assumption that highly natural activities are always better than highly unnatural activities. Experts caution us against this thinking; highly natural activities are preferred *only* when they are effective. If two activities are equally effective, then the more natural activity is preferred. However, if the activity must be modified (i.e., made less natural) to increase effectiveness, the adult modifies the intervention accordingly. Gradually, as the child's skill level improves, the adult adjusts variables to increase naturalness. In the section below, I describe how a practitioner writes goals to reflect the selected language approach.

Table 5.3   **Examples of Focused Stimulation Interventions for Form, Content, and Use**

Communication Domain	Focused Stimulation Activity
Form	• To increase a child's use of negation, the following activity is established: The adult sets up a dollhouse with a man doll, a cat, doll furniture, and a car. The man is sleeping, and the cat is under the bed. ***Adult:*** (Man wakes up) "*Where is that cat? He is <u>not</u> in the kitchen. He is <u>not</u> in the living room. Is he in the car? He is <u>not</u> in the car. I wonder where he is? Is he in the backyard?*" ***Child:*** "*No backyard.*" ***Adult:*** "*He is <u>not</u> in the backyard!*"
Content	• To increase a child's use of superordinate categorization, the following activity is established: The adult shows the child a box containing doll furniture, doll clothes, and vehicles (cars, trucks, bus, taxi, bicycle). ***Adult:*** "*The box is a mess! We are going to organize this box into categories. Some of these objects are <u>furniture</u>, some of these objects are <u>clothing</u>, some of these objects are <u>transportation</u>.*" (Adult lays out a picture of a house, a closet, and a garage) "*Let's figure out where these items should go.*" ***Child:*** "*Okay.*" ***Adult:*** "*This is a hat. It's something you wear on your head. A hat is <u>clothing</u>. I can put it in the closet. We keep <u>clothing</u> in the closet. <u>Clothing</u> is stuff that we wear.*" ***Adult:*** "*This is a bus. We ride on a bus. A bus is used for <u>transportation</u>. Where should we put the bus? Okay, we can park the bus in the big garage. What kinds of things are we going to put in the garage?*" ***Child:*** "*Bus, car.*" ***Adult:*** "*Yes, because a bus and a car are things we use for <u>transportation</u>, we use them to get places.*"
Use	• To increase a child's use of the pragmatic function of *request*, the following activity is established: The adult sets up a picnic, using stuffed animals and plastic food. There are plates, cups, a pitcher for juice, etc. ***Adult:*** "*The bear says, 'I need a plate.' Can you give him a plate? Good. The cat says, 'I need a plate, please.' What does the dog say?*" ***Child:*** (Does not answer, gives dog plate) ***Adult:*** "*Wait, before you give the dog a plate, he has to ask. The dog says, 'I need a plate!'*" ***Child:*** "*Need plate.*" ***Adult:*** "*Good, you made the dog ask for a plate! Let's see who wants some juice.*"

WRITING INTERVENTION GOALS

Making a measurable difference in an individual's everyday interactions is at the heart of efficacious treatment. "It is the ultimate goal, indeed, the gold standard for impairment-based treatment" (Thompson, 2007, p. 5). In order to document changes made during intervention, an interventionist must write goals in which change can be described and measured, select appropriate goal attack strategies, and maintain data to document change. In Figure 5.4 I provide a decision tree illustrating how the goal writing process fits into intervention planning.

When writing intervention goals, a practitioner describes what the student's communication behavior will look like when the skill is mastered. A goal is made up of three components: the *do* statement, the *condition* statement, and the *criterion* statement (Roth & Paul, 2007). The *do* statement describes the behaviors the child will produce. It is important to write the goal with active, observable verbs such as *write, answer, state, imitate, respond,* and *produce*. In contrast, verbs such as *know, understand, realize, comprehend,* and *learn* cannot be measured. Some examples of active verbs in a *do* statement include

- John will <u>initiate</u> . . .
- Xavier will <u>express</u> . . .

Figure 5.4 **Intervention Decision Tree**

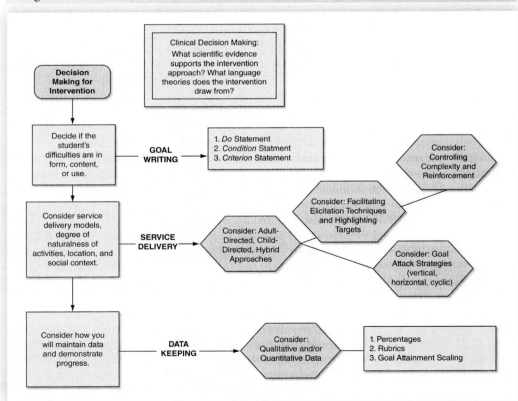

- Sasha will <u>imitate</u> gestures . . .
- Kareem will <u>edit</u> his written work . . .

The second component of the behavioral goal describes the situation or conditions under which the behavior will occur. Remember that a communication goal describes target behaviors as they are produced from the initial learning stage (i.e., the child is provided strong support from an adult in a controlled interaction) to the final stage (i.e., the behavior is produced during natural, spontaneous interactions). Accordingly, the *condition* statement describes the stimuli, where the behavior will occur, and who will be there when the behavior occurs. *Condition* statements often include words such as *following, after, with, in response to, before,* and *during*:

- At the beginning stages of learning, the *condition* statement indicates strong support and cuing. Examples include:
  . . . following an adult model
  . . . with picture cues
  . . . with a written reminder
- In contrast, at later stages the *condition* statement demonstrates the child's increasing independent production of the targeted skill:
  . . . before initiating a written assignment
  . . . in response to peers' questions
  . . . during interactive play routines in the classroom

The final component of the goal statement reflects the criteria determining goal achievement. The *criterion* statement can be measured quantitatively (e.g., with total correct or percentage data) or qualitatively (e.g., with a rubric or description of performance). Quantitative goals often include statements such as:

- *. . . 8 out of 10 times*
- *. . . with 90% accuracy*
- *. . . two times a day for 2 weeks*
- *. . . at least three times in a 10-minute conversation*
- *. . . less than three times during the 20-minute therapy session*

Typically, accuracy levels are set fairly high when they are expected to occur in an adult-directed and less naturalistic setting (i.e., 70–90% accuracy). At the final stages of intervention, when the child is expected to produce the behavior spontaneously, less stringent accuracy levels are expected (e.g., 50–70% accuracy).

A good goal allows a practitioner some flexibility (i.e., is not so specific that it completely limits the choice of therapeutic activity) but is descriptive enough that another professional could reproduce the activity and achieve similar results. An example of an overly limiting goal is "When reading the story *The Three Bears,* John will . . ." This goal limits the therapeutic activities and does not promote generalizability.

SELECTING A GOAL ATTACK STRATEGY

A **goal attack strategy** refers to the way in which multiple goals are approached or scheduled within an intervention session (Cirrin & Gillam, 2008). Three strategies have been identified: (a) a **vertical goal attack strategy** in which one goal at a time is targeted until a predetermined level of accuracy is achieved, (b) a **horizontal goal attack strategy** in which several goals are targeted within every session, and (c) a **cyclic goal attack strategy** in which several goals are targeted with a repeating sequence, each for a specified time period independent of accuracy (Cirrin & Gillam, 2008; Fey, 1986; Tyler et al., 2003).

Each goal structuring method has advantages and disadvantages. Vertical structuring allows a practitioner to work on one goal at a time and a child to achieve a high response rate for a single target in each session. The one-goal strategy may help the child focus attention on the targeted skill. However, vertical structuring may lead to a repetitious and potentially boring intervention.

In a horizontal structure, the practitioner presents two or more goals in the same intervention session. The goals may target related behaviors (e.g., use of the *be* verb as a copula ["The boy is a baseball player"] with a *be* verb as an auxiliary ["The boy is throwing the ball"] or unrelated behaviors (e.g., a goal targeting syntax and a goal targeting semantics). New goals are added as the child reaches predetermined criteria on each goal. The amount of time to reach criteria will vary from goal to goal. One advantage of horizontal structuring is that the intervention session is not too repetitive, and the child is less likely to be bored.

Another advantage of a horizontal strategy is that as a primary goal is achieved in a structured intervention context, the adult can relegate a primary goal to secondary status. The interventionist regularly monitors a student's use of secondary goals during natural, spontaneous speech. In this way, newly learned communication behaviors are generalized to everyday interactions. A disadvantage of horizontal structuring is that presenting multiple intervention targets may cause confusion for children who are easily distracted or more severely impaired.

In a cyclic goal attack strategy, an interventionist moves through a series of targeted goals using a predetermined schedule. For example, in the cyclic approach, Goal 1 is introduced during Week 1 and Goal 2 during Week 2. The interventionist then cycles back to Goal 1 in Week 3 and Goal 2 during Week 4. The cyclic approach has features of both vertical and horizontal attack strategies. When implementing the cyclic attack strategy, a practitioner introduces a different goal each week and then moves from one goal to the next, regardless of the child's progress, or lack of progress, on a particular goal (Williams, 2000). Over time, as the cycle is repeated, the child develops increased competency on individual goals.

Consider the following example of an intervention program that uses the cyclic approach. The interventionist develops three goals for Macauley, a student who has deficits in three areas: (1) third-person verb errors (e.g., "He *walk* to school," "She *drive* the car"); (2) limited use of conjunctions, such as *so* and *but* (e.g., "*The man wants a new car, but he doesn't have enough money*"); and (3) poor comprehension of *why* questions. The interventionist writes a goal for each of the targets:

1. Macauley will produce third-person regular verbs with 70% accuracy in focused stimulation activities in which third-person verbs are contrasted with regular present progressive verbs (e.g., "What is the girl doing? She is walking her dog. What does she like to do? She *likes* to walk her dog? *Does* she do it every day? Yes, she *walks* her dog every day."

2. Macauley will produce four to six sentences using coordinating conjunctions during a retelling of a familiar fairy tale, with access to a written list of coordinating conjunctions.

3. Macauley will produce three different *why* questions and answer at least three different *why* questions during a shared book reading interaction using a first-grade-level book.

The three goals are targeted on a rotating basis, and the interventionist records the child's accuracy for each session. If a child reaches the criteria for a goal, a new goal is brought into the cycle, or the goal is modified to elicit more independent and complex productions. Goals for which the child does not reach criteria continue to be targeted in the cycle. The child learns some skills in a period of a few weeks, but other skills take longer. The cyclic approach has been shown to be effective in teaching morphosyntax skills to preschoolers (Tyler et al., 2003) and in teaching phonological skills (Williams, 2000). A rationale for the cyclic approach is that goal mastery is developmental, and children require varying levels of exposure to meet criteria (i.e., some targets may be acquired with little stimulation, while others take more time). The disadvantage is that generally professionals need more skill and experience to organize and maintain a cyclic intervention schedule.

KEEPING DATA DURING INTERVENTION

An important outcome of EBP is the recognition that all intervention must be evidence based, and there must always be data documenting changes in communication. Although the complex nature of communication means documentation takes organization and planning, it is possible. I tell beginning clinicians, "Don't limit your intervention by choosing goal behaviors that are easy to document; instead, decide what the child needs to practice or learn, and then figure out a way to document change of the needed skill." With that caution in mind, I present strategies for keeping data across the continuum of naturalness: (a) data collection during structured activities (e.g., drill, drill play) and (b) data collection during naturalistic activities. In all cases, the goal of data collection is to track the client's behavior from one session to another, document the efficacy of the intervention, and maximize the professional's effectiveness (Roth & Paul, 2007).

Data Collection during Structured Activities. Data collection in drill and drill-play activities is typically straightforward because the behaviors are adult directed and highly controlled. The interventionist documents the type of child response (e.g., signed, gestured, verbal) and the degree or type of practitioner prompting. Typically, the practitioner compares a child's behaviors before, during, and after intervention. Sometimes a graph is used to document change; a **graph** is a visual representation of the occurrence of a behavior over time. The data obtained prior to intervention is called the **baseline**. In the graph shown in Figure 5.5, the baseline of the child's productions of two-word combinations prior to intervention is documented on the first section of the graph on the *x*-axis (i.e., horizontal axis); the *x*-axis represents the session occurrence (i.e., Session 1, Session 2). The frequency of the child's spontaneous production of two-word combinations is represented by the *y*-axis (i.e., the vertical axis). During the intervention, the practitioner uses strong modeling techniques. The child's increasing production of two-word utterances is shown as higher data points on the *y*-axis.

As shown in Figure 5.5, the interventionist also documents the child's use of two-word phrases in a generalization probe. In the **generalization probe**, the practitioner does not use the strong modeling used during the intervention phase but rather interacts in a typical back-and-forth interaction and documents the child's use of two-word phrases under more natural circumstances. In this case, the child demonstrates continued two-word productions, indicating that he has generalized the behavior following the intervention phase.

As an alternative to graphing the results, sometimes an interventionist counts the occurrences of a behavior and represents them as a percentage. For example, at the baseline phase, a professional might report, "Donald spontaneously produced 2% two-word

Figure 5.5 **Graph of Intervention Data**

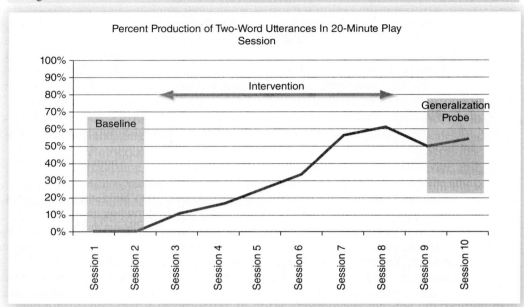

utterances in a baseline probe during a 5-minute drill-play activity." At the intervention and follow-up phases, the professional documents changes in Donald's production levels with percentages. In order to compute a percentage, the practitioner counts all of Donald's verbal productions (one- and two-word productions) and then divides the number of two-word productions by the total number of utterances. Here is an example:

$$\frac{10 \text{ two-word productions}}{30 \text{ one-word and two-word productions}} = 10/30 = 33.3\% \text{ two-word productions}$$

Practitioners often develop simple data sheets to record children's productions as they occur during an intervention session. An example of a recording sheet is provided in Figure 5.6.

Data Collection in Naturalistic Activities. To collect data during naturalistic conditions, an interventionist can videotape interactions. Videotaping allows a practitioner to review an interaction and count behaviors or code the quality of a communication behavior. Alternatively, a practitioner may conduct direct observations. If, for example, a student's communication goal is to increase assertive communication acts, the practitioner may observe the first 10 minutes of the school day and document the student's use of topic initiations and social greetings in the classroom. Sometimes parents and teachers assist in collecting behavioral observations; they provide a summary of the number of times (or the duration of a behavior) the behavior occurred over a class period or conversation. Rubrics are used to evaluate the qualitative nature of behaviors in naturalistic settings. One example is goal attainment scaling a sophisticated use of a rubric. **Goal attainment scaling (GAS)** is an individualized, criterion-referenced approach (Roach &

Figure 5.6 **Data Recording Sheet**

Student			Objectives:		
1.					
2.					
3.					
4.					

Date	Attendance		Objective/Methods/Materials	Notes
	1			
	2			
	3			
	4			
Data Collection				
	1			
	2			
	3			
	4			
Data Collection				

Elliott, 2005). GAS allows a practitioner to document a student's baseline performance and numerically record behavioral changes. Steps in developing GAS include (1) selecting a target behavior, (2) describing the desired behavior or academic outcome in objective terms, and (3) developing three to five descriptions of the probable outcomes from least desirable to most desirable. By using numerical ratings for descriptive levels of functioning, a practitioner documents student progress (Roach & Elliot, 2005).

To complete GAS, a practitioner includes a descriptive word or percentages indicating variation in the child's performance level, ranging in level from −2 to +2. For example, "Johanna never produces possessive pronouns correctly during a grade-level writing activity" is an example of a −2-level goal. In contrast, the goal "Johanna always uses possessive pronouns correctly in a grade-level writing task" is a +2-level goal. Zero on GAS indicates that the student's behavior is unchanged. In other words, zero reflects the student's baseline behavior.

Examples of descriptive vocabulary capturing the −2 to +2 variation include:

- *Frequency* (never—sometimes—very often—almost always—always)
- *Quality* (poor—fair—good—excellent)

- *Development* (not present—emerging—developing—accomplished—exceeding)
- *Usage* (unused—inappropriate use—appropriate use—exceptional use)
- *Timeliness* (late—on time—early)
- *Percentage complete* (0%—25%—50%—75%—100%)
- *Accuracy* (totally incorrect—partially correct—totally correct)
- *Effort* (not attempted—minimal effort—acceptable effort—outstanding effort)
- *Amount of support needed* (totally dependent—extensive assistance—some assistance—limited assistance—independent)
- *Engagement* (none—limited—acceptable—exceptional)

Figure 5.7 documents a student's goal attainment scores over time. In this example, Brittany's initial production of past tense verbs in her written work was 25%. Interventions included one-on-one conversations discussing real-life events and using past tense verbs (teacher uses a nonverbal signal to indicate past tense verb production), guided practice to help Brittany write sentences using past tense verbs, posting of a word list of regular and irregular past tense verbs near Brittany's desk, frequent checks of Brittany's independent work, and monitoring of daily written assignments for past tense verb use. The target (+2) was written as "Brittany uses past tense verbs correctly 70% of the time when writing about a past event in a written assignment of at least 20 sentences." The teacher documented Brittany's use of past tense verbs for approximately 6 weeks. Examination of the GAS ratings demonstrated improvements on the target behavior on 60% of the assessment dates. The practitioner observed that Brittany's conversational use of past tense verbs also improved.

Figure 5.7 Goal Attainment Scaling

Objective: Brittany correctly produces past tense verbs.

+2: Brittany uses past tense verbs correctly 70% of the time when writing about a past event in a written assignment of at least 20 sentences.

+1: Brittany uses past tense verbs correctly 31–69% of the time when writing about a past event in a written assignment of at least 20 sentences.

0: Brittany uses past tense verbs correctly 20–30% of the time when writing about a past event in a written assignment of at least 20 sentences.

−1: Brittany uses past tense verbs correctly 11–19% of the time when writing about a past event in a written assignment of at least 20 sentences.

−2: Brittany uses past tense verbs correctly less than 11% of the time when writing about a past event in a written assignment of at least 20 sentences.

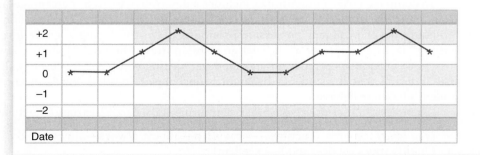

Implementing Effective Interventions

The first part of this chapter discussed intervention techniques in relation to the *why* of intervention decision making, as in *Why am I choosing a particular language facilitation technique or approach?* This second part describes concepts and principles to answer *how*, as in *How do I implement intervention to most effectively impact an individual's communication skills?* You should note that in this section I pull strategies from different theoretical approaches in an eclectic fashion. My goal is to link intervention back to the domains of form, content, and use presented in Chapters 1 and 2.

Thinking about form, content, and use prior to developing an intervention program helps a professional decide which aspects of communication should be targeted. Interventionists use different language intervention strategies, depending on an individual's impairment within pragmatic, semantic, or morphosyntax domains. Basing a student's intervention on his or her abilities in form, content, and use is preferred to designing an intervention based on a child's diagnosis.

EFFECTIVE INTERVENTION: PRAGMATICS DOMAIN

Interventions focusing on pragmatics often are used with individuals who are at an early developing level of communication functioning. Early developing pragmatics skills include turn taking, requesting, and responding to others' communication attempts (see Chapter 2; Subdomain 1). For children who have impairments across multiple domains (i.e., difficulties with pragmatics, semantics, and morphosyntax), family members typically identify the pragmatic impairment as the highest priority.

Communication includes learning to enter into the interactions of others. For children with significant pragmatic difficulties, the practitioner focuses on facilitating a child's turn-taking abilities, encouraging the child to initiate interactions, and increasing the amount of time the child stays in interactions with others. Practitioners use facilitative techniques during their interactions with young children and also train parents to use the techniques at home (Kaiser & Hancock, 2003). Techniques include the following:

- *Be responsive* to child verbal behaviors. Meaningful, related responses encourage child communication.
- *Give a limited number of instructions.* Giving instructions only for important behaviors increases a child's compliance and increases the child's communication.
- Create a *balanced interaction*. Encourage child-initiated utterances, and limit utterances so that the child has time to contribute to the conversation. Wait for the child to take a conversational turn, and then indicate nonverbally and with eye contact that you expect the child to communicate.
- *Expand and extend* the child's utterances; keep language modeling related to the ongoing activity.
- *Follow the child's lead in the interaction.* Watch what the child is interested in doing, and make his or her actions and comments the focus of the conversation. The idea is to be a language responder rather than a leader, teacher, or questioner (Weitzman & Greenberg, 2002).
- *Make the interaction positive.* Praise the child often; limit the number of negative responses or comments. Children's language is enhanced when they interact with positive and warm caretakers who are responsive to their needs and interests (Chapman, 2000).

EFFECTIVE INTERVENTION: MORPHOLOGY AND SYNTAX DOMAINS

Once a child demonstrates social engagement (Communication Subdomain 1), having assimilated concepts and vocabulary associated with everyday activities (Communication Subdomain 2), and begins to regularly produce word combinations demonstrating simple sentence structure (Communication Subdomain 3), it is appropriate to begin interventions focusing on the morphosyntax concepts associated with Communication Subdomain 4. Interventionists target morphosyntax skills using the developmental sequence of children developing typically. Four morphosyntax intervention strategies are highlighted: (a) establishing discourse contexts to elicit specific morphosyntax targets, (b) increasing the "detectability" of targeted morphosyntax features, (c) identifying errors and absent grammatical features, and (d) choosing intermediate language targets.

The first strategy underscores the need to establish an appropriate discourse context to elicit specific morphosyntax features. For example, the third-person singular verb form (verb + s) is used in simple present only in state verbs such as *knows, goes, needs, wants, loves,* or *uses.* **State verbs** describe a person's state of being in contrast to describing an action. The use of third person with state verbs does *not* imply that the condition (or state of being) has lasted over a long period of time. For example, I can say, "She needs a glass of water." This statement does not indicate that she has needed water for a long period of time but rather that she needs water at this moment.

In contrast, when third person is used with action verbs (*drives, cooks, watches*), it is implied that the action occurs every day or over a long period of time. So, for example, if I see a girl studying in the library, I say, "She is studying." If I know she goes to the library regularly, I say, "She studies at the library." In the latter case, with the action verb *studying,* I changed the verb to third-person regular (i.e., *studies*) to indicate that the action happens regularly.

Skilled practitioners are careful to set up discourse contexts that require the targeted form when establishing a morphosyntax intervention. In the above example, the adult must create an appropriate context to elicit a third-person action verb by demonstrating that the action occurs frequently or consistently (Oetting & Hadley, 2009). For example, the child and adult could create a play routine with a toy school bus and comment, "The boy rides to school every day." Conversely, the adult avoids asking the child to use a third-person verb in an inappropriate discourse context.

A second strategy underscores the need to make targeted morphosyntax features easily detectable. Children are more likely to attend to new morphosyntax features if they are embedded within sentences containing familiar vocabulary and include familiar tasks (i.e., functions).

Accordingly, if an interventionist is teaching present progressive verb use *is + ing,* the form is first embedded into a sentence with simple vocabulary (e.g., "The girl is riding a bike."). The interventionist realizes that complexity is increased with unfamiliar vocabulary (e.g., "The veterinarian is examining the dog.").

Similarly, interventionists teach new forms within familiar functions (Slobin, 1973). For example, children learn to produce statements (e.g., "That is Mother's purse.") before question forms ("Is that Mother's purse?"). Consequently, teaching the possessive morpheme ('s) is facilitated when it is produced in a statement rather than a question. Skilled practitioners realize that form, content, and use are interconnected. At the initial stage of learning, when form (i.e., morphosyntax) is the intervention target, content and use should be familiar. Learn more about the relationship between form, content, and use in Focus 5.3.

FOCUS 5.3   *Learning More*

In this chapter, I have stated that when form is the intervention target, content and use should be familiar at initial learning stages. This statement was first expressed by Slobin (1973) in his adage, "New forms first express old functions and new functions are first expressed by old forms" (p. 184). In other words, children first learn new behavior (i.e., form, content) in a familiar context (i.e., function) and vice versa. So, for example, when children are learning to request an action, they are likely to use familiar words. They are unlikely to use new words (i.e., content) or new form (i.e., syntax) while practicing a new function.

For example, Mary (age 21 months), says, "Hold you!" which means "Pick me up now!" She has heard her parents ask the familiar question "Do you want me to hold you?" so she uses part of the familiar form and content to produce a new function (Sara Jones, personal communication, January 23, 2009).

A skilled professional considers Slobin's adage when developing an intervention program. If the goal is to have a child learn new words (i.e., content), ask him or her to produce new vocabulary within a familiar pragmatic task. Keep the syntax simple by embedding new vocabulary in simple sentences instead of complex sentences.

The interventionist should modify the pragmatic and syntax demands as the child's new vocabulary is established. Alternatively, if the goal of intervention is to teach new syntax, the inteventionist initially minimizes the pragmatic and semantic demands of the task.

The third strategy suggests that interventionists must note the absence of particular morphosyntax forms, in addition to noting error patterns. I have observed that beginning students readily identify some morphosyntax deficits but have difficulty identifying other error patterns. For example, even beginning students cringe (along with the child's parents and teachers) when they hear "Her do it" or "Me go outside now?" Beginning students clearly identify the pronoun errors—in this example, the child's substitution of possessive or object pronouns (*her* = possessive pronoun, *me* = object pronoun) for subject pronouns (e.g., *she, he, I*).

However, in addition to making pronoun errors, the child is failing to produce an important morphosyntax feature. Morphosyntax deficits also include the lack of grammatical features. Take a look at the example above, ignore the pronoun errors, and identify something the child is not producing. Did you notice that the child is lacking auxiliary verbs? In both cases, the child omits the use of an auxiliary verb: "Her *can* do it" and "*Can* me go outside now?" The verb *can* is a form of auxiliary verb called a modal verb (e.g., *can, do, will*). Children with language impairments frequently have difficulty with auxiliary verb forms; they exhibit difficulty with modal verbs as well as auxiliary *be* verbs (e.g., *is, was, are*). Auxiliary verb deletion should be a focus of intervention because complex sentence construction requires auxiliary verb production (Justice, 2002). As a result, a skilled interventionist targets auxiliary verbs in addition to—or before—pronoun errors. The interventionist notes grammatical features that are *not* used, in addition to noting morphosyntax features used incorrectly.

The fourth strategy underscores the need to choose intermediate vs. beginning-level morphosyntax targets. An **intermediate-level intervention goal** is a goal that highlights grammatical categories, operations, or processes (Swanson et al., 2005). For example, an intermediate pronoun intervention context for a child with subject pronoun errors potentially contrasts the use of subject pronouns with possessive pronouns: "This is *her* book. *She* is reading. Is *she* reading? *She* is reading *her* book!" The contrastive use of the subject and possessive pronouns is an intermediate target highlighting the relationship of pronouns to underlying sentence structure.

In the previous example, along with intermediate pronoun intervention targets, the adult also demonstrated two different intermediate verb targets. First, the adult contrasted auxiliary verbs in both the statement form and interrogative form. The statement form was produced as "She is reading," and the interrogative form was produced as "Is she reading?" Second, the adult contrasted two forms of the *be* verb—the copular *be* verb ("This *is* her book") and the auxiliary *be* verb ("She *is* reading"). Contrasting verb forms is an intermediate goal as it highlights underlying verb-related operations. Note that in the example above, I included both pronoun and two different verb form contrasts to demonstrate different intermediate-level morphosyntax goals. In actual practice, a practitioner carefully considers a child's ability level and typically focuses on only one structural contrast at a time. Practitioners often focus on early verb learning for children with language impairments; learn more about this in Focus 5.4.

FOCUS 5.4   *Learning More*

Why do children with language impairments have difficulty learning verbs?

- Verb use is connected to the subject and object of a sentence. This syntactic relationship impacts verb argument; *verb argument* refers to a phrase that appears in a syntactic relationship with the verb in a clause. In English, the two most important arguments are the subject and the direct object. The properties of verb argument result in verbs carrying more syntactic information than nouns.
- Correct verb use demands noun–verb agreement; there must be agreement in person. For example, I say "She *walks*," but I change the verb with a plural noun, "They *walk*." I can say, "I *am* a girl" but must change the copula verb with a third-person singular pronoun, as in "She *is* a girl." The speaker must change the verb in relation to the subject; this makes verb learning complex.
- Verbs also require varying relationships with direct objects. Consider the verbs *smile* vs. *move*. *Move* is a transitive verb,

meaning that it requires a direct object (e.g., "John moves the car"). *Smile*, in contrast, is an intransitive verb; it does not require a direct object (e.g., "John smiles"). Other verbs require a noun phrase + prepositional phrase sequence or a noun phrase + noun phrase sequence in the direct object position. The verb *give* is an example of such a verb. I can say, "I give the present to the boy" or "I give the boy a present." The speaker must know if a verb is transitive or intransitive; this also makes verb learning complex.

- Children must process a lot of information to use verbs effectively. Research indicates that children with language impairment use fewer argument types in spontaneous speech than children developing typically.

Source: Based on information from "Verb Argument Structure Weakness in Specific Language Impairment in Relation to Age and Utterance Length" by E. T. Thordardottir and S. E. Weismer, 2002, *Clinical Linguistics and Phonetics, 16*, pp. 233–250.

A practitioner chooses intermediate goals to foster systemwide change. An intermediate goal highlights the processes or operations behind a morphosyntax form and increases generalization. To further enhance generalization, a practitioner also embeds intervention targets into meaningful social contexts and includes multiple modalities (i.e., oral, writing, reading).

EFFECTIVE INTERVENTION: SEMANTIC DOMAIN

Semantic deficits are an early sign of language impairment; young children with LI are typically delayed in their rate and quantity of word learning. Semantic deficits continue to limit academic performance in older students with LI (McGregor, 2009). As a consequence, practitioners target semantic skills (Communication Subdomains 2 and 3; see Chapter 2) for many children with language impairments.

When selecting semantic goals for young children, interventionists consider semantic transparency. **Semantic transparency** refers to words or phrases in which meaning is easily observed or intuited. For example, the verb *pour* (said as "one *pours* water into a glass") is semantically transparent, while the word *know* (e.g., "I *know* I want water") is less transparent. Children learn vocabulary more easily when the referent is connected to the label provided by the adult. In semantic interventions, a practitioner chooses words and manipulates the context to increase semantic transparency.

In order to learn new words, children with language impairments need more frequent exposure than children developing typically (Gray, 2004). To provide increased exposure to word meaning, a practitioner provides (a) repeated models of the new word within a play context, (b) prompts the child to produce the word, and (c) provides feedback on word accuracy. Adding semantic and phonological cues appears to enhance word learning for children with language impairments (Gray, 2005). Semantic cues include describing the physical characteristics, providing item function, and providing the word category (e.g., "This is a muffler; it is something you wear; it's clothing.") Phonological cues include emphasizing the initial sound or first syllable, clapping out syllables in the word, or providing a rhyming word (e.g., "The word is wheat; it sounds like your brother's name, Pete!").

At older ages, the practitioner works to increase the breadth (i.e., number of new words) and depth (i.e., nuanced vocabulary to express familiar concepts) in a student's semantic lexicon. McGregor (2009) indicates that the practitioner should work on:

- Idiomatic phrases (e.g., "What does *flipping her lid* mean?").
- More subtle vocabulary (e.g., *morose, depressed,* or *glum*) to replace a familiar word (e.g., *sad*).
- Alternative meanings to a familiar word (e.g., "At night we can say it is dark. What do I mean when I say 'He has a dark personality'?").
- Compound word construction (e.g., "When we make a compound word, the describing word [i.e., adjective] goes first. We say *blue + berry*, not *berry + blue*, and *mail + box*, not *box + mail*."
- Prefixes (*readmit, bidirectional, autopilot, disappear*) and suffixes (*transition, presentable, nutritious*). **Prefixes** and **suffixes** are groups of letters attached to the beginning (prefix) or end (suffix) of a word to form a new word; prefixes and suffixes sometimes change the grammatical function of the original word. (Learn more about prefixes and suffixes in Focus 5.5.)

FOCUS 5.5 *Learning More*

Prefixes and Suffixes

- Teaching students to find a base word along with a suffix and prefix is considered an intermediate-to-advanced word study strategy generally appropriate for children in third to fourth grades (Bear et al., 2007). Word study should relate to words children use while reading and writing.

- During word study, children learn to complete the following sequence when they come to an unfamiliar word while reading: (1) Take off the prefix; (2) take off the suffix; (3) look at the base word to determine whether it is familiar; (4) reassemble the word and make a hypothesis about word meaning; (5) try the hypothesized meaning in the sentence; (6) if the sentence does not make sense, look up the word in the dictionary; (7) record the word in a word study notebook.

- Suffixes and prefixes are learned in a developmental sequence.

- Early suffix skills include identification of plural endings (*s* and *es*), suffixes related to size (*er, est*), compound words (*snowman, pancake*), and spelling rules such as changing the final *y* to *i* and adding *ed* or *s* (*cry–cries*). Simple prefixes include *un-, re-, sub-,* and *in-*.

- Middle-level affixes include advanced rules that govern spelling, such as producing plurals by changing *y* to *i* (*babies* vs. *toys*). Other middle-level suffixes include -*such, -ship, -ity, -ment,* and -*ic.* Middle-level prefixes include *dis-, mis-, pre-, pro-,* and *con-*.

- Late-developing word study focuses on teaching students to recognize common roots in English such as *port* (to carry; *portable, transport*), *duct* (to lead; *conduct, tear duct*), *spec* (to look at; *spectator, spectacles, inspect*).

In addition to the suggestions above, Beck and her colleagues (Beck, McKeown, & Kucan, 2002) provide a helpful perspective for vocabulary intervention. They suggest that a well-developed vocabulary consists of three tiers. Tier 1 words consist of basic vocabulary used on a daily basis (e.g., *climb, sofa, man, close*). Tier 1 words rarely require instructional attention for most school-age students.

Tier 2 words are used across domains by skilled speakers, writers, and readers. Tier 2 words occur within academic settings and in books but are difficult for students to learn in daily interactions. Consequently, Tier 2 words should be the focus of vocabulary intervention. Examples of Tier 2 words include *merchant, required, tend, maintain, identified, fortunate,* and *unscrupulous* (Beck et al., 2002).

In contrast, Tier 3 words are words related to a specific domain (e.g., science [*acceleration, hibernation*], occupation [*lathe, stethoscope*], social studies [*peninsula, lava*]). Beck argues that domain-specific words are used infrequently and are most appropriately learned when a specific need arises—such as when a learning unit is introduced in class.

A practitioner decides which words to target for vocabulary instruction by determining whether a student has old, familiar words to describe a new Tier 2 word. So, for example, if the student knows the word *dishonest* or *cheating*, the practitioner may choose to teach the Tier 2 word *unscrupulous*. A strategy to enhance a student's vocabulary knowledge is described in Focus 5.6.

FOCUS 5.6   *Clinical Skill Building*

There are four guiding principles for vocabulary instruction. Effective instruction should help students (1) relate new vocabulary to background knowledge, (2) develop elaborated word knowledge, (3) become active participants in learning new words, and (4) develop strategies for learning new vocabulary (Nelson & Van Meter, 2007). Keep the following ideas in mind when thinking about high-quality vocabulary instruction.

- A method called *robust vocabulary instruction* has been evaluated in research studies; it is an effective approach to helping students learn the meanings of words and improve reading comprehension (Beck & McKeown, 2007). With robust vocabulary instruction, students learn how a novel word is similar to and different from related concepts and how the word is used in a variety of situations. Storybook reading is an effective context for robust vocabulary instruction. A language facilitator uses a storybook interaction to introduce new vocabulary, provide a child-friendly definition of a word, give an example of the word in a different sentence, and provide follow-up activities in which children choose between words, relate words to known concepts, and ask questions using the new words.
- Robust vocabulary instruction is effective with low-income and middle-class European American children but also is an effective and culturally sensitive strategy for improving vocabulary in African American students. Storybooks with cultural themes are used to connect the vocabulary to children's lives (Lovelace & Stewart, 2009).

Summary

- Speech-language pathologists (SLPs) and educators consider a variety of issues with regard to intervention stimuli. Stimuli can either be nonlinguistic or linguistic and can be presented via pictures, objects, or computers. Prompts, shaping, and fading techniques are used in conjunction with stimuli to provide varying levels of support. Reinforcement can be primary (i.e., food) or social; reinforcement schedules are varied based on the child's needs and the behaviors being trained.
- Language facilitators use modeling techniques that are contingent on child interests and behaviors to facilitate children's language production. *Self-talk* is language in which the adult describes what he is thinking, feeling, or seeing. In contrast, an adult uses *parallel talk* to describe a child's actions. Both self-talk and parallel talk facilitate child language output. Once a child produces a phrase or sentence, the adult uses *expansions* and *extensions* to modify the child's simple sentences into more sophisticated sentence constructions and to add related information. When using *sentence recasts*, the adult changes the sentence modality to highlight specific linguistic features. In *focused stimulation*, a child is exposed to multiple examples of a linguistic target within a meaningful communication context. Modeling techniques are based on social interactionist theory. Social interactionist theory maintains that children benefit from the support of a more skilled language user; with repeated supported exposure, children internalize underlying concepts and become independent language producers.

- The *assertiveness–responsiveness scheme* helps an interventionist profile an individual's ability to initiate conversational turns and respond to others' communication attempts. An effective communicator is both assertive and responsive. A practitioner uses the scheme to determine whether a child has the needed skills to be an effective communicator. The *continuum of naturalness* describes the activities, location, and social aspects of intervention. A practitioner considers these variables when developing an intervention program. Intervention varies from highly unnatural (e.g., adult directed, drill activities) to highly natural (e.g., child directed, in the child's home or classroom, with the child's family or peers). The practitioner chooses between natural and unnatural variables, depending on the intervention goal and the child's abilities.

- A goal is made up of three components: the *do* statement, the *condition* statement, and the *criterion* statement. The *do* statement describes the behaviors the child will produce. The *condition* statement describes the situation or conditions under which the behavior will occur; the *criterion* statement reflects how the goal will be measured.

- Data collection can be either qualitative or quantitative. Qualitative measures include rubrics, goal attainment scaling, and rating naturalistic interactions. Quantitative data are often computed with percentages or represented on graphs.

- Practitioners make intervention decisions based on a child's abilities with regard to form, content, and use. If a child has errors in form, the professional uses strategies to make certain the discourse facilitates the child's production of the required form, makes certain that targeted features are easily detected, notes a child's errors and absence of linguistic features, and chooses intermediate-level targets. Intervention related to content focuses on highlighting the semantic transparency of vocabulary and choosing Tier 2–level vocabulary with older children. Pragmatic intervention focuses on a child's ability to take conversational turns and initiate conversation. Pragmatic intervention with young children often includes parent training; parents learn to facilitate optimal parent–child conversations.

Discussion and In-Class Activities

1. In a small group, role-play intervention sessions for a 4-year-old child with (a) a pragmatic deficit, (b) a semantic deficit, and (c) a morphosyntax deficit. In each case, demonstrate the use of a variety of stimuli (i.e., pictures, objects, computers), reinforcements (i.e., primary, secondary), and prompts. Evaluate the different techniques and discuss the strengths and weaknesses of the demonstrated approaches.

2. Your instructor will show you videotapes of language intervention. After watching the session, identify the intervention goal, the prompts used by the adult, and the adult's evaluation of the child's responses. Discuss whether you believe this was a successful session. Why do you think it was or was not successful? What could have been changed to make the session more effective? As a second activity, develop a strategy for recording the child's behaviors. Watch the session a second time and record and evaluate the child's responses. Did everyone in the class evaluate the child's behaviors in the same way? How could the data collection procedure be modified to increase the reliability of the scoring method?

3. Brainstorm Tier 2 vocabulary that could be introduced to (a) a first-grader who needs to use more interesting verbs, (b) a third-grader who writes only sentences with Tier 1 vocabulary (e.g., "The boy walks to his house"), or (c) a fifth-grader who is writing a report on Native Americans. Use a thesaurus or the Internet to develop a word list.

4. Write intervention goals for (a) a 3-year-old child, (b) a 6-year-old child, and (c) a 12-year-old child. Make sure each goal contains a *do* statement, a *condition* statement, and a *criterion* statement. Indicate whether each goal is focused on form, content, or use. Describe where the goal would be placed on the continuum of naturalness.

Chapter 5 Case Study

You are an SLP in a community speech-language-hearing clinic. Your department supervisor assigns two new children to your caseload. You review their files: The first child, Cole, is 2 years, 6 months old; the second child, Maria, is 5.

Cole has no known developmental delays other than his language delay. His hearing is normal, and his physical development is within normal limits. He appears to understand most of what is said to him but uses only a few words spontaneously (i.e., *pizza, no*). During communication interactions, he responds to what others say with physical actions and some word imitations, but he rarely initiates communication. Cole's parents are anxious to work with their son at home and want to be involved in the intervention program.

Maria is in kindergarten and is learning to read but is at the low end of academic performance compared to other children her age. She is a personable child and makes friends easily. She produces a variety of grammar errors in her spoken language. Most noticeable is her incorrect use of prepositions (e.g., *on, under, in*) and her lack of possessive forms ("Mother dress" instead of "Mother's dress").

Questions for Discussion

1. Does Cole's primary language deficit represent form, content, or use? Does Maria's primary language deficit represent form, content, or use?

2. How would you describe (a) Cole's and (b) Maria's communication patterns using Fey's assertiveness–responsiveness scheme? How would you use this information to frame your overall intervention plans?

3. Using the continuum of naturalness, (a) what kind of intervention will be most appropriate for Cole, and (b) what kind of intervention will be most appropriate for Maria (i.e., child directed, hybrid, adult directed)? Provide a rationale for each of your answers.

4. What kinds of suggestions will you give (a) Cole's parents and (b) Maria's parents? Role-play the session in which you explain the language techniques you would like the families to use.

5. Your department supervisor asks you to provide a rationale for your intervention plans for Cole and Maria. Explain your rationale for (a) Cole's intervention and (b) Maria's intervention; use one or more language theories (e.g., behaviorism, social interactionist, cognitive theory) to support your intervention programs. Write language goals for the two students. How will you document change in their intervention programs?

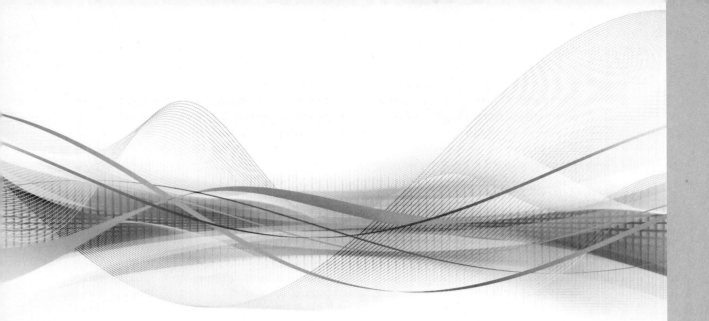

6 Children with Specific Language Impairment

Chapter Overview Questions

1. What criteria are used to diagnose a child with specific language impairment (SLI)? How does SLI differ from the term *late language emergence*?

2. What are the primary language deficits of children with SLI? Give examples.

3. What are some intervention approaches used as part of social communication intervention?

4. How does language theory guide assessment? Explain two assessment protocols and describe their theoretical framework.

5. Describe three different intervention approaches appropriate for children with SLI. How do the interventions differ in theoretical stance and approach?

In this chapter, I present information about children who have **specific language impairment (SLI)**. One of the most common reasons children are referred to a speech-language pathologist (SLP) is delayed expressive language development (Rescorla & Lee, 2000). Children with SLI have a language deficit, but without accompanying factors such as hearing loss, low intelligence scores, or neurological damage. While most children appear to learn language effortlessly, children with SLI struggle to become effective language users.

This chapter is an important component of your clinical training. Many children—those with SLI and those with other diagnoses—have significant difficulties with syntax and morphological skills, as well as associated deficits in semantics and pragmatics. The information in this chapter will be widely applicable to your future clinical work.

Definition, Prevalence, Causation, and Major Characteristics

DEFINITION

SLI is a diagnosis based on **exclusionary criteria**. This means that other possible causes of language impairment must be eliminated as possible reasons for a child's language delay. The exclusionary characteristics of SLI include (a) a language test score −1.25 standard deviations or lower (corresponding to a standard score of 81 or lower on a test with a mean of 100); (b) nonverbal IQ of 85 or higher, indicating that intellectual function is within normal limits; (c) normal hearing, as determined by a hearing screening; (d) no oral structural or oral motor abnormalities; (e) no evidence of neurological disorder; and (f) within-normal social ability (i.e., the child is not on the autism spectrum). As you can see, many possible deficits must be excluded before a child is diagnosed as having SLI.

The terminology related to language impairment can be confusing because practitioners use a variety of terms to describe this population of children; in addition to *SLI*, the terms used include *language delay, language disorder* (as in the DSM-5 description below), *developmental language disorder,* and *language-learning disability* (*LLD*). The term *LLD* typically is used to refer to school-age students with a primary language impairment and associated literacy deficits (i.e., dyslexia and poor reading comprehension; Paul & Norbury, 2012). Further, it is a clinical dilemma that some children do not meet all the criteria for SLI but also do not fit into any other diagnostic category. Approximately 15% of children who are clinically considered to have SLI do not meet all the SLI criteria (Tomblin, 1996).

The **Diagnostic and Statistical Manual of Mental Disorders, Fifth Edition** (DSM-5; American Psychiatric Association, 2013) is the published set of standards used for developmental and psychiatric medical diagnosis in the United States. The DSM-5 uses the term *language disorder* to classify children with receptive, expressive, or mixed receptive-expressive language disorders. The DSM-5 diagnostic criteria for *language disorder* include persistent difficulties in the acquisition and use of language across modalities (i.e., spoken, written, sign language) due to deficits in comprehension or production. To qualify for the DSM-5 diagnosis of language disorder, an individual's language abilities must be substantially and quantifiably below age expectations. Read about the DSM-5 position regarding language dialects in Focus 6.1.

In addition to the diagnostic category language disorder, DSM-5 also has a category called *social (pragmatic) communication disorder*. This category is used to classify individuals who demonstrate significant pragmatic language deficits but not the repetitive or restrictive behaviors associated with autism spectrum disorders. You will be learning more about social (pragmatic) communication disorders in Chapter 9. Both DSM-5 categories language disorder and social (pragmatic) communication disorder may be applicable to children with SLI.

Some literature refers to a young child under age 5 with a language delay as evidencing **late language emergence (LLE)**. LLE is sometimes called **delayed language development,**

FOCUS 6.1   *Multicultural Issues*

DSM-5 indicates that regional, social, or cultural/ethnic variations of speech should be considered before making a diagnosis of language disorder. DSM-5 also states that standardized measures must be relevant for the individual's cultural and linguistic experience. This language conforms with ASHA's recommendation that neither regional, social, cultural, nor linguistic language variation (e.g., dialect) should be considered a language disorder.

or the child is referred to as a **late talker**. LLE is diagnosed when language development is below age expectations (e.g., less than 50 words at 24 months, inability to follow verbal instructions, limited use of gestures and sounds to communicate, limited symbolic play, and few word combinations at 30 months). The term *LLE* is used instead of SLI in recognition of the fact that not all children with early language delay continue to have language impairment; in fact, only 25–50% of children who are language delayed as toddlers go on to have long-term language impairments (Weiss, 2001). However, the fact that some late talkers catch up with their peers does not minimize the importance of early intervention for young children with language delay.

Prevalence and Causation. The prevalence of SLI is 7% (Fox, Dodd, & Howard, 2002). There are discrepancies in the findings related to gender and SLI. While some experts report that SLI occurs more frequently in males than females, at a ratio of 3:1 (Leonard, 1998), other researchers have not found a greater occurrence in males (Tomblin et al., 1997).

In recent years, there has been a major breakthrough in genetic research: A gene locus that is linked to individuals with speech and language impairments has been identified (Marcus & Fisher, 2003; Rice, Smith, & Gayán, 2009). This finding corroborates other literature indicating that a child with SLI is more likely than a child who is not language impaired to have a family member with language impairment. Consequently, most experts now believe that there is a genetic basis for SLI (Rice, 2000).

Along with genetic factors, a child's environment also affects language development. While it is true that limited language stimulation negatively impacts children's language development, a lack of language stimulation is not typically the reason for most language impairments. Instead, experts believe that children with SLI require more intense and focused stimulation to become language proficient than do children who are developing typically.

Although the environment typically is not the cause of SLI, a practitioner knows that parent–child communication patterns should be monitored and sometimes modified to foster language. Communication is a two-way street; when a child fails to produce language, it is easy for parents to develop nonfacilitating communication patterns. For example, parents may be more conversationally directive with children who are language impaired. **Directive language** occurs when a parent requests that a child say or do something, or when the adult asks many questions. The overuse of directive language is a concern because children with language impairments respond less positively to maternal use of commands and questions than do typical peers (Rabidoux & MacDonald, 2000).

In your work as an SLP or educator, you will determine whether parents should modify their communication patterns as part of the overall intervention program. The play-based assessment described below is one approach often used to assess parent–child communication patterns. The enhanced milieu approach, also discussed below, is an intervention approach that targets parent–child interactions.

MAJOR CHARACTERISTICS

The morphosyntax features of language are the primary deficit for children with SLI. While children with SLI generally develop morphosyntax features in the same developmental sequence as their peers, they take longer to reach the same linguistic milestones (Rescorla & Lee, 2000). Refer to Chapters 1 and 2 for a review of the terms *syntax*, *morpheme*, and *morphosyntax*.

Specific morphemes are particularly problematic for children with SLI. Challenging morphemes include (a) verb forms (e.g., third-person singular *s*, past tense *ed*, copula verbs [*is, are*], auxiliary verbs [*is, are, do, can*]), (b) articles (*a, the*), (c) possessive *'s,* and (d) pronouns (Rescola & Lee, 2000). Table 6.1 provides an expanded list of morphosyntax features frequently delayed in children with SLI. Practitioners should remember that in some homes, children do not hear or use General American English dialect (sometimes called Mainstream American English); dialects in some homes are characterized by

Table 6.1 **Morphosyntax Deficits in Children with SLI**

Morphosyntax	Example of error
• *ing* (present progressive verb)[1]	"Dog eat him food." (The dog is eat*ing* his food.)
• Plural /s/[2]	"Me got two cat." (I have two cats.)[3]
• *Wh-* questions	"What we can make?" (What can we make?) "What do you think what the boy broke?" (What do you think the boy broke?)
• Prepositions *in* and *on*	"Mommy put table, my book." (Mommy put my book *on* the table.)
• More likely to use demonstratives (*this, that, these, those*) without a paired noun	"This mine!" (*This book* is mine!)
• Pronoun usage, particularly the nominative (subject) case	"Her sleeping." (*She* is sleeping.) "Me want it." (*I* want it.)
• Difficulty using auxiliary verbs (e.g., *is, do, can*)	"Sara do it!" (Sara *can* do it!)
• Difficulty with adverbials (omits adverbial in obligatory context)	"We left." (We left on Saturday.)
• Produce three-element noun phrases (determiner + adjective + noun) less frequently than typically developing peers	"The girl here. The girl big." (The big girl is here.)
• Difficulty with copula *be* verb	"Me Batman today!" (I *am* Batman today!)
• Difficulty using articles (*a, the*)	"Give me cookie, Okay? (Give me *a* cookie, Okay?)
• Pronoun case marking	"Her do it." "That him bike." (*She* can do it. That is *his* bike.)

Morphosyntax	Example of error
• Possessive *'s*	"That mommy coat." (That is *Mommy's* coat.)
• Regular past tense[1]	"He push him." (He *pushed* him.)
• Third-person singular verbs[2]	"Daddy fix cars." (Daddy *fixes* cars.)
• Difficulty with embedded clauses in *wh-* questions	"What do you think what Sara broke?" (What do you think *that she broke?*)

[1]In general, children with SLI use more bare-stem verbs (verbs without markings) than typically developing peers; consequently, they have difficulty with a variety of verb tense markers.

[2]This is controversial; some investigators have reported that plural forms are not deficient in children with SLI.

[3]Plural deletions with the use of a numerical word (*two*) also can be a dialectal error, but in this example, it is meant to illustrate the omission of the plural form.

distinct variations in morphosyntax structure. A child who is using his or her home dialect (and demonstrating the variations consistent with that dialect) should not be erroneously classified as having SLI. Learn more about dialectal morphosyntax variations in Focus 6.2 and in Appendix E.

As you might expect, when there is a primary deficit in morphosyntax, there is a trickle-down effect that impacts other aspects of language ability and academic functioning. This is certainly the case for children with SLI. For example, as children with SLI enter school, they have difficulty with the more sophisticated language needed for academics. Written language has more compound and complex sentences than spoken language. Children with SLI have difficulty with syntactically complex sentences and use embedded clauses less often than children who are developing typically. Figure 6.1 demonstrates how the morphosyntax of children with SLI lags behind that of their typically developing peers.

Semantic skills also are affected. Children with SLI have difficulty with vocabulary development. This pattern of slower vocabulary growth is seen in children at very young ages. Children with SLI often produce word combinations up to 3½ years behind their peers and have difficulty learning to use verbs. Children with SLI use a smaller variety of verbs and rely on a handful of high-frequency verbs, such as *want, get,* and *like.* Experts believe that the lexical problems of children with SLI relate to (a) the additional time needed for word retrieval, (b) decreased ability to expand new object names to objects in

FOCUS 6.2 *Multicultural Issues*

It can be difficult for an SLP who does not use African American English (AAE) to differentiate a child with a language disorder from a child with a language difference (e.g., a child who uses AAE). Sometimes children who speak AAE are misdiagnosed. There are a number of AAE linguistic patterns that can be viewed as language errors if AAE linguistic variations are not understood. For example, a speaker who uses AAE might say, "What do this mean?" instead of "What does this mean?" Learn more about how an SLP can avoid misdiagnosing a child who uses AAE in Appendix E in this book.

Figure 6.1 **Comparison of Development of Children with and without Specific Language Impairment**

	Years			
	2	3	4	5
	Months			
	18 20 22 24 26 28 30 32 34	36 38 40 42 44	46 48 50 52 54	56 58 60

Children developing typically (Typical age of development)

- 2-word phrases produced
- Plural s; auxiliary *be* emerges
- *in/on, ing, 's* > 80%
- MLU of 4.2
- Mastery of copula and auxiliary *be* and auxiliary *do*

Children who are SLI (Evidence of delayed production)

- 2-word phrases
- MLU 2.6
- Auxiliary *be* emerging for some children with SLI
- Prepositions *in/on*
- 50% of children with SLI still having difficulty with copula and auxiliary *be* and *do* at 5–6 years

the same semantic category, and (c) the need to learn new words embedded within simple versus complex sentences (Ravid, Levie, & Avivi Ben-zvi, 2003).

The trickle-down effect also affects pragmatic development in children with SLI. For example, when communicating with adults, preschoolers with language impairment are less likely than their typically developing peers to initiate topics. Their conversational turns are more likely to merely acknowledge the communication partner's utterance instead of offering new information.

Pragmatic difficulties continue as children with SLI reach school age, with resulting social communication problems. **Social communication problems** are limitations in an individual's social, cognitive, and language skills necessary for contextually appropriate, meaningful, and effective interpersonal communication (Adams, 2005).

As an example of social communication problems, older children with SLI have difficulty entering into peer-group conversations and struggle to make conversational repairs such as clarifying their communication when there is a conversational breakdown. Children with SLI have less opportunity to practice their communication skills because their typically developing peers tend to dominate shared interactions. Consequently, an unfortunate situation begins when children with poor language ability have reduced opportunity to practice and improve their communication performance. A negative cycle is created in which children with SLI fall further and further behind their peers in their social communication.

Research on the social challenges associated with SLI has influenced many professionals to include social and pragmatic interventions for children with language impairments. Data show that many adults who were diagnosed as having SLI as children continue to experience serious problems with employment, independent living, and personal relationships (Clegg et al., 2005). Early intervention can help prevent this negative cycle of social and academic failure. I discuss a social peer-based approach to intervention later in this chapter.

Children with SLI also have more frequent phonological impairments than their typically developing peers (Conti-Ramsden & Durkin, 2012); it has been estimated that up to 40% of children with SLI have phonological deficits. The phonological differences emerge at an early age. For example, toddlers with SLI have smaller consonant and vowel inventories and use a more restricted and less mature variety of syllable shapes than do their typically developing peers. An example of a simple syllable shape is a consonant–vowel (CV) combination (e.g., *toe*); a more complex syllable pattern is a CCV (e.g., *play*) or a CVC (e.g., *hat*). Phonological and articulation deficits continue to be problematic in later years, resulting in reduced speech intelligibility.

ASSOCIATED PROBLEMS

Research demonstrates that children with SLI need more time to process information than do children developing typically; this finding supports the claim that children with SLI have capacity limitations in their cognitive processing resources (Weismer & Thordardottir, 2002). The slower rate of processing results in reduced ability to rapidly name pictures and recognize words. The rate of **nonword repetition tasks** (i.e., repetitions of nonsense words) also is reduced in children with SLI; the use of a nonword repetition task has been proposed as a way to differentiate children with and without SLI (Weismer & Thordardottir, 2002).

A higher-than-expected proportion of children with SLI are diagnosed with **attention-deficit/hyperactivity disorder (ADHD)**. In fact, children with SLI are about two times more likely to show ADHD symptoms than children developing typically (Yew & O'Kearney, 2012). Children with SLI who have significant levels of receptive language impairment appear to be the most likely to exhibit behaviors of impulsivity, high activity, and distractibility associated with the ADHD diagnosis. Attention deficits likely contribute to language learning difficulties for many children with language impairment. Practitioners compensate for diminished attention capacity by providing repeated and focused stimulation of targeted linguistic structures and facilitating increasingly longer periods of sustained attention.

Approximately 80% of school-age children with SLI experience reading problems (Botting, Simkin, & Conti-Ramsden, 2006; Catts et al., 2002). It has been suggested that SLI and dyslexia are linked, with SLI forming a dyslexia subgroup. In this theory, children with SLI exhibit a severe form of dyslexia in that they have phonological awareness difficulties associated with dyslexia in addition to morphosyntax problems (Bishop & Snowling, 2004). **Phonological awareness deficits** result in problems detecting, segmenting, and blending sounds in words, hindering children's **reading decoding** (e.g., sounding out and spelling words while reading and writing). Children's reading and academic difficulties can persist throughout the students' academic years. For example, researchers followed 200+ children who had received language intervention prior to age 7. When the students were 17 to 18 years old, they were retested; 89% of the students still experienced significant difficulty on one language test, and 63% exhibited widespread difficulties (i.e., poor performance on three or more tests; Conti-Ramsden et al., 2001). The majority were not proficient readers.

Writing, along with reading, poses challenges. Children with SLI demonstrate frequent grammatical errors in their writing and have difficulty with written verb morphology (Scott, 2002; Scott & Windsor, 2000). Complex sentence formation difficulty also affects writing performance. Children with SLI rarely write sentences that have more than one subordinate clause. Spelling difficulties also are common and may be linked to underlying phonological, morphological, and semantic deficits (Apel, Masterson, & Niessen, 2004).

FOCUS 6.3 *School-Age Children*

Reading demands coordinated use of high-level language skills. Children need a more sophisticated vocabulary and must be able to comprehend low-frequency syntax structures (e.g., passive sentences, embedded subordinate clauses, elaborated noun phrases) that occur more frequently in written language than oral discourse (Wright & Newhoff, 2001). Other skills such as phonological awareness, print concepts, alphabetic knowledge, and spelling conventions also impact literacy development. In recent years, SLPs and educators have begun to directly support children's reading and writing development. During intervention with school-age children with SLI and associated reading and writing deficits, practitioners should do the following (American Speech-Language-Hearing Association [ASHA], 2001):

- Integrate spoken and written language targets; students should alternate between reading, writing, and oral productions.
- Assist children in decoding/encoding and comprehending language at the sound, syllable, word, sentence, and discourse levels.
- Help children form associations between how groups of letters look, sound, and feel in the mouth and link this awareness to word recognition and spelling skills.
- Develop children's meta-awareness of spoken and written language and facilitate students' use of computers and software to strategically support written language.

Focus 6.3 gives more information about supporting reading development in school-age children I specifically address reading, writing, and spelling interventions for students with language impairments in Chapter 10.

Connections

Children with SLI do not function socially like children with typical language development. Throughout this book, I describe the fact that social interactionist theory provides the theoretical base for many aspects of language intervention. Once again, this theory underscores the need to focus on the peer relationships of children with SLI. I describe peer-mediated intervention in this section because peer-mediated social communication intervention is a form of intervention appropriate for students with a variety of disorders, such as students with cognitive disability and students who are on the autism spectrum (Goldstein, Schneider, & Thiemann, 2007).

CHILDREN'S SOCIAL COMMUNICATION

Peer-mediated treatment is a form of intervention that focuses on a student's social communication. To facilitate social communication, practitioners follow one of three basic treatment paradigms (Machalicek et al., 2008). The first, **social intervention** with peers, involves identifying a social skill hierarchy, teaching the student with the communication disorder specific social skill strategies, and facilitating the student's use of social strategies with his or her peer group. The second paradigm is called **peer confederate training**. In confederate training, students with typical language development are trained to use social strategies to encourage communication from students with communication disorders. The third paradigm, **sociodramatic script training**, involves engaging children in opportunities to role-play **social scripts**. A social script is a repeated social interaction that is likely to occur in daily life; examples of social scripts include greeting, interactions over lunchtime or during recess, asking a friend to play, and joining in a group activity. During script training, an adult uses role-play and cuing to familiarize the student with daily discourse routines. Below I describe two important social interactions for young children with communication impairments: peer entry and cooperative play. Following this information, I discuss issues of peer interaction for older students with communication impairments.

Peer Entry. In order for a child to enter into a group-play situation, he or she must display a combination of verbal and nonverbal skills. Typically, children demonstrate 10 or more entry behaviors before being included in a group-play activity (Timler, Olswang, & Coggins, 2005b). Entry behaviors include low-risk behaviors such as engaging in a similar activity as the other children in the group and high-risk behaviors such as commenting on the activity or requesting to join the activity. It is interesting that positive comments about the activity have been identified as being a more successful means of gaining entry than asking to join the activity (Timler et al., 2005b). The hovering behavior often demonstrated by children with SLI is not a successful strategy; neither is directly demanding to be included, responding negatively to a peer's communication or activity, or ignoring others' comments and requests. Figure 6.2 is an example of a positive peer entry strategy.

Cooperative Play. During cooperative play, children take on specific roles that are maintained with play organizer statements such as "Let's say this house is on fire, and we'll both be firemen." When there are disputes, effective communication strategies involve

Figure 6.2   **Child Entering Peer Group**

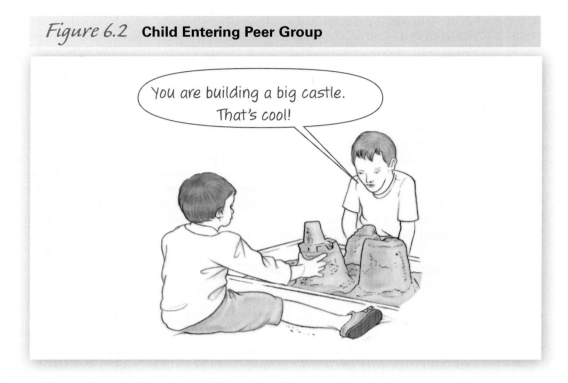

giving a reason for the problem ("No, this is the house because, see, here's the roof."), making a polite request, or suggesting a compromise. In order to be successful during cooperative play, children with SLI must be able to answer peer questions, acknowledge comments, ask for needed information, and comment about the activity.

Peer Interactions for School-Age Students. At older ages, students with language impairments continue to exhibit communication difficulties stemming from pragmatic deficits. Young adults with a history of SLI have few close friends and less-rewarding social relationships (Howlin, Mawhood, & Rutter, 2000). Students with a history of language impairment often have difficulty negotiating conflict and have lower social self-esteem than their typically developing peers (Wadman, Durkin, & Conti-Ramsden, 2008). Consequently, practitioners continue to facilitate social communication skills for school-age children.

Before initiating a social communication intervention for an older child, a practitioner considers the student's environment by discussing patterns of social communication with the student's teachers, parents, siblings, and peers. Sometimes communication partners unconsciously develop nonfacilitative patterns of communication, such as excessively asking direct questions or answering questions for the student. A practitioner also talks directly to a student with language impairment about the need for social communication intervention. Teamwork makes it possible to alter the student's environment comprehensively. There is more likely to be a positive outcome when all team members realize changing social behavior is complex and social communication intervention demands significant time and effort (Brinton & Fujiki, 2005).

PEER-MEDIATED INTERVENTION APPROACHES

Intervention Strategies for Young Children. When working with a young child with communication impairments, a practitioner facilitates the child's assertive communication strategies while minimizing ineffective or disruptive strategies (Fujiki & Brinton, 2009). For example, a child with communication impairments may attempt to join a peer group by grabbing group members' toys or without making sufficient eye contact. The following example represents observational notes completed on a child with difficulty during social interaction:

> J outside; running circles around perimeter of the playground. Stops to go down the slide. Then runs to sand area and attempts to pour sand in a bucket with two other girls. Girls tell him to leave (J looks upset), begins to run around the playground again. (Timler et al., 2005b, p. 171)

Timler et al. (2005b) identified intervention targets for children to facilitate (a) peer entry into groups and (b) cooperative play:

- To facilitate peer entry, the practitioner teaches the child to:
  - Approach peers physically.
  - Watch what peers are doing and imitate the activity.
  - Make a positive statement about the group activity.
- To improve cooperative play, the practitioner teaches the child to:
  - Establish eye contact.
  - Share play materials.
  - Take turns.
  - Make a play organizer statement, compliment peers, request assistance, and offer assistance.
  - If a conflict arises, state a reason for the disagreement or suggest a compromise.
  - Answer when a peer asks a question, respond to peers' comments, and maintain the ongoing topic.

The behaviors listed above can be a starting point for identifying the social behaviors potentially limiting a child's peer interactions. Once deficits are identified, the adult continues the intervention by (a) teaching a specific social communication behavior, (b) practicing the behavior with the child in small-group activities, and (c) supporting the child as he or she begins to use the strategy independently.

Intervention Strategies for School-Age Students. Experts have proposed a number of intervention approaches to guide social communication interventions for school-age students (Adams, 2005; Timler, Olswang, & Coggins, 2005a). Techniques include increasing the student's ability to take another's perspective, practicing social routines, and understanding hidden meanings.

To facilitate a student's ability to take others' perspectives, a practitioner helps the student use and define emotion words to encourage understanding others' emotions. Some students with communication impairments need to be taught to evaluate a social situation from others' perspectives and to appropriately describe what others may be thinking or feeling.

For example, if you viewed two individuals engaged in a confidential discussion, it is unlikely that you would attempt to enter the interaction. In contrast, a student with poor social communication skills may not consider others' nonverbal cues or emotions and may attempt to join the discussion. In this case, the professional encourages the student to verbalize what others are thinking or feeling. Following role-playing social scenarios, the student with communication impairment practices answering questions such as "What was my friend thinking?" and "How did my friend feel?"

A practitioner also uses sociodramatic script training to improve school-age students' communication. The practitioner and the student practice established social routines first during role-play and then in everyday situations. As the student gains competence, the practitioner establishes more flexibility by regularly adding small changes to the established routine.

A final intervention goal with older students is to help a student use and understand hidden meanings. Indirect communication is an example of a hidden meaning. For example, if you are at a party and you want to leave, you might say to your partner, "Wow, it's getting late!" You use an indirect statement as a subtle indicator that you want to leave the party. Indirect communication can be challenging for an individual with social communication impairments; he or she may not understand or act on the social implications of indirect statements.

Practitioners target indirect language by improving a student's meta-awareness of indirect communication. The practitioner and the student might view videotaped examples of indirect communication and discuss rules for deciphering hidden meanings. Practitioners sometimes use comic strips as a source of discussion. Students practice interpreting the hidden meanings of a comic strip; learning to explain "what makes it funny" helps a student understand implied meanings behind words.

Assessment

Assessment for an individual with SLI typically includes an in-depth language sample analysis and norm-referenced assessments such as the Preschool Language Scale, Fifth Edition (PLS-5; Zimmerman, Steiner, & Pond, 2011), or (for older school-age students) the Clinical Evaluation of Language Fundamentals–5 (Semel, Wiig, & Secord, 2013). More examples of norm-referenced assessments appropriate for students with SLI are provided in Chapter 3.

Criterion-referenced assessments also contribute important information with respect to deficits in language form, content, and use in everyday interactions. In this section, I discuss two different criterion-referenced assessment approaches: (a) parent–child toy play and book reading observational assessments and (b) curriculum-based language assessment.

Parent–child interaction assessment and curriculum-based language assessment are two forms of criterion-referenced assessment in an overarching category called naturalistic assessment. **Naturalistic assessment** provides multiple opportunities for an individual to perform skills across domains (i.e., social, cognitive, motor, communication). Naturalistic assessment can be a planned activity (as when the adult sets up toys and observes a child during play) but also includes observation of a child in the classroom or home. It is important to note that the naturalistic approaches described in this chapter also are appropriate for individuals with other types of communication disorders (e.g., children with hearing loss, children with cognitive disability, children on the autism spectrum). Learn more about naturalistic assessment by viewing the video clip at http://www2.cde.state.co.us/media/ResultsMatter/RMSeries/WhatIsAuthenticAssessment_SA.asp.

PARENT–CHILD INTERACTION ASSESSMENTS

Throughout this book, I emphasize the fact that language theory underlies clinical decisions. The relationship between clinical procedures and theory also plays a role in the assessment process. Language theory guides the assessment protocols used in an assessment battery.

Consider, for example, a professional who believes that social interaction theory plays a strong role in language acquisition. Social interactionist theory is based on the theories of Lev Vygotsky. According to Vygotsky, children's development results from social interactions with more capable peers. Within this perspective, as adults identify and interact within children's zone of proximal development, children's development is stimulated. Observations of parent–child book reading and toy play align with the social interactionist approach.

To begin a parent–child observation, an assessor supplies appropriate books and toys and asks the child's parents to interact as typically as possible with their child. The assessor includes a variety of books (e.g., alphabet books, storybooks, simple books without text). The assessor also includes a variety of toys to prompt a range of play behavior; toys should include thematic toys (e.g., a farmyard, small "people" figures, vehicles, animals), toys for sociodramatic play (e.g., dishes, dish pan, sponge, baby doll, doll clothing), and toys stimulating motor play (e.g., stacking rings, mailbox with different-sized blocks to be inserted in "mail slots").

There are several advantages and disadvantages to parent–child interaction assessments (Losardo & Notari-Syverson, 2001). Advantages are that (a) young children are more likely to use complex language in child-initiated familiar routines, (b) children are more likely to interact in ways that represent their true abilities, and (c) children are more likely to be highly engaged during play activities than during more formalized assessment procedures. Disadvantages include the fact that play-based assessments, like other naturalistic assessment protocols, require more planning and more expertise than does administration of norm-referenced assessment.

One area of expertise required to complete an effective observation is the assessor's ability to identify the parent's scaffolding strategies and to assess the effects of varying strategies on the child's communication. As you recall, scaffolding refers to the graduated assistance provided to novice learners in order to help them achieve higher levels of conceptual and communicative competence. The assessor may use a criterion-referenced assessment tool to document observed parent scaffolding behaviors.

An example of a parent–child observational form used to document book-reading behaviors is shown in Table 6.2. The assessor notes the parents' scaffolding strategies that are elaborative (i.e., expanding child utterances) or directive (i.e., asking the child to repeat words or asking the child to "fill in the blank"; Crain-Thoreson, Dahlin, & Powell, 2001). When used most effectively, scaffolding is faded from levels of high support (e.g., providing an imitative model, limiting the child to two choices) to minimal levels of guidance (e.g., asking open-ended questions).

While the assessor is noting parental scaffolding, the assessor also observes the child's responses to the adult's different conversational strategies. Variations in the child's communication and engagement suggest parent language approaches that should be facilitated or reduced. For example, if the child responds more when the parent follows the child's conversational lead—in contrast to the child's response to direct questions—parents can be coached to increase their use of the former conversational strategy.

Table 6.2 **Parent Scaffolding Behaviors during Parent–Child Book Reading**

Child's name: Book used: Date:		*Book type* (alphabet, narrative, rhyming, etc.)
Scaffolding behaviors observed	**Child response**	**Behavioral observations**
1. Labeling and commenting	Positive/Negative	
2. Oral dialogue to explain/elaborate text	Positive/Negative	
3. Pauses	Positive/Negative	
4. Sentence recasting or language expansion (i.e., elaborative strategy)	Positive/Negative	
5. Simplifying the book's text by simplifying syntax	Positive/Negative	
6. Tag questions (e.g., *"He's big, isn't he?"*)	Positive/Negative	
7. Direct questions (*"Where is the man going?"*) or asking the child to "fill in the blank" (i.e., *"The man is wearing a yellow _____."*) (i.e., directive strategy)	Positive/Negative	
8. Following the child's comment by making a linked comment	Positive/Negative	
9. Retelling story by making up own words	Positive/Negative	
10. Other forms noted:	Positive/Negative	

Did the child evidence enjoyment of the book interaction? YES NO

Did particular parent scaffolding strategies work well to engage the child? YES NO List:

Did the child react negatively to particular scaffolding strategies? YES NO List:

If the child evidenced a lack of engagement or interest in the interaction, what scaffolding strategies might be most effective? List:

Further recommendations to improve the quality of book-reading interactions: (book type, length of interaction, contextual demands, etc.)

Source: From *Parent-Child Joint Book Reading: An Observational Protocol for Young Children* by J. N. Kaderavek and E. Sulzby, 1998, American Journal of Speech-Language Pathology, 7, pp. 33–47. Used with permission.

An assessor also carefully considers a child's play behaviors during an observation. The assessor may choose to apply a cognitive-constructivist framework to a parent–child observation. An observation based on the cognitive-constructivist approach is likely to consider the child's ability to use means–end behavior, imitate motor behaviors, manipulate objects in functional ways, and use objects symbolically. (See Chapter 2 to review the behaviors associated with Piaget's cognitive constructivist theory.) The cognitive constructivist perspective helps an assessor focus on behaviors associated with a child's level of cognitive development. An example of a criterion-referenced assessment documenting a child's use of sensorimotor, presymbolic, and symbolic play behaviors is shown in Table 6.3.

Last, but not least, a parent–child observational assessment can be framed within a behaviorist perspective. A professional coming from a behaviorist position is likely to take note of slightly different aspects of a child's behavior. With this perspective, the assessor documents the occurrence of target behaviors and notes the antecedent events and reinforcements that precede and follow each behavior.

Table 6.3   **Play and Language: Observation Checklist (9–24 months)**

Play behaviors observed	Communication and language behaviors observed
9 to 12 months	
_____ Awareness that objects exist when not seen; finds toy hidden under scarf	_____ Sounds rather than language; may have words that are associated with actions
_____ Means–end behavior: crawls or walks to get what he/she wants; pulls string toys	Exhibits following communicative functions:
_____ Does not mouth or bang all toys (some used appropriately), manipulates objects	_____ Request
	_____ Command
13 to 17 months	
_____ Purposeful exploration of toys; discovers operation of toys through trial and error; uses variety of motoric schemas	_____ Context-dependent single words; for example, child may use the word *car* when riding in a car; words tend to come and go in child's vocabulary
_____ Hands toys to adult if unable to operate	Exhibits following communicative functions (linguistically or nonlinguistically):
	_____ Request
	_____ Protesting
	_____ Command
	_____ Interactional
	_____ Response
	_____ Personal
	_____ Greeting
	_____ Label
17 to 19 months	
_____ Beginning of pretending (early symbolic) play behaviors with himself/herself as agent (e.g., child pretends to go to sleep or pretends to drink from cup or eat from spoon)	_____ Beginning of true verbal communication. Words have following functional and semantic relations:
_____ Beginning social play; child plays same or similar activity while engaging in social interaction with peer	_____ Recurrence
	_____ Agent
	_____ Existence
_____ Uses most common objects and toys appropriately	_____ Object
	_____ Nonexistence
_____ Tool use (uses stick to reach toy)	_____ Action or state
	_____ Rejection
	_____ Location
	_____ Denial
19 to 22 months	
Symbolic play extends beyond the child's self:	_____ Refers to objects and person not present
_____ Plays with dolls; brushes doll's hair, feeds doll a bottle, or covers doll with blanket	Beginning of word combinations with following semantic relations:
_____ Performs pretend activities on more than one person or object; for example, feeds self, a doll, mother, and another child	_____ Agent–action
	_____ Action–locative
	_____ Action–object
_____ Combines two toys in pretend play; for example, puts spoon in pan or pours from pot into cup	_____ Object–locative
	_____ Agent–object
	_____ Possessive
	_____ Attributive (*many, dirty, big*)
	_____ Dative (*that, this*)

(continued)

Table 6.3 **(continued)**

Play behaviors observed	Communication and language behaviors observed
24 months	
_____ Represents daily experiences; plays house—is the mommy, daddy, or baby; objects used are realistic and close to life size; beginnings of make-believe play	_____ Uses earlier pragmatic functions and semantic relations in phrases and short sentences
_____ Completes short routines (e.g., puts food in pan, stirs, and eats; stacks and knocks down blocks; pours and dumps sand and water)	Beginning use of morphological markers appear:
_____ Beginnings of cooperative social pretend play; child plays with others (but is not likely to use verbal communication while doing so)	_____ Present progressive (*ing*) on verbs
	_____ Plurals
	_____ Possessives

Sources: From *Assessment of Cognitive and Language Abilities Through Play* by C. E. Westby, 1980, Language, Speech, and Hearing Services in Schools, 11, pp. 154–168. Copyright© 1980 by American Speech-Language-Hearing Association.

You might be thinking that all this observation takes a very long time! In actuality, a professional moves back and forth between theoretical perspectives and identifies the most relevant aspects needed for each child. But, as I continue to emphasize throughout this book, a skilled professional understands the *why* that drives every clinical activity. Your understanding of the theoretical basis of varying protocols also helps you explain the assessment results to a child's parents and teachers.

CURRICULUM-BASED LANGUAGE ASSESSMENT

Curriculum-based language assessment is another naturalistic assessment process; in it, an assessor considers the academic content and social interaction demands of the curriculum, assesses the language skills a student brings to the curriculum, determines the knowledge and language skills the student needs to succeed academically, and identifies instructional modifications to enhance the student's academic success (ASHA, 2001). Curriculum-based language assessment requires an assessor to (a) observe a child in the classroom, (b) identify (with the classroom teacher) aspects of the curriculum that are problematic, (c) consider aspects of the instruction (e.g., Are instructions provided verbally? In writing? What is the language complexity of the instructions?), (d) evaluate student work samples (e.g., evaluate written work for error patterns), (e) evaluate textbooks and classroom materials to identify vocabulary and/or morphosyntax that is poorly comprehended by the student, and (f) identify strategies that the student can use to organize his or her work or improve performance. I provide more information on curriculum-based reading assessments in Chapter 10.

It is important for practitioners to use curriculum-based language assessment to develop effective interventions for school-age students. To be successful in the classroom, students must learn to identify the most important components for a specific academic task. Good students take this for granted, but it can be challenging for students with language impairments and learning deficits.

For example, imagine that you are conducting a classroom observation as part of your curriculum-based language assessment. You observe that, during a science unit, the teacher asks students to "summarize what we have learned about butterflies and moths." The students developing typically immediately begin listing the two categories and noting similarities and differences between the two species. However, a student with language impairment does not use this underlying strategy, and his answer is disorganized and incomplete. The information you obtained during the assessment provides data documenting the need to improve the student's organizational strategies and semantic categorization skills.

In another example, you note that a student with language impairment is unable to produce a coherent response to a classroom story-writing assignment. Her story has no clear plot, lacks descriptive words, and does not indicate cause and effect with conjunctions such as *because*. You note this difficulty, do some more assessment probes on the student's narrative abilities, and develop goals to target narrative production. (See Chapter 10 for more information about narrative interventions.)

As a final example, you may have a student complete a writing probe. A writing probe is an appropriate assessment protocol for a student whose written work consists of simple sentences, lacks descriptive words, and demonstrates poor punctuation and spelling. You supply a story starter (e.g., *One day I landed on a desert island and . . .* and ask the student to write for 10 minutes). At the end of the 10-minute period, you count the number of complex and compound sentences, evaluate the student's use of descriptive words, and count the number of punctuation and spelling errors. You target some or all of these areas in your intervention and periodically readminister the writing probe to assess progress.

As the examples above demonstrate, an advantage of curriculum-based language assessment is that the assessment procedure results in meaningful intervention goals. Another advantage is that curriculum-based language assessment requires close collaboration between the SLP and the classroom teacher; professionals work together to identify areas of academic weakness and develop remediation strategies. This collaboration is likely to improve student outcomes. The disadvantages of curriculum-based language assessment mirror the challenges of other forms of naturalistic assessment. Curriculum-based language assessments are more time-consuming than, for example, norm-referenced assessments. Curriculum-based language assessment procedures also require professional expertise to evaluate curriculum materials and identify student weaknesses within the classroom.

Intervention

I present three interventions in this chapter on SLI: enhanced milieu teaching (EMT), conversational recast training (CRT), and sentence-combining (SC) intervention. EMT and CRT are most appropriate for young children with language impairment, while SC intervention typically is implemented with students who are 5 to 12 years of age.

Many different approaches can be implemented for children with language impairments. I have chosen these three approaches for this chapter because they (a) are based on clear theoretical positions, (b) have results published in peer-referred journals, and (c) have data demonstrating efficacy. These three approaches illustrate variations in interventions for children with SLI; there are dozens of other viable approaches. If you are a member of the National Student Speech-Language-Hearing Association (NSSLHA), you can access the American Speech-Language-Hearing Association website to find additional intervention approaches for children with language impairments: www.asha.org /members/ebp/compendium/.

Remember that language interventions are not necessarily specific to a particular language diagnosis. Interventions designed to be used with children with autism or children with intellectual disability may also be appropriate for a child with SLI. A practitioner does not choose a treatment because a child with communication impairment has a particular diagnosis; instead, a professional matches the intervention to the child's deficits within the language domains of form, content, and use.

Imagine that you are working with a child, Samuel, who is 3 years old and has significant social interaction deficits. He has not been diagnosed with an intellectual disability or autism. However, you know that enhancing social interaction skills is a primary intervention goal, and you consider using the *Developmental, Individual Difference, Relationship-based (DIR®) Floortime* approach (Wieder & Greenspan, 2003). Floortime builds parent–child interactions and facilitates child-initiated communication; it was developed for children on the autism spectrum. You may hesitate to use Floortime because Samuel has language impairment without a diagnosis of autism. If Samuel has not been diagnosed with autism, does that mean that Floortime is inappropriate? Absolutely not! As a professional who understands (a) how to evaluate a child's communication disorder within the domains of form, content, and use and (b) how to evaluate a specific intervention program, you may well decide that Floortime is a very appropriate approach to develop Samuel's social communication skills. You can find out more information about Floortime at www.icdl.com/dirFloortime/overview/.

In the same vein, you may decide to use an approach described in this chapter with an individual who has a diagnosis other than SLI. Children with SLI talk less than their typically developing peers, have more difficulty learning vocabulary words, and struggle to learn grammatical morphemes. Other children with different communication disorders have similar communication challenges. For example, you might decide to use the sentence-combining approach with a high-functioning student on the autism spectrum. A skilled professional understands the specific language skills targeted within each approach and chooses an intervention based on this knowledge.

INTERVENTION APPROACH: ENHANCED MILIEU TEACHING (EMT)

Enhanced milieu teaching (EMT) is a naturalistic approach appropriate for children who (a) are able to imitate sounds and words, (b) have a vocabulary of at least 10 words, and (c) have an MLU between 1.0 and 3.5 words (Hancock & Kaiser, 2006). This MLU level is the language stage when children learn lexical items (i.e., words) and semantic relational combinations (e.g., agent + action ["Mommy go"]; agent + action + object ["Daddy throw ball"]). In the EMT approach, parents are trained to be their child's primary language teacher. EMT also is implemented in preschool classrooms and small-group sessions, where the practitioner uses EMT language teaching strategies.

On the continuum of naturalness, EMT is considered a hybrid midway between highly child-directed and adult-directed approaches. EMT uses simple questions and requests for child imitation, along with adult language modeling techniques; the adult uses the language techniques in response to the child's focus of attention. The EMT hybrid approach differs from (a) highly child-directed modeling-only approaches where the adult models language without placing response demands on the child and (b) adult-controlled interventions where intervention often is skill based with adult-controlled stimuli presentation.

EMT is particularly effective for children with relatively low receptive or expressive language levels (i.e., beginning language learners), while children with higher language ability benefit from either a more didactic (i.e., direct teaching and adult controlled) approach or a responsive teaching approach in which adults model and expand language forms and promote topic-continuing talk (Carta & Kong, 2009; Kaiser & Trent, 2009). Three points clarify why EMT is effective for children at the earliest stages of language learning.

First, EMT is appropriate for beginning language learners because it implements language teaching during familiar routines and everyday activities (Delprato, 2001). Beginning language learners learn new language forms most easily in familiar and frequently occurring interactions. A beginning language learner is less likely to be able to generalize language forms learned in decontextualized settings; EMT promotes generalization of newly learned communication strategies.

EMT also is an appropriate intervention for beginning language learners, because language teaching episodes are initiated in response to the child's focus of attention. In a didactic, adult-directed approach, stimulus items are preselected (e.g., the adult decides on the targeted vocabulary). In contrast, EMT language facilitation techniques are linked to the child's interest and motivation. For example, if the child points at an item, the adult begins the mand-model teaching sequence by saying, "What do you want?" (See Table 6.4 for the definition of *mand-model*.) Beginning language learners benefit from seeing how communication provides real benefits in everyday interactions. Children with SLI learn a language target most efficiently when they are asked to say the target word to gain access to a favorite toy or activity in contrast to just listening to the language model.

The third and final reason that EMT is appropriate for a beginning language learner is that EMT primarily focuses on vocabulary development and early semantic combinations (e.g., Brown's Stage I). In contrast, the other approaches described here focus more on grammatical morphological acquisition (e.g., Brown's Stage II and beyond). A more advanced language learner is likely to have mastered the vocabulary and early word combinations emphasized during EMT.

Theoretical Foundations and Teaching Strategies in EMT. EMT is based on a number of strong theoretical principles. I have emphasized the naturalistic, child-centered focus of EMT. I hope you have reflected back on your knowledge of language theory and connected this approach to the social interactionist theory presented in Chapter 2 (e.g., Vygotsky, Bruner).

EMT has other theoretical roots as well. It has a connection to behaviorial theory in that parents prompt a child's language using an antecedent–behavior–consequence (A-B-C) behavioral sequence. The mand-model teaching technique uses this A-B-C progression. For example, a child who is developing typically looks at a cookie jar and says, "I want cookie." A child with SLI may fuss or attempt to climb up and open the cookie jar but may not have the language skill to ask for a cookie. In EMT, the practitioner uses the child's attention on the cookie jar (the antecedent event) to model and prompt a mand: "Tell me what you want" (the behavior). Obtaining the cookie is the naturally occurring consequence, along with providing an opportunity for a language expansion: "Wow, what a yummy cookie!" Modeling, with three additional strategies, **mand-model, time delay,** and incidental teaching—is the primary language training method in EMT. As I described in Chapter 5, modeling includes the adult behaviors of expanding, elaborating, and buildup/breakdown. In addition to the modeling terminology already familiar to you, in Table 6.4, I provide new definitions for mand-model, time-delay, and incidental teaching.

A practitioner generally needs between 20 and 30 sessions to train parents to effectively implement EMT tasks. The following steps outline the parent training sequence (Hancock & Kaiser, 2006):

Table 6.4 **Enhanced Milieu Teaching (EMT) Definitions and Strategies**

Term	Explanation	Use of technique in EMT to facilitate language for child with language impairment
Modeling (see also Chapter 5)	The language trainer notes the child's focus of attention and provides a language model reflecting the child's interest.	The child wants a block to put into the toy mailbox. (The mother has the blocks in her lap.) The mother says, "Do you want block?" and motions to the blocks. If the child imitates the model, the mother provides the block and gives a language expansion: "I want the red block!" An incorrect response or lack of child response triggers a second language model. After a third incorrect child response, the mother restates "want the block" and then gives the block to her child.
Mand-model procedure	The language trainer uses a verbal prompt in the form of a question ("What do you want?"), choice ("Do you want _____ or _____?"), or mand ("Tell me what you want.")	The child is focusing on an object or activity (in this example, he has a piece of paper but nothing to write with); the language trainer provides a prompt connected to the child's interest. Examples include saying "What do you want?" or providing a choice, such as "Do you want a crayon or a marker?" or providing a mand, such as "Tell me what you want." If the child does not respond, the trainer provides a model: "Say 'want a crayon.'" If the child does not repeat the model, the trainer provides a verbal model ("want a crayon") and provides the crayon.
Time delay	The language trainer uses a nonverbal prompt and waits before providing the desired object or action.	The child and his teacher are tossing a ball back and forth; the teacher says "throw the ball" when the child is throwing. After a few throws, when the teacher has the ball, she stops, looks expectantly at the child, and waits. If child does not say "throw (the) ball," the teacher says, "Tell me what you want!" or models "Say 'throw the ball.'" If the child does not imitate, the teacher provides the model ("throw the ball") and throws the ball.
Incidental teaching	The language trainer manipulates the environment so that the child is more likely to talk.	It is snack time, and the children are pouring juice. The child is given a cup but no juice. The adult waits for the child to ask "*juice?*" before pouring juice in the cup. If the child does not respond, the adult provides a model or mand-model training sequence.

Source: From "Enhanced Milieu Teaching," by T. B. Hancock and A. P. Kaiser, 2006. In R. J. McCauley and M. E. Fey (Eds.), *Treatment of Language Disorders in Children* (pp. 203–236). Baltimore, MD: Brookes.

- Parents are trained to choose materials to capture their child's interest and attention. They learn to manage toys so that their child stays engaged and to maximize child communication.
- Parents learn to follow their child's lead, pause to wait for a child's conversational turn, and maintain balanced adult–child interactions. Interaction balance is documented by computing the following formula: [number of parent verbal turns] – [number of child verbal and nonverbal turns] = X. A balanced interaction results in $X = 0$.
- Parents practice the EMT training strategies of modeling, mand-model, time-delay, and incidental teaching. By the end of the parent training sessions, parents should be implementing EMT strategies more than 80% of the time.

A decision tree example of an EMT treatment sequence is shown in Figure 6.3.

Figure 6.3 **Enhanced Milieu Teaching Decision Tree**

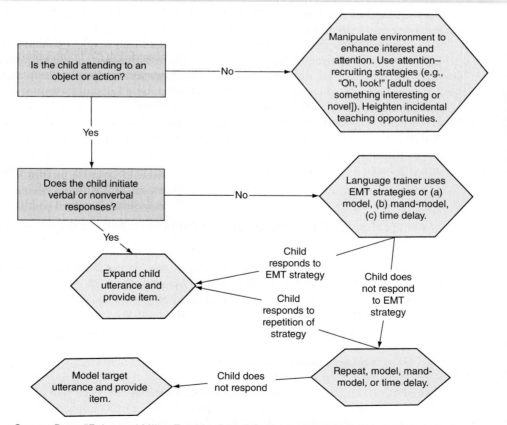

Source: From "Enhanced Milieu Teaching" by T. B. Hancock and A. P. Kaiser, 2006. In R. J. McCauley and M. E. Fey (Eds.), *Treatment of Language Disorders in Children* (pp. 203–236). Baltimore: Paul H. Brookes.

Data collection is an important part of EMT; data help a professional modify appropriate intervention treatment goals as a child's communication improves. For example, documentation of parent behaviors might include recording the percentage of parent expansions of child utterances, the average length of parent utterances, and the number of times the parent fails to pause after taking a conversational turn. After analyzing the data, the practitioner sets parent intervention goals. Examples of EMT parent goals are shown in Figure 6.4; Goals 1 and 2 are potential goals developed to enhance parent language teaching strategies. Goals 3 and 4 in Figure 6.4 reflect child intervention goals. Goals 3 and 4 facilitate specific word combinations, while Goal 5 targets utterance length.

Child performance data are also recorded on a regular basis. Table 6.5 demonstrates how child language data could be organized; documentation includes recording the child's utterance length (i.e., the number of 1-, 2-, 3-, and 4-plus-word utterances) in addition to the child's spontaneous and imitative use of various semantic combinations (e.g., action + object, modifier + noun).

Evidence Supporting the EMT Approach. Researchers in more than 30 studies have examined the effects of EMT. Several single-subject studies (e.g., Hancock & Kaiser, 2002; Kaiser, Hancock, & Nietfeld, 2000) have shown clear effects on children's use of target language and evidence of generalization to parent–child interactions at home.

A recent study that used randomization resulted in Level I evidence supporting the EMT approach (Kaiser, & Roberts, 2013). Although this particular study focused on children with intellectual disabilities, EMT is appropriate for children with a range of language impairments (e.g., children with LI, children who use augmentative communication devices). In this study, 77 children were each randomly assigned to one of two treatments (Treatment #1 = parent-delivered + SLP-delivered EMT; Treatment #2 = SLP-only EMT); children received 36 intervention sessions. Results supported the use of parents as language trainers; children receiving Treatment #1 had longer utterances, more vocabulary, and produced 16% more language targets than children in the SLP-only intervention.

Figure 6.4   **Example Goals for Enhanced Milieu Teaching (EMT)**

Goal 1   Hana's mother will use 3-word utterances during 20-minute shared play interactions with Hana ≥ 80% of her utterances.

Goal 2   Todd's father will pause 5 seconds after an initial model or mand ≥ 80% of his utterances in 4 out 5 consecutive 20-minute play routines.

Goal 3   Abel will produce introducer + X (e.g., "Hi Mamma," "Hi Pooh-Bear") in response to mand ("What do you say?") and visual stimulus (e.g., mother walks in room, playing "peek-a-boo" with stuffed Pooh-Bear) ≥ 90% of opportunities for 8 out of 10 days.

Goal 4   Jackson will spontaneously produce negative + X (e.g., "No outside," "No ball") within appropriate contexts during preschool outdoor play ≥ 70% of opportunities for 8 out of 10 days.

Goal 5   Odell's length of utterance will average 2.5 words when provided an adult model during a 20-minute play intervention for 8 out of 10 days.

Table 6.5 **Example of Data Documentation to Establish EMT Intervention Goals**

Measure	Data
Mean length of utterance	1.83
Total number of words	145
Number of different words	62
Number of one-word utterances	51
Number of two-word utterances	27
Number of three-or-more-word utterances	22

Target	Number of utterances produced spontaneously	Number of times prompted
1. Two-word request (e.g., "Want milk," "Give bubbles")	4	2
2. Action + object (e.g., "play ball," "blow bubbles")	5	1
3. Modifier + noun (e.g., "red ball," "little bubble")	2	1

Source: From *Enhanced Milieu Teaching* by T. B. Hancock and A. P. Kaiser, 2006. In R. J. McCauley and M. E. Fey (Eds.), *Treatment of Language Disorders in Children* (pp. 203–236). Baltimore: Paul H. Brookes.

INTERVENTION APPROACH: CONVERSATIONAL RECAST TRAINING (CRT)

Practitioners need effective interventions to teach grammatical targets to children with SLI. There is strong evidence that conversational recast training (CRT) is an effective approach that facilitates grammatical development in children with SLI (Fey, Long, & Finestack, 2003; Hassink & Leonard, 2010). CRT is appropriate for children from age 2 up to early elementary age (Camarata & Nelson, 2005); it is most effective with children above the two-word level and when the child has at least some ability to produce the targeted form (Fey & Loeb, 2002).

A primary technique of CRT is the use of sentence recasts. As I described in Chapter 5, a sentence recast is an adult response to a child's utterance that modifies the child's utterance while maintaining the child's meaning. A recast is similar to an expansion; however, CRT varies from traditional language expansion in two ways: (1) Sentence recasts vary the sentence modality to heighten the child's awareness of the targeted form, and (2) CRT facilitates a higher rate of production than more traditional language expansion techniques.

Consider the following example of an adult using a sentence recast. In this example, the child omits the *be* auxiliary form (e.g., says *noun* + [*verb* + *ing*] instead of *noun* + *is* + [*verb* + *ing*]):

Child: "Man running."

Adult: "Yes, the man is running."
(Adult points to a picture of a man sitting)

> *Adult:* *"Is the man running?"*
> *Child:* *"No, man sitting."*
> *Adult:* *"Oh, I see, the man is sitting. The man is not running. The man is sitting!"*

In this example, the adult alternates between statements and interrogative reversals (e.g., "Is the man running?") and also embeds negative sentence forms ("The man is not running."). It is hypothesized that using alternating sentence modality heightens a child's awareness of the targeted grammatical feature and encourages comparison of sentence forms (Fey & Proctor-Williams, 2000). In order to increase a child's exposure to the target forms, an SLP should include recasts formed as questions (ADULT: "What *is* the man *doing?*" CHILD: "Man sitting." ADULT: "Yes, the man *is sitting.*"), false assertions (ADULT: "Oh, I think that man is running!" Child: "No, is sitting." ADULT: "Oh, you are right, the man is sitting!"), and forced-alternative questions (ADULT: "Do you think the man is eating or the man is sitting?"). Note also that recasts can be corrective (i.e., recasting to correct a child's error or omission), as in CHILD: "The duck swimming" ADULT: "Yes the duck is swimming," or noncorrective as in CHILD: "The duck's swimming" ADULT: "Yes, the duck swims in the lake." In this example of a noncorrective recast, the adult builds on the grammatically correct child utterance in order to emphasize third-person regular verb use (i.e., *swims*).

CRT sometimes is implemented via a cyclic goal attack strategy; in this case, a practitioner selects multiple grammar targets after analyzing the child's error patterns (e.g., a verb form, *wh-* questions, noun modification). After initially introducing one target during a single session, the practitioner cycles through the remaining grammar targets, presenting one or two targets per session. An example of an intervention session in which the practitioner uses CRT is demonstrated in Figure 6.5. An example of CRT intervention goals is demonstrated in Figure 6.6.

A second feature of CRT is that the targeted grammatical feature is produced very frequently during the intervention session—as often as one recast per minute. The example above illustrates how this high target frequency is achieved. It is suggested that the exposure rate should be even more frequent—as much as two recasts per minute—to obtain good results (Proctor-Williams, Fey, & Loeb, 2001).

On the continuum of naturalness, CRT is a hybrid approach. Children are engaged in playlike routines; however, the activities are modified to maintain the child's attention on a specific language target. Activities are selected, and the adult output is carefully designed to facilitate specific linguistic targets. An illustration demonstrating a practitioner using CRT is shown in Figure 6.7.

An important theory of language learning, the **transactional model**, underlies CRT. Like the social interaction perspective, the transactional model considers a child's utterances as the antecedent event triggering an adult response (Camarata & Nelson, 2005). The cyclic links between child verbal initiations and adult response is considered a primary feature promoting child language learning.

Implementation of CRT requires that a practitioner target developmentally appropriate grammatical features. During pretreatment assessment, the adult determines the grammatical forms and sentence structures that a child does and does not produce (e.g., Does the child use an auxiliary form in the initiation of a question? ["Is Daddy outside?" versus "Daddy outside?"]). Because children with SLI frequently have difficulty with verb forms, verb production often is a focus of intervention. However, other grammatical forms including gerunds, passive voice, relative clauses, and *wh-* questions also are possible CRT targets.

Figure 6.5 Example of CRT Sequence

The adult sets up the zoo. The adult says, "*The animals are hungry and tired. Let's help the zookeeper feed the animals and put them to sleep.*"

Dialogue:

> **Adult:** "*Every day, the zookeeper* feeds *the animals. He* feeds *the giraffe. He* feeds *the giraffe every day. What* does *he do?*"
>
> **Child:** "*He feed giraffe.*"
>
> **Adult:** "*He* feeds *the giraffe, doesn't he? Let's ask the giraffe what he* wants *to eat. What* do *you want to eat? What* do *you want to eat, giraffe? You ask the giraffe what he* wants *to eat.*"
>
> **Child:** "*What you eat?*"
>
> **Adult:** "*What* do *you eat, giraffe? Oh, he* says *he* eats *hay. Does he eat bananas? No! The giraffe* eats *hay! The monkey* eats *bananas, doesn't he? Who do you think* eats *these bananas?*"
>
> **Child:** "*Monkey eats bananas.*"
>
> **Adult:** "*Yes, the monkey* eats *these yellow bananas. Let's help the zookeeper put the giraffe to sleep. Where does the giraffe sleep? Does the giraffe sleep in a pond?*"
>
> **Child:** "*No, the frog sleep in pond. The giraffe sleep under tree.*"
>
> **Adult:** "*Oh, I see; the giraffe* sleeps *under this tree and the frog* sleeps *in a pond! You make the zookeeper ask the giraffe where he sleeps.*"
>
> **Child:** "*Where you sleep?*"
>
> **Adult:** "*Where* do *you sleep, giraffe? The giraffe* says *he* sleeps *under the tree.*"

Figure 6.6 Example Goals for CRT

- Gavin will spontaneously produce the copula *is* in yes-no questions ("*Is the boy happy?*") to obtain information in obligatory contexts ≥ 50%[1] of the time in a naturalistic[2] 30-minute interaction. Preintervention baseline on (date) was 10%.
- Suzanne will spontaneously produce the possessive (*'s*) to describe ownership ("*This is mommy's purse,*" "*I want the girl's hat*") ≥ 50% of the time in a naturalistic 30-minute interaction in obligatory contexts. Preintervention baseline on (date) was at 12%[3].

[1]Once a child reaches 50% spontaneous production in a naturalistic setting, it is not necessary to emphasize the target as a primary goal. The target can, however, be embedded into other activities and monitored to determine continued mastery (Fey, 1986; Lee, Koenigsknecht, & Mulhern, 1975).

[2]An interaction is considered "naturalistic" even if the adult has to provide stimulus items making it more likely that the target form will be required. Some grammatical forms are low frequency and, without environmental manipulation, the child is not obliged to produce the target. The stimuli should be novel.

[3]Fey (1986) suggests that grammatical forms used between 10–50% in a preintervention baseline should be considered primary intervention targets.

Figure 6.7 **CRT**

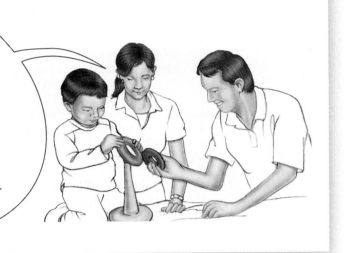

Ilan: Me get it!

SLP: You <u>got</u> the ring!

Ilan: Me throwed it.

SLP: You <u>threw</u> it, you <u>threw</u> the ring. Did Daddy hide the ring? No, Ilan <u>hid</u> the ring!

Ilan: Me putted it on.

SLP: Did you <u>put</u> the ring on the post? You <u>put</u> the ring on the post. What did Daddy do?

Ilan: Daddy <u>put</u> ring on!

Communication Challenge and Intervention Goals: Ilan does not use irregular past tense verbs. The adult uses sentence recasts maintaining Ilan's meaning but incorporating past tense verbs. The SLP sometimes alternates sentence modality between declarative and interrogative sentence construction.

CRT is most frequently implemented in individual or small-group sessions. Parents have been trained to use sentence recasts. However, CRT techniques require significant training—up to 10 sessions of training—for effective implementation. Data keeping in CRT consists of regular probes to monitor a child's production of the targeted grammatical form in spontaneous, untrained interactions. In Figure 6.6, preintervention baseline data are incorporated within the intervention goals.

Sentence recasting may be effectively combined with more adult-directed didactic therapy approaches (Fey & Proctor-Williams, 2000). The adult first teaches the grammatical form through modeling and imitation procedures. After a brief period of imitation and modeling practice, the adult introduces sentence recasts during conversational and book-reading interactions. The adult then alternates between modeling/imitation and CRT activities until the child spontaneously produces the target in novel interactions.

Evidence Supporting the CRT Approach. In the 1990s, a number of Level II studies documented CRT as effective; experts concluded that recast intervention helps children with language impairment acquire grammatical forms. More recently, researchers have investigated specific CRT techniques to learn how recasting can be used most effectively. For example, Hassink and Leonard (2010) examined the transcripts of recasting interventions provided for 17 preschoolers; the grammar target was third-person regular verbs. They reported that both noncorrective recasts and corrective recasts facilitate children's grammar. Data also suggested that using a recast when the child's utterance lacks a subject is not facilitative. The authors argue that when the child's utterance lacks a subject, the practitioner may misinterpret the child's intent. Consider the following example: CHILD: "Drive in the garage" ADULT: "The man drives in the garage." In this example, the child may have intended to say "I am driving in the garage," so the adult's misinterpretation is counterproductive and may draw the child's attention away from the grammar target. In the future, additional studies like this one will help SLPs understand how they can use recasting most appropriately with different populations and grammar targets.

INTERVENTION APPROACH: SENTENCE COMBINING (SC) INTERVENTION

During a sentence combining (SC) intervention, students are supported to (a) combine smaller related sentences into a compound sentence using the conjunctions *and, but,* and *because*; (b) embed an adjective or adverb from one sentence into another; (c) create complex sentences by embedding an adverbial and adjectival clause from one sentence into another; and/or (d) make multiple embeddings involving adjectives, adverbs, adverbial clauses, and adjectival clauses. In one approach, students work collaboratively in pairs while the adult provides support and modeling (Graham & Perin, 2007).

To understand how this is done, consider the following examples:

Simple Sentence #1: *The boy is running fast.*

Simple Sentence #2: *The boy wears a red hat.*

Simple Sentence #3: *The boy finished the race first.*

Complex Sentence #1: *The boy* who is wearing a red hat *is* running fast and finished *the race in first place.*

Complex Sentence #2: Because *the boy with the red hat is running fast, he finished the race in first place.*

In the examples above, *who is wearing a red hat* is a relative clause; *running fast and finished* demonstrates a compound sentence (i.e., two verbs joined with the conjunction *and*); and *because* is a subordinating conjunction. It is interesting to note the two complex sentences vary slightly in meaning: Complex Sentence #1 emphasizes the description of the boy (*wearing a red hat*), while Complex Sentence #2 emphasizes the boy's speed (*because he is running fast*).

Students' ability to use complex grammar is improved when they understand how using more sophisticated sentence structure conveys meaning. Sentence manipulation and sentence combining help students see how words can be put into varying patterns. Eisenberg (2006) describes two different forms of sentence combining: **open combining** and **sentence expansion**. During open combining, the student experiments with different ways of combining simple sentences to make a longer, more complex sentence (as shown in the examples above). During sentence expansion, the adult provides the student with a kernel sentence and then asks the student to elaborate the sentence. The example below demonstrates this process:

Adult: "*The kernel sentence is* The clown is happy. *Now expand the sentence and tell me why the clown is happy.*"

Student: "*The clown is happy* because *the dog is doing funny tricks.*"

Adult: "*Nice job! Now tell me where the clown is standing; remember to use descriptive vocabulary!*"

Student: "*The clown is happy* when *he stands under the* giant *tent.*"

Adult: "*Good job. Now make a complex sentence; this time use the word* but."

Student: "*The clown is happy,* but *he knows it's almost time to leave the circus.*"

You should note that the examples above demonstrate a sophisticated level of language production. It is unlikely that students with language impairment could spontaneously produce sentences at this level. Before asking a student with SLI to complete sentence expansions, generally a practitioner provides a variety of supportive techniques. Examples of supports include (a) showing pictures to help stimulate possible complex sentences, (b) providing several models before asking the student to produce a sentence, and (c) providing the student with written "scrambled sentences" and asking the student to combine words into varying combinations.

SC is an appropriate technique for school-age students and has even been used to improve grammar skills in college students. SC also has been documented as an intervention approach for remedial and at-risk students. Generally, brief sessions are better than semester-long drilling on SC (Eisenberg, 2006). The recommended practice is to provide shorter sessions of SC in combination with reminders to use longer sentences during writing practice. SC (as illustrated above) is an example of an adult-directed intervention technique.

Scott and Nelson (2009) describe the use of SC during the writing process for students with language impairment; the use of SC with student writing samples reflects a hybrid approach on the continuum of naturalness. In this hybrid model of intervention, SC is embedded within the writing process as students are asked to plan, draft, and revise original written stories.

A practitioner initiates a curriculum-based language assessment prior to implementing an SC intervention. To obtain baseline data, a practitioner has a student complete a writing probe. The practitioner then computes the occurrence of complex and compound sentences within the writing sample. The T-unit analysis (see Chapter 3) is a particularly appropriate qualitative approach to document sentence complexity. Periodic writing probes document the student's progress in the SC approach.

Evidence Supporting the Sentence-Combining Approach. A number of studies document the effectiveness of the SC approach (Andrews et al., 2006). For example, Saddler and Graham (2005) randomly assigned 44 fourth-grade writers to either SC or traditional grammar instruction groups. Practitioners taught the SC group to (a) combine sentences with *and, but,* and *because*; (b) embed adverbs or adjectives into sentences (e.g., simple sentences = *They eat food. They eat a lot*; more complex sentence = *They eat a lot of food*); and (c) create complex sentences by creating subordinate clauses. Students practiced the SC skills with their teacher and with a peer.

The control group was called the *grammar instruction group*. Practitioners taught the control group students the parts of speech and encouraged students to use descriptive nouns, verbs, adjectives, and adverbs. To assess students' writing development, students (a) provided a first- and second-draft writing sample to a picture prompt, (b) completed a sentence-combining task, and (c) were assessed with a norm-referenced test of writing ability (Test of Written Language–3 [TOWL-3]; Hammill & Larson, 1996). Results demonstrated that the students in the SC group were twice as likely to produce complex sentences during the SC task and scored significantly better on the SC subtest of the TOWL-3.

Analysis of the students' writing samples resulted in a more nuanced result. There was no treatment effect for the quality ratings of first drafts; however, the students in the SC group performed better on improving writing when they revised their papers. This result suggests that the SC approach improved the students' metaskills in terms of revising and rewriting. Overall, this level of evidence is consistent with the Level I hierarchy of intervention evidence.

Summary

- Specific language impairment (SLI) is a diagnosis based on exclusionary criteria. A child with SLI has a significant language impairment *without* associated hearing loss, cognitive deficit, or neurological or motor impairments. About 15% of children who are clinically considered to have SLI do not meet all of these exclusionary characteristics.

- Before age 5, children who are language delayed are sometimes referred to as having late language emergence (rather than SLI) because many children who are language delayed as toddlers catch up with their peers in late preschool. It is very important, however, to identify language delay at an early age. The prevalence of SLI is 7%.

- A primary focus of intervention is the development of morphosyntax, which is a primary area of difficulty in children with SLI. Young children with SLI have difficulty with verb forms (including auxiliary verbs), possessives, and pronouns, in addition to difficulty learning complex syntax and vocabulary. Pragmatic problems often occur because of problems with interactive communication. Children with SLI more frequently have phonological impairments than do their peers. A higher than expected percent of children diagnosed with SLI also are diagnosed with attention-deficit/hyperactivity disorder. Parent–child interactions sometimes require intervention to facilitate language learning for children who have SLI. During the school year, children with SLI often have difficulty with reading and writing development and peer interactions.

- Peer-mediated treatment is a form of intervention that focuses on children's social skills. Three basic paradigms for social skill building are social intervention with peers, peer confederate training, and sociodramatic script training. Interventionists can facilitate children's ability to (a) enter into play with other children, (b) play cooperatively, and (c) interact socially with school-age peers.

- A critical component of the assessment process is language sample analysis (LSA); in addition, assessors complete norm-referenced and criterion-referenced assessments on children with SLI. Two criterion-referenced assessments are parent–child interaction observations and curriculum-based language assessments. Both are forms of naturalistic assessment providing multiple opportunities for an individual to perform skills across domains (i.e., social, cognitive, motor, communication).

- Three intervention approaches for children with SLI include enhanced milieu teaching (EMT), conversational recast training (CRT), and sentence combining (SC). EMT includes the mand-model, time-delay, and incidental teaching strategies, along with adult modeling. CRT uses a strategy called sentence recasting. SC is an intervention appropriate for school-aged students who need to improve sentence complexity.

Discussion and In-Class Activities

1. In a small group, role-play a scenario in which you present the results of an assessment to a parent. Imagine that the child is age 4 and is talking in two- and three-word combinations; he demonstrates a number of syntax and morphological errors (e.g., "Me do it!"). His receptive language is better than his expressive language, but his receptive language is slightly delayed. He has a number of phonological errors but is

about 60% intelligible. He is within normal limits in IQ and has normal hearing. The parent wants to know what is causing his child's impairment. Role-play your answer. Make sure you explain in a way that is meaningful to a parent without background knowledge of language development.

2. Role-play a social group and have one student use poor social communication skills to enter the group interaction. Discuss problems and write one or two goals that could be implemented to improve the student's peer interaction.

3. View a videotape of a child with SLI. Use the utterance-level worksheet in Chapter 3 (Table 3.3) to analyze the child's language. Discuss the ways that the child is pragmatically successful or unsuccessful. Discuss the errors demonstrated in morphosyntax. How do these two language domains operate independently in the communication of young children? Write an intervention goal for the child as a result of the language sample analysis.

4. Obtain a case example with a conversational transcript or a videotape of an older student with SLI. Refer to the information in Chapter 3 on topic control, conversational repair, informativeness, and conjunctive cohesion. Write an intervention goal based on the decision-making process.

5. Obtain a case example with a conversational transcript or a videotape of a young child at Brown's Stage I. Use the enhanced milieu decision tree in Figure 6.3 to determine a possible EMT strategy. Write intervention goals based on the decision-making process.

6. Write two to three additional goals that are consistent with the CRT and the SC approaches. Determine a language target appropriate for either younger children (e.g., present progressive verbs, third-person regular verbs, pronoun use, regular past tense) or older students (e.g., subordinate conjunctions, embedded clauses). Also use objects for younger children (e.g., dolls, trucks, balls, bubbles, bean bags) or pictures for older school-age students. Role-play an adult–student interaction representing the two approaches with the items provided.

Chapter 6 Case Study 1

Zachary is a 10-year-old fifth grader. He is social and well liked by his peers. He is a natural athlete but doesn't enjoy organized sports. He doesn't easily follow the coaches' verbal instructions, and this interferes with his participation. Zachary's interests are rap music and video games. He enjoys talking about his favorite topics but loses interest when the conversation changes to other topics.

Zachary's parents are both attorneys; they work with him daily to help him complete his homework. He was in third grade before he could decode grade-level text. Now, in fifth grade, Zachary is a slow reader and does not easily comprehend what he reads. He works diligently to complete his schoolwork, but his work is generally low average. His writing consists of simple sentences and is produced slowly. Zachary is well behaved in class but generally doesn't participate in classroom discussions.

Zachary's parents are not sure what, if anything, they should do to help Zachary participate more in class and improve his reading and writing. Zachary has not been previously assessed for language impairment or learning disabilities.

Questions for Discussion

1. What do you think might be the underlying cause of Zachary's communication style (e.g., avoiding unfamiliar topics)?
2. What classroom-based assessments might you consider to obtain more information about Zachary's abilities?
3. What kinds of information could you provide to Zachary's parents to help them understand their son's abilities?
4. What educational or communication goals could be included in an intervention program for Zachary?

Chapter 6 Case Study 2

In this chapter, I discussed how a primary deficit in morphosyntax may trickle down, resulting in associated semantic and pragmatic deficits. The following case study discusses how a morphosyntax delay can impact other language domains.

Logan is in second grade and has been diagnosed with SLI. He has difficulty with morphosyntax, particularly in complex sentences that contain causal conjunctions such as *because* and *if*.

Logan's class is completing a science unit on "states of matter" (i.e., liquid, solid, gas). In one experiment, the students heat water, record water temperature, and make predictions regarding when they believe the water will start to evaporate. Along with the prediction, each student is expected to provide a rationale—to explain why the water evaporates faster at a higher temperature. Logan is frustrated during this science activity. He misbehaves during the experiment; he does not interact well with his peers, does not follow the inquiry process "rules" (i.e., asking questions, explaining the rationale for his prediction), and struggles to learn the required science vocabulary (e.g., this science unit includes target vocabulary such as *condense, evaporate, hypothesize,* and *investigate*).

Questions for Discussion

1. What language skills are needed for science inquiry?
2. How might Logan's morphosyntax deficits impact his semantic development?
3. How might Logan's morphosyntax deficits impact his pragmatic development?
4. How might an SLP support Logan's academic skills?

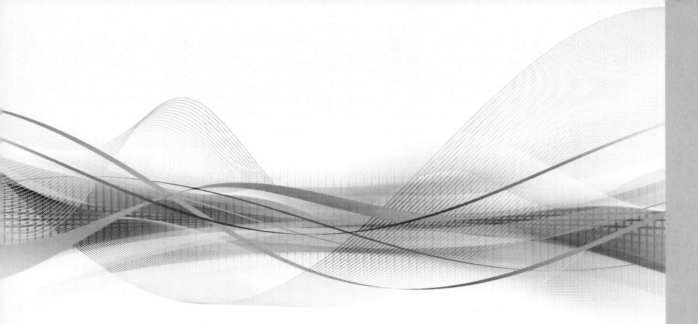

7 *Children with Hearing Loss*

—Lori A. Pakulski

Chapter Overview Questions

1. What are the differences between hearing losses (HLs) classified as sensorineural, conductive, and mixed?
2. What are APD and AN/AD? How are they different from other types of hearing impairments?
3. What language domains are potentially affected by HL?
4. What paradigm shift has radically changed intervention for children with HL? How might

outcomes be different for children with HL who have co-occurring conditions?
5. What factors are of concern at early stages of HL identification?
6. What facilitative counseling strategies are used when working with a family?
7. What are the Cottage Acquisition Scales and the Ling Sound Test?
8. What are "Learning to Listen" sounds, and how are children exposed to these sounds?

This chapter focuses on language learning in the presence of a hearing loss (HL). You will learn about the language challenges associated with hearing loss. In addition, I will discuss issues surrounding your role as a practitioner as you work with a child with HL, his or her family, audiologists, and educators.

Children with HL are a heterogeneous group, meaning that the cause and severity of HL varies significantly. The ways that children learn to communicate also vary. For example, many young children will experience fluctuating and temporary hearing loss caused by infection in the middle ear (known as **chronic otitis media**); other children have permanent hearing loss due to damage in the inner ear. Some families choose to teach their children to listen and talk; other families communicate through sign language. People often assume that if a child has a significant and permanent hearing loss, he or she must learn sign language to communicate. However, today many, if not most, children can learn to listen and talk effectively thanks to early identification and intervention that includes high-power digital hearing aids and **cochlear implants**. This chapter will help you explore the impact of HL on language. The information I present will allow you to help children and their families maximize their language potential.

Description of the Disorder

PREVALENCE

An increasing number of children are born each year in the United States with significant permanent hearing loss (4 out of every 1000), making it one of the most common disabilities (Alexander Graham Bell Association [AG Bell], 2011). Hearing loss also occurs after birth. Middle ear infection, or **otitis media,** is the most common reason U.S. children are seen by a physician. Otitis media may cause HL in as many as one-third of affected children in kindergarten and first-grade classrooms on any given day. The prevalence of HL increases with age; 20% of the U.S. population aged 12 years and older has hearing difficulties severe enough to impact communication (Lin, Niparko, & Ferrucci, 2011). Because most children learn language by hearing it, a child's early exposure to language is critical in building communication skills. Children with HL are at risk for delays in speech, language, and intellectual development.

TYPES OF HEARING LOSS

Hearing loss is identified by type (**conductive, sensorineural,** or **mixed**) and severity. When the hearing loss occurs in the outer and middle ear, it is called a conductive loss. A conductive loss is typically the result of a medical problem, such as a fluid-filled middle ear (otitis media), or damage, such as a perforated eardrum. Because most conductive disorders are amenable to medical treatment, the hearing loss is typically temporary. Despite the temporary nature of the loss, fluctuating or inconsistent hearing in early childhood may cause problems in the development of auditory brain centers and language (Ucles et al., 2012).

Three out of four children will experience at least one episode of otitis media by the time they are 3 years old; many will experience repeated episodes. Children who experience repeated (chronic) otitis media are at risk for other problems. Emerging data suggest that recurrent otitis media has a considerable negative impact on the quality of life of children and causes concern to their caregivers. These effects are proportional to the severity of the condition (e.g., Dubé, De Wals, & Ouakki, 2010).

Sensorineural losses are caused by damage to the inner ear structures or auditory nerves. When a child has both a sensorineural hearing impairment and a conductive disorder (e.g., permanent hearing loss due to a genetic disorder co-occurring with a middle ear infection), the loss is called *mixed.*

Sensorineural hearing loss can be caused by a number of factors, including genetic disorders, birth defects, premature birth, and infections such as meningitis. Typically,

Table 7.1 **Co-occurring Conditions**

Condition	Percentage of children
Autism	1.7%
Attention-deficit/hyperactivity disorder	5.4%
Visual impairment	5.5%
Learning disability	8.0%
Other	10.2%
Intellectual disability and/or developmental delay	13.6%
No additional disorders	61%

one-third of congenital losses are attributed to genetic disorders, one-third to nongenetic disorders, and one-third to unknown causation. Disorders that can co-occur with HL are presented in Table 7.1. As you can see in Table 7.1, because 40% of children with profound hearing loss have additional disabilities (Gallaudet Research Institute, 2011), it is important to note that not all children with HL will respond to similar treatment strategies in the same way.

Before you read the rest of this chapter, you might need to learn more or review information about the anatomy of the hearing system. There is an excellent series of video presentations on ear anatomy on the web at www.nebraskamed.com/health-library/3d-medical-atlas/topic/16/ear.

VARIATIONS IN HL BY RACE/ETHNICITY

Various types of hearing problems impact race or ethnic groups differently. There are more European Americans with HL (47%) than Hispanic/Latinos (25%) or African Americans (15%; Gallaudet Research Institute, 2011). European Americans also are more susceptible to noise-induced hearing loss than are African Americans, whereas Alaska Natives and American Indian populations experience more frequent otitis media (Singleton et al., 2009).

DEGREE OF HEARING LOSS

One way to think about HL is to consider the sounds a person can and cannot hear. A person with normal hearing can detect very soft sounds, ranging from low-frequency sounds to high-frequency sounds. Sound **frequency** relates to the perceptual quality we call **pitch**. Most hearing tests measure pitch by exposing the listener to sounds ranging from 250 Hz to 8000 Hz. The sound of a bullfrog is a common example of a low-frequency sound, while a bird tweeting is a high-frequency sound. In terms of human speech, *oo* is low frequency and *s* is high frequency.

The **degree of hearing loss**—that is, the severity of the HL—determines which sounds will be inaudible to a person. The degree of hearing loss is determined by measuring the **intensity** level at which a person can detect sounds. Intensity level relates to the perceptual quality of loudness. The degree of loss is determined by identifying an individual's **hearing threshold** and is measured in **decibels (dB)**. A person with normal hearing acuity can

Table 7.2 **Categorizing Degree of Hearing Impairment in Children**

Degree of loss	Decibel level (dB)
Normal	−10 to 15
Slight	16 to 25
Mild	26 to 40
Moderate	41 to 55
Moderately severe	56 to 70
Severe	71 to 90
Profound	91+

Source: American Speech-Language-Hearing Association (ASHA), 2013.

hear very soft sounds and has hearing thresholds in the range of 0 dB to 15 dB across the frequency range. When a person requires more intensity or loudness to hear a sound, the person is said to have HL. A degree or severity rating (from slight to profound loss) is assigned according to the intensity (in decibels) necessary for a person to detect a particular sound (see Table 7.2). The degree of impairment may vary across the frequency range or between ears. HL can also be characterized in terms of temporary or permanent, fluctuating or progressive, and unilateral (one ear) vs. bilateral (both ears). As you can already see, the reasons for and implications of a hearing loss are complex. It is important to consider the kinds of questions and concerns parents will bring to you as a professional. Begin to build your clinical skills by considering the issues posed in Focus 7.1.

AUDITORY PERCEPTUAL PROBLEMS

There is an additional disability type that is related to auditory perceptual problems rather than hearing loss. Auditory perceptual problems are generally caused by **auditory processing disorder (APD)** or **auditory neuropathy/dys-synchrony (AN/AD)**. APD and AN/AD are auditory problems, but they cannot be categorized within the domains described above. APD, also sometimes called **central auditory processing disorder (CAPD)**, refers to the efficiency and effectiveness by which the central nervous system uses auditory information. APD/CAPD includes the auditory mechanisms underlying the skills of sound localization and lateralization; auditory discrimination; auditory pattern recognition; temporal aspects of audition, including temporal integration, temporal discrimination, temporal

---

FOCUS 7.1 *Clinical Skill Building*

What parent concerns might you learn of that could indicate a potential hearing loss? How might the concerns differ for a mild hearing loss, a severe hearing loss, or an auditory processing problem?

ordering, and temporal masking; auditory performance in competing acoustic signals; and auditory performance with degraded acoustic signals (Buehler, 2012). Children identified as having APD typically are referred for assessment or intervention because they have difficulty with hearing in noisy situations, remembering spoken information (i.e., auditory memory deficits), maintaining focus on an activity if other sounds are present, reading and/or spelling, and processing nonverbal information (e.g., recognizing variations in pitch or duration of sounds).

Current research suggests that APD is caused by malfunctioning of the auditory pathway to the brain or small defects in the brain's auditory cortex and/or the language learning centers of the brain (Miller & Wagstaff, 2011; Sharma, Purdy, & Kelly, 2009). The auditory-neural defects do not result in a true loss of hearing sensitivity; the outer, middle, and inner ear function well. However, the neural or auditory pathway deficits make it difficult for an individual with APD to comprehend spoken language. In other words, the loss is not due to access to sound or audibility—so hearing aids do not help. Instead, the individual may benefit from an assistive device to help highlight the desired signal (speech) so that it can be differentiated from background noise. In other cases, an individual with APD may need to learn speech-decoding strategies. As you can imagine, auditory processing disorders are difficult to identify and may not be diagnosed until a student is school age.

AN/AD is another auditory processing deficit; in this case the auditory signal is impeded as it travels from the cochlea to the brain. Like APD, AN/AD is not due to a malfunction in the outer, middle, or inner ear. However, it can be diagnosed early with an appropriate test battery.

The treatment for children with APD and AN/AD can be either different from or in some ways similar to intervention programs for children with HL. For example, some children with AN/AD are provided a cochlear implant to bypass malfunctions in the auditory system. However, a cochlear implant is not appropriate for children with APD.

Environmental management *is* important for children with APD and AN/AD. If listening is challenging, improving the intensity level of the desired sound signal so that it can be differentiated from background noise benefits both APD and AN/AD listeners. The ratio of the desired sound to background noise level is called the signal-to-noise ratio (SNR). SNR is important for all listeners, but it is particularly important for children with auditory perceptual problems. In most cases, intervention focuses on remediation of the language disorders resulting from the child's auditory processing difficulties. See Focus 7.2 for more information regarding the results of a systematic review of the APD literature.

Causation, Risk Factors, and Communication Impairments

Many factors affect language development in children with HL. The most important factors include the age when the hearing impairment occurs (e.g., congenital, or acquired before or after the child learns to speak), the age when the hearing loss is identified and treated, the child's auditory and language experience, and the level of parental involvement. I present more information about these factors within this chapter.

It is important to remember that a child's language development will vary in relation to the severity and type of hearing loss (e.g., mild conductive loss vs. severe sensorineural loss) and other less critical factors. Normal hearing allows auditory access to spoken

---

FOCUS 7.2   *Clinical Skill Building*

Evidence-Based Systematic Review of APD Studies

As noted elsewhere in this book, it is important for practitioners to continually evaluate the research evidence that does (or does not) support the implementation of specific intervention approaches. Fey and his colleagues (2011) evaluated all available peer-reviewed literature on the efficacy of interventions on school-age children with APD. Searches of 28 electronic databases yielded 25 studies for analysis; the studies were categorized and ranked on a standard set of quality features evaluating the methodology and results of each study. After evaluating the scientific evidence, the experts concluded that there was little indication that observed improvements were due to the auditory listening tasks included in these programs. Examples of auditory listening tasks included listening to sounds in competing noise or listening to speech with modified rate or intensity. In sum, there was not enough evidence to provide clear guidance to speech-language pathologists faced with treating children diagnosed with APD.

Fey and colleagues recommended that practitioners who decide to use auditory interventions should be aware of the limitations in the evidence and take special care to monitor the spoken and written language status of their young clients. Based on these recommendations, and until there is more research, many practitioners are choosing to focus on the language and literacy deficits evidenced by children rather than include auditory listening tasks as part of the intervention approach.

It will be important to monitor the research evaluating the effectiveness of APD interventions in the coming years.

---

language from birth and even before birth (i.e., prenatal development). When a permanent hearing loss exists, language acquisition is affected because children cannot access everyday communication interactions. The lack of auditory access also results in a lack of self-monitoring of speech and language productions. For example, children with HL (who are not exposed to amplified sound) begin to make babbling sounds, but their babbling does not continue due to a lack of self-monitoring. The "feedback loop" between sound production and auditory stimulation does not maintain the babbling behavior.

Extensive research has documented the impact of hearing loss on children's language development. Studies have investigated the language proficiency of children with HL who use spoken language and children with HL who use manual communication (e.g., American Sign Language [ASL]). Most recently, research has focused on the benefits of early intervention and early cochlear implantation. Due to technological advances in auditory amplification, the field of deafness and HL has undergone a **paradigm shift**: a radical change in thinking, leading to new approaches.

The paradigm shift that has occurred in the area of deafness and HL can be summarized in this way:

> When family and environmental support are in place and when appropriate and high quality amplification and early intensive intervention is provided, a child with HL who is identified and treated in the first few months of life has the potential of developing language commensurate with normal hearing peers when no other disorders exist. (Moeller, 2000, p. E43)

Table 7.3 **Language Problems of Children with Hearing Impairment**

Dimension	Concern
Phonology	Child experiences difficulty with (a) managing breath stream for speech, (b) rotating tongue forward and backward to establish vowel postures, and (c) moving articulators smoothly and continuously from one articulatory posture to the next.
Pragmatics	Child has difficulty due to inexperience (e.g., limited conversational partners).
Semantics	Child may not have sufficient vocabulary variety; may not have complex vocabulary; may not understand subtle differences or figurative language.
Syntax	Child demonstrates unsophisticated grammatical forms and sentence structures; may have a reduced mean length of utterance.

This paradigm shift has changed family decision making regarding communication options. An example of this shift was reported in a program in North Carolina in which parents are given unbiased information about all communication options. In 1995, 60% of the families chose to use sign language, while only 40% chose spoken language options. In contrast, by 2005, 85% of the families chose spoken language options, while only 15% chose sign language (Brown, 2006). We will discuss the implications of the different communication modalities later in this chapter.

It is also important to remember that some children with HL do not access services at early ages or their hearing loss is complicated by other associated conditions (see Table 7.1). In this situation, children with HL are likely to demonstrate language deficits similar to those of other children with language impairment. The additional risk factors may result in selecting sign language as the most appropriate communication option.

The categories of language impairment for children with HL reflect the domains of language that by now are familiar to you. Language domains include morphological and syntax deficits as well as semantic, pragmatic, and speech production problems (i.e., articulation and phonological deficits). A summary of specific language problems is provided in Table 7.3. Children who have been identified at older ages as having HL or who have associated deficits may experience language problems ranging from mild to severe.

Factors Influencing Outcomes for Children with Hearing Loss

A number of factors strongly affect language outcomes for children with hearing loss. In this section, I discuss three factors: (a) early identification and audiological management, (b) choice of **communication modality,** and (c) family involvement in the remediation process. In 1993, the National Institutes of Health's (NIH) Consensus Development Conference concluded that all infants should be screened for hearing loss, preferably before hospital discharge. More than a decade later, most states have adopted universal newborn hearing screening (UNHS) as part of an early detection of hearing impairment (EDHI) program. EDHI programs provide two critical improvements: (1) Children are now identified at birth as opposed to 2 or 3 years of age, and (2) intervention can begin within critical windows of opportunity in the first few months of life. In short, the educational outlook for children born with hearing loss is remarkably better today due to universal screening.

EARLY DETECTION

Early detection underlies the paradigm shift that has occurred in the field of deafness and hearing loss. Left untreated, children with HL will have delays in auditory and language development (Ching et al., 2013; Fulcher et al., 2012), and this language gap will widen over time (Huber & Kipman, 2012; Sininger, Grimes, & Christensen, 2010). However, new evidence demonstrates that children who are identified and treated within the first year of life can achieve language levels equivalent to their hearing peers (Fulcher et al., 2012). It is important to note, however, that achievement of typical language levels is not guaranteed; children with HL who have the best chance of achieving a within-normal-limits language levels (a) do not have other risk conditions, (b) are diagnosed at birth and receive amplification by 3 months, (c) are enrolled in interventions that focus on listening and speaking by 6 months, and (d) receive a cochlear implant by 18 months, if required. However, the fact that a child with HL can reach a typical level of language development is important because it demonstrates that hearing impairment in and of itself does not diminish a child's learning and communication ability. However, late identification paired with lack of treatment has profound negative consequences and may limit a child's ability to learn to listen and talk.

NEUROPLASTICITY

The ability to achieve language levels consistent with hearing peers is based on the fact that the auditory system, which supports language development, is "plastic." This phenomenon is known as **neuroplasticity** of the auditory system. Auditory plasticity means that despite damage or disease, the auditory system can develop appropriately with early stimulation. If we remember that we hear with our ears and listen with our brain, it makes sense that if sound does not reach the brain (auditory deprivation), the auditory system development in the brain will be arrested (Kral & Sharma, 2012).

However, with early stimulation, the brain grows and refines the auditory neural connections needed for spoken language development (Kral & Sharma, 2012; Sharma, 2007). Importantly, if auditory skills are mastered as close as possible to the typical "biological clock," the neural system experiences **developmental synchrony** (Robbins et al., 2004). Developmental synchrony is the brain's ability to take advantage of developmental "windows of opportunity" (Flexer et al., 2005; Robbins et al., 2004). Researchers have reported that without auditory stimulation, the human central auditory system remains maximally plastic for only 3.5 years; this period of time is considered the sensitive period for auditory development (Sharma, Dorman, & Spahr, 2002). To summarize this important information: A child who receives intervention, particularly auditory stimulation, in the first year of life outperforms children who are identified at later ages (Kral & Sharma, 2012; Miyamoto et al., 2007). More importantly, children who are identified early are likely to have language quotients (language age/chronological age) consistent with their hearing peers by kindergarten (Kral & Sharma, 2012). For a more in-depth look at language development in children with HL, review the following articles and books:

- Cole, E. B., & Flexer, C. (2012). *Children with hearing loss: Developing listening and talking, birth to six* (2nd ed.) San Diego: Plural Publishing.
- Easterbrooks, S. R., & Beal-Alvarez, J. (2013). *Literacy instruction for students who are deaf and hard of hearing.* New York: Oxford University.
- Paul, P. (2009). *Language and deafness* (4th ed.). Sudbury, MA: Jones & Bartlett.

CHOOSING A COMMUNICATION MODALITY

One of the most controversial aspects of working with children with HL relates to issues surrounding the choice of communication modality. You might be aware that there is a controversy between proponents of **Deaf culture** and professionals who believe that children with HL can learn to talk and listen. The situation is complex because 95% of children born with significant hearing loss are raised by parents who can hear (Mitchell & Karchmer, 2004). If parents consider the language used in their home and community, spoken language is chosen as the preferred communication modality. On the other hand, if parents consider the philosophy of the Deaf community—whose members believe that that deafness is not a disorder to be fixed but a culture to be embraced—parents may consider using sign language as the child's native language and focus on teaching English in its written form as a second language (bilingual). Additional information about the Deaf culture is presented in Focus 7.3.

In order to bridge this difference of opinion, many families choose **total (or simultaneous) communication**, a mode of communication combining spoken language with sign language. Regardless of the specific communication mode a family chooses for a child,

---

FOCUS 7.3   *Multicultural Issues*

Deaf Culture

For those of us who are hearing, it is sometimes difficult to imagine a culture that celebrates deafness—something we might consider to be a deficit or disability. *Culture,* by definition, is a set of learned behaviors of a group of people who have their own language, values, rules of behavior, and traditions. When we consider this definition, it makes sense that a culture may develop when a group of like individuals forms a community around a shared experience such as deafness. If they define themselves by their deafness, they may find that they have common interests, shared norms of behavior, and similar techniques for facing life challenges. A culture provides social interaction and emotional support.

The cornerstone of Deaf culture is American Sign Language (ASL). Members of the Deaf culture have a sense of pride about their language and its rich culture. Mastery of ASL and skillful storytelling are valued; wisdom, values, and heritage are passed from generation to generation through ASL. When ASL is the primary language for social interactions, written language (English) must be learned as a second language. For this reason, those in the Deaf culture often consider themselves bilingual-bicultural. You can learn more about Deaf culture by going to the website www.gallaudet.edu and searching for "Deaf culture."

critical components of intervention must be realized, whether the child is taught to listen and talk, to use sign language and learn English as a second language, or to use total communication.

A professional provides information to families to help them make important decisions about their child's communication modality. Each communication modality has positive and negative considerations, and efficacy data must be considered when presenting data to families. Efficacy data represent research-based documentation of intervention outcomes. Below, I discuss approaches and highlight research data pertaining to two communication modalities: spoken communication (talking and listening) and sign language (total communication approach).

Approaches Focusing on Talking and Listening. Historically, when practitioners implemented talking and listening interventions with HL children, they used either an auditory-verbal or auditory-oral approach. Today, auditory-verbal and auditory-oral approaches have more similarities than differences and lead to similar outcomes (AG Bell, 2013). The AG Bell Academy now recommends using a newer term, **listening and spoken language specialists (LSLS)**, rather than categorizing practitioners with labels such as auditory-verbal specialist or auditory-oral specialist. The guiding principles and philosophies guiding listening and spoken language (LSL) terminology are summarized in Table 7.4.

LSL intervention emerged primarily from parallel work done in the mid-20th century by Doreen Pollack in Colorado and Helen Beebe in Pennsylvania. These pioneers believed that with intensive and appropriate intervention, children could learn to listen and talk. In the early years of the approach, their methods were not consistently supported, as some educators considered that LSL approaches "forced" children who were deaf to use their senses in unconventional ways. In reality, their methods were somewhat ahead of their time, considering that at the time hearing aids were less than adequate and children were typically not identified with an HL until age 2 or 3. The cornerstone of the LSL approach is that children can and must be taught to develop listening function and, with intensive intervention, will be able to develop spoken language.

LSL goals include integration of listening, speech, language, and cognition, following the normal developmental sequence. Much as with typically developing children, with LSL approaches, children with HL learn to listen before learning to talk. Early intervention includes development of prespeech and language skills with listening as the foundation, without regard for the child's age. In other words, if Johnny's hearing loss is identified and treated beginning at age 2, his LSLS begins by teaching Johnny to listen to sounds just as if he were a baby. The LSL principle is that Johnny's hearing is like that of an infant. This concept, called **hearing age**, refers to the amount of time that a child has had exposure to sound. In other words, the number of years between the time a person is treated for hearing impairment (e.g., hearing aids fitted and intervention initiated) and his chronological age is his hearing age. Learn more about hearing age in Focus 7.4. In order to engage a child, LSL activities must be interesting and motivating so that the child will attend to and persist in the LSL tasks.

Research Evidence for LSL Approaches. It is important that your recommendations to parents reflect recent studies that support (or refute) a particular intervention approach. Prior to 2010, most research supporting the LSL approach was retrospective data obtained by evaluating records or interviewing prior students to determine outcomes. Retrospective

Table 7.4 **Philosophy and Principles for Listening and Spoken Language Specialists (LSLS)**

Philosophy:

a. LSLS professionals help children who are deaf or hard of hearing develop spoken language and literacy, primarily through listening.
b. LSLS professionals focus on education, guidance, advocacy, family support, and the rigorous application of techniques, strategies, and procedures that promote optimal acquisition of spoken language through listening by newborns, infants, toddlers, and children who are deaf or hard of hearing.
c. LSLS professionals guide parents in helping their children develop intelligible spoken language through listening and coach them in advocating their children's inclusion in the mainstream school. Ultimately, parents gain confidence that their children will have access to the full range of educational, social, and vocational choices in life.

Designations of certification for LSLS professionals:

a. Certified Auditory-Verbal Therapist (LSLS Cert. AVT; the LSLS Cert. AVT works one-on-one with the child and family in all intervention sessions).
b. Certified Auditory-Verbal Educator (LSLS Cert. AVEd; the LSLS Cert. AVEd involves the family and also works directly with the child in individual or group/classroom settings).

The two types of LSLS have similar knowledge and skills and work on behalf of the child and family.

Principles:

- Specialists from both designations follow developmental models of audition, speech, language, cognition, and communication.
- Specialists from both designations use evidence-based practices.
- Specialists from both designations strive for excellent outcomes in listening, spoken language, literacy, and independence for children who are deaf or hard of hearing.

Source: Adapted from *AG Bell Academy for Listening and Spoken Language*, Alexander Graham Bell Association, 2013, retrieved May, 2013, from www.listeningandspokenlanguage.org/AcademyDocument.aspx?id=541. Used with permission.

FOCUS 7.4   *Intervention*

Hearing Age

When comparing children with hearing loss to their typically hearing peers, it is common to compare their developmental skills based on hearing age as opposed to chronological age, much as a premature infant might be compared by gestational age. Hearing age, sometimes called *listening age,* is used to recognize the important role of audition in the development of language and underscores the expected delay in language until auditory concerns are properly addressed. The closer the chronological age is to the hearing age, the more likely a child's language skills are to be on target by the time he or she reaches school age.

studies are considered Level III research. (See Chapter 1 for a review of the levels of evidence.) Since 2010, there have been high-quality nonrandomized studies supporting the LSL approach that have provided more rigorous Level II evidence. The studies listed below are examples of recent research regarding the effectiveness of the LSL approach:

- Hickson and colleagues (2010) completed a longitudinal study in which they examined outcomes for 29 children with HL (ages 2–6 years) enrolled in speaking and listening interventions. They compared the children with HL with typically hearing children at 9, 21, and 38 months. An assessment battery was used to measure speech and language ability, reading, mathematics, and self-esteem. Results showed no significant differences between the groups for speech, language, and self-esteem. Reading and mathematics scores were comparable between the groups, although there was not enough data for statistical analysis. The authors concluded that the speaking and listening intervention was effective for their sample of children with hearing loss.

- Fulcher and colleagues (2012) considered whether a group of 45 children with HL, who were identified prior to 1 year of age, could achieve age-appropriate speech and language outcomes at 3, 4, and 5 years of age. The children had a range of levels of hearing loss but had no other developmental risk factors. Fulcher et al. compared the development of the children identified early with those identified later. The children identified early significantly outperformed those who were identified later at all ages and for all severities of HL. Importantly, by 5 years of age, 96% of the children identified early achieved typical levels of performance in speech, and 100% of the children identified early had typical levels of language ability.

One of the factors contributing to successful outcomes for children with HL learning to speak and listen is the increased use of cochlear implants. Approximately 188,000 people worldwide have received cochlear implants. In the United States, approximately 41,500 adults and 25,500 children have received cochlear implants (NIDCD, 2013), and it is estimated that about 1 million individuals in the United States could benefit from them (Parisier, 2003). Faster rates of language learning and higher overall language achievement levels are consistently documented in children who use cochlear implants compared to their deaf peers who use hearing aids (Svirsky et al., 2000). The basis for improving the language-learning trajectory when children receive cochlear implants at early ages relates to sensitive periods and neural plasticity (Ganek, Robbins, & Niparko, 2012).

Cochlear implants have external (outside) components and internal (surgically implanted) parts that work together to allow the user to perceive sound. The external components of the cochlear implant include a microphone, a speech processor, and a transmitter. The microphone picks up sounds and sends them to the speech processor. The speech processor is a computer that analyzes and digitizes the sound signals and sends them to a transmitter that in turn sends these to an implanted receiver just under the skin. The receiver takes the coded electrical signals from the transmitter and delivers them to electrodes that have been surgically inserted in the cochlea. The electrodes (i.e., internal components) stimulate the fibers of the auditory nerve so that the listener perceives sound sensations (Carlson et al., 2012). Results indicate that children who access auditory stimuli through a cochlear implant early in life can develop spoken language and literacy competence commensurate with their hearing peers (Eisenberg, Fink, & Niparko, 2006; Moog, 2002; Nicholas & Geers, 2006; Spencer, Barker, & Tomblin, 2003; Svirsky et al., 2000). An illustration of a child wearing a cochlear implant is shown in Figure 7.1.

Figure 7.1 **Child with a Cochlear Implant**

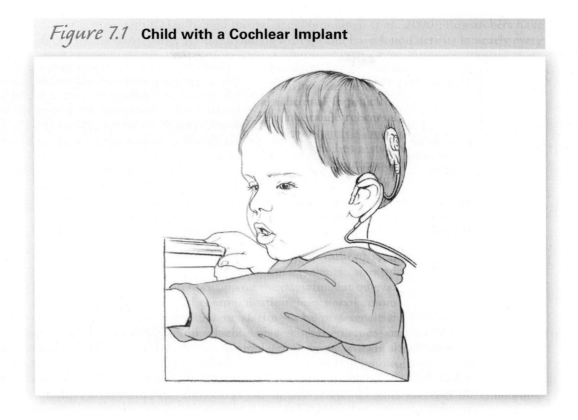

Family and Educational Issues for LSL Communicators. Before selecting any communication modality, families should receive unbiased information about the range of options for children with HL, including information about ASL, total communication, and interventions focusing on speaking and listening. Families also should have a chance to interact with individuals who are members of the Deaf culture; individuals who communicate orally with the benefit of hearing aids or cochlear implants; and individuals who have been educated in typical classrooms, center-based classrooms, or residential schools. As mentioned previously in this chapter, because of current hearing technology, increasingly more families are choosing an LSL approach.

The LSL philosophy is founded on the belief that strong auditory skills are critical for language development. In order for children to obtain sufficient auditory experience, parents must (a) maximize auditory input by accessing high-quality and ongoing audiological services, (b) implement all available technology (e.g., hearing aids, cochlear implants), and (c) provide intensive auditory and language experiences in age-appropriate and natural contexts. All this intervention and management is, of course, guided by professionals.

Once a parent decides to commit to an LSL approach, finding qualified professionals to manage the intensive intervention program is challenging. While the LSLS certification is becoming widely recognized, there are still relatively few certified LSL specialists. The LSLS certification process, begun in 2008, helps more specialists receive the appropriate training. Check out the AG Bell website, at www.agbellacademy.org/certification.htm, for more information on the certification process for LSL specialists.

Table 7.5 **Tips for Collaborating with Teachers**

Make sure teachers are well informed. Help teachers understand . . .	• a child's auditory and language-learning needs. • which classroom situations will be challenging. • how to identify auditory and language problems. • how to read an audiogram and understand its implications on classroom performance.
Coordinate inservice training with the audiologist and SLPs so that teachers . . .	• can recognize and troubleshoot amplification device problems. • improve classroom acoustics (e.g., put pads or old tennis balls on table and chair legs).
Provide teachers with instructional tips that improve auditory access to the high language demands in the classroom.	• Outline each day's schedule on the board. • Send home materials for prelearning. • Always face the class when speaking.

Because the overarching goal of LSL is full participation in society for children with HL, inclusion in regular education is expected in LSL approaches. This principle is consistent with the Individuals with Disabilities Education Act (IDEA, 2004). However, achieving complete educational inclusion can be challenging. Common barriers to full inclusion include lack of understanding of the approach on the part of the administrators and educators, lack of an appropriate auditory learning environment, and failure to use all available auditory technology. Table 7.5 and Focus 7.5 provide suggestions and highlight issues pertaining to working with teachers.

Approaches Focusing on Visual Learning and Manual Communication. Sign language has received a great deal of attention as a means of improving the early communication skills of typically developing (normal hearing) infants (e.g., Seal, 2010). The popular press has dubbed this approach "baby signs."

In addition to being used with typically developing infants, sign language sometimes is used to enhance the expressive language of children with communication disorders other than HL (e.g., autism, Down syndrome). However, the use of sign language for

FOCUS 7.5   *Issues for School-Age Children*

Inclusion for Children with Hearing Loss: Working with Teachers

Inclusion is an educational option that allows children with HL to be in the classroom with their typically hearing peers. In this model, support is provided to both students and teachers in order to facilitate optimal access to learning. To improve your clinical decision-making skills, give some examples of how an SLP could work with a teacher if a child with a hearing loss were in a general education classroom.

children with intellectual disability (ID) or autism spectrum disorder (ASD) must be considered separately from its use related to HL. The underlying cause of language delay in ID or ASD is completely different from the language challenges of children with HL. Consequently, the rationale for choosing sign language as a alternative means of communication for a child with autism or intellectual disability is very different from the rationale for choosing manual communication for children with HL.

Sign language as a communication approach for children with HL is based on an underlying philosophy: Children who are deaf use sign language because they can see but not hear. Deaf students are primarily visual learners because "they use their eyes as their primary learning channel. They can process some language and environmental information aurally, but this auditory channel is secondary to the visual channel" (Maryland School for the Deaf [MSD], 2009, pg. 11). If you compare this statement to the findings presented earlier related to the development of auditory channels of the brain and the impact on spoken language, it should be evident that there is a clear difference of opinion. The conflicting views in the field of HL challenge parents to make decisions based on the best approach for their own child.

There are a number of sign language choices. Children with HL who are born to deaf parents are typically immersed in the Deaf culture and learn ASL. As described earlier, ASL is often thought of as a **bilingual-bicultural approach**. According to the Gallaudet (2011) annual survey, approximately 21% of deaf children use sign language as their primary mode of communication.

Total (simultaneous) communication (TC) combines auditory and visual learning and communication strategies; it is the more common manual approach. TC is used more frequently than ASL. TC may incorporate a variety of different forms of sign language, including ASL, **Signing Exact English (SEE)**, and **Pidgin**. TC was developed by educators at The Maryland School for the Deaf; currently, the school advocates that children (a) use ASL to learn language and (b) learn written English as a second language. This approach represents the bilingual-bicultural philosophy.

Family and Educational Issues for Manual Communicators. Some families choose to have their child communicate primarily with sign language because their child has concomitant risk factors for language learning, because they want their child to participate in Deaf culture, or because their child's language development is not progressing, even with high-quality speaking and listening intervention. As in every other case, a practitioner should support the family in understanding the implications of their decision. Most importantly, family members, friends, and others who wish to communicate effectively with a child with HL should realize that they must either (a) learn to sign or (b) rely on an interpreter.

Families should consider the requirements needed to support their child's communication skills over time. Initially, communication partners can communicate with basic sign language picked up from sign language courses, videos, or books. However, as a child's language develops, the child will need to interact in a sign-language-rich environment. Parents who choose sign language as the primary communication mode for their family will need to devote considerable time and effort to achieve the best possible outcome.

Research underscores the importance of intensive immersion in sign language to achieve good results. For example, when children with HL are brought up in a home with deaf parents who use ASL (i.e., native speakers), the rate and pattern of the children's early ASL development parallels early spoken language development of children with typical hearing. This contrasts with outcomes for individuals who are raised in homes where family members are not skilled ASL communicators. Data indicate that non-native ASL communicators have significant language deficits compared to native signers—even after using ASL as their primary communication mode for 20 to 40 years (Lederberg, Schick, & Spencer, 2013).

When parents choose a manual communication modality, they should also consider the greater community and academic system in which their child will be raised. If a child relies primarily on sign language, he should use an interpreter for many routine events (e.g., ordering food at a local restaurant, asking for directions). Initially, a parent may serve as the interpreter, but as the child becomes more independent, the parents should consider ways to increase the child's independence through the use of other interpreters.

Academic placement for children who use manual forms of communication typically depends on local programming. Some school districts have special schools or classes exclusively developed for children with HL who communicate with sign language. In areas where there are fewer students with HL, children often are mainstreamed with an interpreter.

FAMILY INVOLVEMENT IN THE REMEDIATION PROCESS

Both IDEA (2004) and the Division of Early Childhood (DEC; Sandall et al., 2006) emphasize the importance of family involvement and parental competence in supporting children's language learning. I will discuss these important factors, which have recently been explored by researchers, only briefly here because they are also covered later in this chapter.

When a child is diagnosed with HL, his or her parents must learn to maximize early language experiences (Cruz et al., 2013; Frush Holt et al., 2012; Quittner et al., 2013). Parents should be taught to use scaffolding, imitation, and closed-ended questions during the first year of life (Yoder et al., 2001). As a child enters the preschool years, parents should use facilitative language techniques that reflect the child's zone of proximal development (Cruz et al., 2013). See Chapter 5 for descriptions of facilitative language techniques consistent with social interaction theories of language development. Parents should be trained to use everyday interactions to explicitly teach important language concepts (Cruz et al., 2013; DesJardin, 2006; Quittner et al., 2013). Parents also should be supported to engage their child with HL in frequent storybook reading interactions (Kaderavek & Pakulski, 2007).

Connections

Each of the *Connections* sections throughout this book highlights information relevant to a particular domain or disability group. But the information in *Connections* also has broader implications across the speech-language pathology field. In this section, I present information about (a) the role of a counselor and the process of helping families through emotions triggered by the identification of their child's hearing loss and (b) the important role of family participation in educational decision making and language intervention. While reading this information about children with HL, you should consider the application of this information to children with other disabilities. Almost all parents, even if their child is only mildly impaired, will be affected to some degree by psychological stress after discovering that their child has special educational needs. Families with children who are diagnosed with specific language impairment, autism, intellectual disability, and reading/writing deficits also will experience emotional distress and grief. As a speech-language pathologist (SLP), you will play an important role in helping parents cope with their feelings, regardless of their child's diagnosis.

In this section, I also discuss issues related to family participation in the intervention process. It is important to remember that families play a critical role in the habilitation of all children, whether they have autism, intellectual disability, specific language impairment, or hearing loss. Therefore, the information presented in this section will apply to many different families in your professional career.

COUNSELING PARENTS OF CHILDREN WITH SPECIAL NEEDS

Parents of children newly diagnosed with hearing impairment (or other disabilities) often indicate feeling overwhelmed and inadequate to manage their children's special educational needs (Bosteels, Van Hove, & Vandenbroeck, 2012). These feelings of inadequacy can trigger feelings of anger. In fact, the cycle of emotions triggered by the identification of a child's disability is similar to the grief process triggered by the death of a loved one. The parent mourns the loss of the hoped-for "perfect" child and cycles through phases of emotions before accepting the fact that his or her child has a disability. Stages of the grief process are briefly described in the next section.

Because understanding a person's psychological state is so important to the habilitation process, SLPs and special educators should develop excellent counseling skills so they can support family members' emotional and psychological concerns. However, in my teaching experience, I have found that beginning clinicians often have difficulty implementing effective counseling skills. One of the difficulties in becoming a good counselor is that counseling behaviors are quite different from typical conversational exchanges.

Several counseling techniques make counseling different from regular conversation, including (a) tolerating conversational silence, (b) reflecting feeling, and (c) asking open vs. closed questions. These techniques are based on humanistic theory and are useful in that they assume that, given support, individuals will work through emotional crises. The counseling techniques of waiting, listening instead of talking, reflecting feeling, and asking open-ended questions encourage families to talk about their emotions. Family's emotional responses and their coping strategies are directly related to child outcomes.

Tolerating Pauses and Listening. In order to help an individual work through his or her emotions, SLPs and special educators employ a client-centered focus (Shames, 2000). This means that when family members are talking about their feelings, an SLP listens to what they are saying without interjecting their own thoughts and feelings. This sounds easy, but it is harder than you might think. In typical conversations, we are used to a back-and-forth verbal exchange, like this:

Speaker 1.A: *"I had a terrible day today. I could not find a parking place on campus. I must have driven around for 20 minutes looking for a place to park—and I was late for class."*

Speaker 1.B: *"I know what you mean. Monday mornings on campus are terrible; I can never find anything either!"*

Speaker 2.A: *"He makes me so mad. He always thinks he's right [KW1]and I'm wrong!"*

Speaker 2.B: *"I've been telling you he's a loser. I think you should dump him!"*

In the first example, Speaker B responds with a shared experience; in the second example, Speaker B gives advice to her friend. Both of these responses are appropriate for a typical conversation, but counseling is different. The counselor stays focused on the speaker's emotional reactions.

The first counseling technique is to learn to wait after an individual begins to talk about his or her emotions. Waiting with relaxed arms and legs (i.e., avoid crossing your arms across your chest) and maintaining a forward-leaning body position (i.e., leaning slightly toward the speaker rather than leaning back in your chair) are nonverbal signals that you are comfortable and open to listening. In U.S. culture, we typically wait only a few seconds between conversational turns. It will feel very uncomfortable for you to wait after a speaker shares his or her feelings. You will find, however, that if you wait a few more seconds (I recommend slowly counting to 5), the speaker often continues to share feelings and emotions. Sharing negative emotions to a sympathetic listener helps families psychologically adjust to their child's diagnosis.

Reflecting Feeling. Right about now, you might be saying to yourself, "So, I'm just sitting there, not talking, and waiting for the family member to say something? What if he doesn't say anything else?" When it is apparent to you that the client needs to express emotions, it is helpful to use a technique called **reflecting feeling**. When a professional reflects feelings, he or she responds to the client's emotional expressions rather than to the content of the message. Reflecting emotions is important because family members often hide negative emotional reaction. The use of feeling-related comments is one of the most significant illustrations of empathetic listening and is a powerful means of letting family members know that their feelings are valid and that you are there to support their adjustment to the new situation (Kaderavek, Laux, & Mills, 2004). Here is an example of a reflection of feeling:

> *Family Member:* *"I thought that something was wrong, but I was afraid to tell anyone about it. I didn't want to accept the fact that he couldn't hear me. But now I feel guilty that I didn't get him tested earlier."*
>
> *Professional:* (After a long pause) *"It's hard not to feel guilty as a parent, isn't it?"*
>
> *Family Member:* *"Yes, it's hard not to feel responsible, but I know that I have to let go of the guilt; it doesn't do any good now."*

In the example above, the typical conversational response might be to immediately reassure the family member, "There's no reason to feel guilty!" However, by reflecting feelings, you indicate that you understand that families feel a range of emotions, including anger, fear, and sadness. Reflecting feelings rather than providing advice in response to expressed emotions also indicates your understanding that parents must work through their feelings in their own way.

Open-Ended Questions. Open questions allow family members to respond in a number of different ways, while closed questions require a specific response (Cormier & Nurius, 2003; Seligman, 2004). Professionals often use closed questions during an initial interview to obtain specific information. Examples of closed questions include "When was your child's hearing loss identified?" and "How many words does your child use?" and "Is your child using amplification all the time?" Closed questions often are comfortable for beginning students because closed questions are aimed at obtaining factual information rather than emotional responses.

When a professional wants to help a family explore the emotions connected with their child's hearing loss, an important technique is to use open-ended questions. Open-ended questions provide more opportunity for a family member to "just talk" and discuss the relevant issues in a way that is most meaningful to him or her. Some examples of open-ended questions include "Tell me how your family reacted when you told them about your child's hearing loss" and "Tell me about your child's experiences at school so far" and "What is a typical day like for you at home with your child?" Open-ended questions provide an opportunity for family members to reveal feelings and communicate that the professional is willing to listen. After posing an open-ended question, the professional waits before responding, tolerates pauses in the conversation, and reflects feelings as appropriate.

THE GRIEF PROCESS

A classic model describing the emotions triggered by death and bereavement is called the *stages of grief model*. This model also has been used to describe the emotional reactions of parents after learning that their child has a disability. In a survey of parents, researchers found that parents reported feeling shock (42%), anger (23%), confusion (42%), fear (52%), sadness (16%), frustration (31%), depression (37%), loneliness (16%), and blame (16%) after their child's initial diagnosis of hearing loss (Yoshinaga-Itano & de Uzcategui, 2001). Many of these feelings are associated with the grief model. Keep in mind that parents typically do not pass through emotional stages in a step-by-step fashion. Instead, parents alternate between emotions, with a gradual progression toward acceptance, optimism, and hope (Kearney & Griffin, 2001).

The emotions associated with the grief model include the following:

- *Denial:* Denial is a conscious or unconscious refusal to accept the facts; it is a normal response to a significant negative event.
- *Anger:* Sometimes family members are angry with themselves or focus blame on one of the professionals working with their child. Family members may react with anger in ways that appear inappropriate.
- *Depression:* Depression is an overwhelming feeling of sadness and loss.
- *Acceptance:* While many individuals pass through periods of grief and loss, in the long term, most parents of children with disabilities report that they are "better people" and "feel strengthened" by their experiences, and they describe the joy their child brings to the family (Kearney & Griffin, 2001).

As you perfect your counseling skills and become a sympathetic and supportive listener, you will help families move toward the acceptance stage.

FAMILY ROLE IN INTERVENTION

No matter what communication modality a family chooses—teaching the child to listen and talk, sign language, or total communication—parents play a critical role in their child's growth, development, and overall outcomes (Cruz et al., 2013; Frush Holt et al., 2012; Quittner et al., 2013). To develop language, children must be immersed in language—and parents are the child's primary language teachers. The following are some considerations in working with families:

- Parents are encouraged to develop the skills and knowledge they need to foster their child's communication. A professional avoids taking on the role of an expert who can fix the child's communication. Instead, from the outset, the SLP, an audiologist, medical personnel, an educator, and family members work together to develop the child's intervention program.

- A professional recognizes that each family has a unique structure. As a professional, you will work with single-parent families, foster families, families with two parents of the same gender, parents who both work full time, fathers who provide most of the child care, and families headed by grandparents. A professional demonstrates sensitivity and respect for the various values and customs of each child's family (Schirmer, 2000).

- Professionals consider all of a child's daily experiences as potential opportunities for language learning. Encourage everyone possible, including teachers, babysitters, church-school teachers, preschool teachers, coaches, and the child's peers to become involved in communicating with a child with HL.

Assessment and Progress Monitoring

Children with HL experience a great deal of testing during their early years. Audiologists periodically evaluate and monitor the level of hearing loss and evaluate the benefits provided by different amplification systems. The practitioner concentrates on assessing and monitoring a child's speech and evaluating the child's language and literacy development. The practitioner also assesses the influence of the child's amplification device on the home and educational environments.

ASSESSMENT TOOLS

There are a number of approaches to assessment for children with HL (see Table 7.6). One frequently used measure is the MacArthur Inventory (Fenton et al., 2007). The MacArthur-Bates Communicative Development Inventory: Words, Gestures, and Sentences includes a questionnaire format and asks parents to identify various words that their child either says or signs. It includes vocabulary related to home, people, action words, description words, pronouns, prepositions, and question words. The McArthur Inventory also documents a child's use of sentences and grammatical forms. The McArthur scale was not developed specifically for children with HL but is an effective tool for documenting vocabulary growth.

Another assessment tool, the Cottage Acquisition Scales for Listening, Language, and Speech (CASLLS; Wilkes & Sunshine Cottage School for Deaf Children, 1999), includes a developmental checklist for assessment and planning for diagnostic therapy. The language section includes steps from preverbal to complex sentences, including pragmatic development. The CASLLS was specifically designed for children with HL and is based on a developmental approach. A developmental approach describes the child's abilities along a continuum of language milestones.

In contrast to the developmental approach used in the CASLLS, other assessment tools take an identification-of-deficit position typically documented via a norm-based test. This approach typically is used with older children with HL, particularly when the HL has significantly impacted language development. With the deficit approach, the professional compares the language ability of the child with HL to other children with HL and the language development of typical peers. An example of a normative-referenced instrument is the Clinical Evaluation of Language Fundamentals–Preschool–Second Edition (CELF-P-2; Semel, Wiig, & Secord, 2004). The CELF-P-2 evaluates expressive and receptive language

Table 7.6   **Sample Tools for Assessment and Monitoring**

Test	Description
Boehm Test of Basic Concepts— Third Edition (Boehm-3; Boehm, 2000)	Measures the understanding of basic positional concepts of young children and provides information about conceptual development.
Bracken Basic Concept Scale— Third Edition (BBCS-3; Bracken, 2007)	Evaluates concepts essential to early communication development and school readiness.
Preschool Language Scale—Fifth Edition (PLS-5; Zimmerman, Steiner, & Evatt Pond, 2011)	Measures language and developmental milestones.
Structured Photographic Expressive Language Test–3 (SPELT-3; Dawson, Stout, & Eyer, 2003)	Provides a means for analysis of specific language structures (e.g., syntax) that may not occur in spontaneous language samples.
Test of Auditory Comprehension of Language (TACL-3; Carrow-Woolfolk, 1999)	Measures receptive spoken vocabulary, grammar, and syntax.
MacArthur-Bates Communicative Developmental Inventories— Second Edition (CDI-2; Fensonet al., 2007)	Standardized, parent-completed report assists professionals in screening young children's emerging language and communication skills.

ability, focusing on word meanings, word and sentence structure, and recall of spoken language. It is standardized for children with normal hearing abilities from ages 3 years, 0 months to 6 years, 11 months, and it uses pictures as stimuli for all three areas of language development. In its standardized administration procedure, the CELF-P-2 requires a child to listen to auditory instructions.

Example of an Assessment Using the CASLLS. Let's look at an example of a student and think through the process of assessment. Imagine that you are a practitioner who must assess a transfer student with HL midway through the school year. How can you ensure that the child's learning needs are met while simultaneously assessing communication skills?

First and foremost, when working with a child with HL, you (in conjunction with the educational audiologist and other members of the educational team) must ensure that auditory learning is accessible. This can be done by completing a **Ling Six Sound Test** (Ling, 1989) at various distances in and across contexts. The Ling Test can be completed by anyone (e.g., parents, SLPs, teachers, audiologists) and is an easy tool for determining whether a child is hearing sounds in the speech frequency. The Ling test is further described in Focus 7.6. The Ling sounds are shown in Figure 7.2.

Next, you must assess the child's communication skills. Diagnostic testing can take weeks to complete, so it is often useful to think of assessment as an ongoing process interspersed with trial intervention. We will start by using the Cottage Acquisition Scales to complete an observation of a child with HL.

FOCUS 7.6 *Clinical Skill Building*

Ling Test

When a child presents with an apparent communication deficit, hearing impairment must always be ruled out. Screening is often the first step. A hearing screening can be completed in a physician's office but is more commonly completed as part of a speech and language evaluation unless the child is under 3 years of age. Before age 3, a child must be screened/assessed by an audiologist. An audiologist also diagnoses and quantifies a child's hearing loss.

Before initiating a diagnostic evaluation (or therapy session), the professional must determine that the child with HL has auditory access. In other words, you must determine whether the child's amplification device is working. A simple evaluation tool, developed by Daniel Ling (2002), is called the Ling Six Sound Test. The Ling test evaluates a child's ability to detect and discriminate sounds across the speech spectrum. Figure 7.2 illustrates the relationship between the six Ling sounds (*m, ah, oo, ee, sh,* and *s*) and the speech spectrum. When a child is able to repeat each sound in response to a clinician's request, the adult can be certain that the child has auditory access. In order to ensure that the child is hearing and not seeing the sounds, an acoustic hoop is used to cover the clinician's mouth without interfering with the acoustics of the signal. A simple embroidery hoop with speaker cloth is typically used for this purpose.

A second component of this test is referred to as *circle of hearing* or *listening distance.* Once it is established that the child can hear each sound, the adult determines the distance (usually in feet) at which the child is still able to detect the sound, by repeatedly asking the child to discriminate a sound as he or she moves away from the child.

Figure 7.2 **Approximate Frequency Distribution of Ling Sounds**

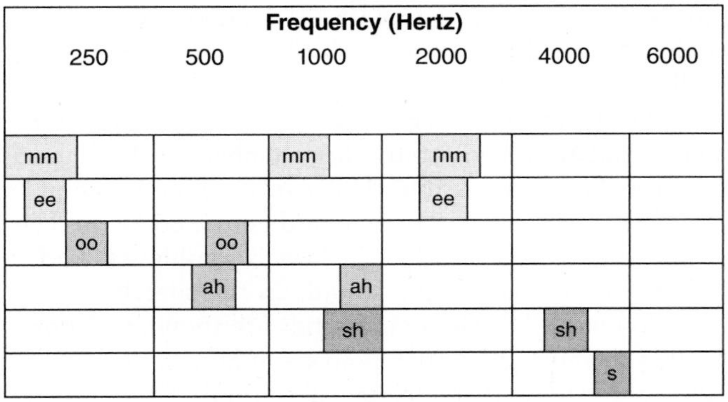

Frequency (Hertz)					
250	500	1000	2000	4000	6000
mm		mm	mm		
ee			ee		
	oo	oo			
		ah	ah		
			sh	sh	
					s

Mary, age 7, was born with a mild, bilateral, sensorineural hearing loss that was not diagnosed until she was a toddler. She is shy but interacts with peers when they initiate the interaction or to meet classroom demands. She uses courtesy language (i.e., "thank you," "hello") without prompting but does not repair communication breakdowns. (Communication repairs are a child's efforts to clarify communication when he or she is not understood as a communicator.) For example, a classmate approaches Mary and comments, "Mary, I'd like to use the pencil sharpener," to which Mary replies, "Hi." When the first child clearly does not respond to Mary's interaction, Mary does not attempt to continue the conversation or clarify that she did not understand the first child's communication.

Mary speaks softly and is moderately intelligible. Her language is approximately a year delayed but is consistent with her hearing age of 5 years, 9 months. Mary has bilateral behind-the-ear hearing aids that should be coupled with a frequency modulation (FM) system for maximal audition. An FM system is an assistive listening device that delivers the teacher's voice, via a microphone and receiver, directly to Mary's hearing aids. An FM system improves Mary's ability to hear the teacher at a distance and over background noise. However, like many other school-age children with mild hearing loss, Mary resists using the assistive listening devices (Walker et al., 2013).

As you complete your classroom observations, you observe the following:

- Mary has difficulty with plurals, possessives, and past tense, often omitting the final consonant and using incorrect grammar. For example, when asked, "How did you get to school today?" Mary answered, "I walk."
- On her spelling and vocabulary assignments, Mary has trouble with simple words. Mary drew a sled when asked to make a picture of a flag.
- After reading aloud to the class, the teacher asked Mary to answer some basic comprehension questions. When the teacher asked Mary, "Who did the dog belong to?" and "Where did the dog sleep?" Mary had difficulty describing the central characters in the story and did not understand the story's events.

Despite the language difficulties displayed, Mary also demonstrated communication skills consistent with her hearing age. Age-appropriate communication skills included (a) use of subordinate clauses, (b) use of indirect discourse (e.g., "Mom said I can go."), and (c) adverb formation using *ly*. Based on what you know about speech perception, the level of Mary's hearing loss, and her age of identification, do the errors described above seem more or less severe than expected?

To answer this question, again consider Mary's hearing age of 5 years, 9 months. Mary's hearing age suggests that her speech and language age will be equivalent to a younger child's. Table 7.7 provides Mary's expected language use, based on the Cottage Acquisition Scales. When considering Mary's hearing age of 5:9, however, we see that Mary is making unexpected errors. Plurals, possessives, and past tense are typically mastered between 3 and 4 years of age; vocabulary and her ability to answer questions also should be more developed. Mary is experiencing communication problems that are not consistent with her hearing age.

To understand Mary's difficulties, we must consider again that language development and use are dependent on listening. If someone asks, "Do you want two or three book?" (omission of the plural morpheme [*books*]) or states, "I would like to borrow Emily book" [omission of possessive morpheme [*Emily's*]), a typical listener is able to fill in the missing

Table 7.7 **Select Language Use of 5- to 6-Year-Olds, Based on the Cottage Acquisition Scales**

Dimension	Description
Nouns, noun modifiers, and relative clauses	Uses superlative *est*; uses *er* to form nouns (*teach–teacher*); uses gerund ("*Teaching* is fun"); uses relative clauses.
Prepositions and pronouns	Uses reflexive pronoun (*themselves*); uses possessive nominative (*its, ours*); uses *this* and *that* to stand for entire ideas; uses adverbs of time (*within*).
Verbs, adverbs, and infinitives	Uses *ly* to form adverbs; uses specific times (*1* A.M.); uses indirect discourse; uses infinitive with *wh-* words ("What *to do?*").
Tense, negation, and modals	Uses present perfect, negative + perfect tense, future progressive, present perfect progressive, modal progressive, and negative with *say, ask,* and *tell*.
Coordination, nominals, and adverbials	Produces clauses (e.g., *as soon as, before*); uses *or* to indicate inclusion; uses *neither, do, do too,* and *whether (or not)*; uses subordinate clauses and nominal clauses.
Questions	Asks *wh-* questions with *do* verb ("What does it *do?*").
Discourse	Uses focused chains for narratives; gives threats; issues promises and praise; stays on conversational topic; uses pronoun reference as cohesive device.

Source: Sunshine Cottage School for Deaf Children is the author of the Cottage Acquisition scales for Listening, Language and Speech (CASLLS)

plural or possessive morpheme. In contrast, children with hearing loss are unable to fill in the missing information. Because a child with HL has reduced auditory experience, he or she often is not able to produce or self-monitor important language components.

Vocabulary comprehension also can be challenging for children with HL. In the example of Mary's confusion with *flag* and *sled,* you may have concluded that Mary did not know the words or was inattentive during the task. While these may be causal factors, there are other issues to consider. First, children with mild hearing impairment may mistake one word for another if the sounds (phonemes) in the words are similar. When we think of similar sounds, we might think of *bat* and *pat.* The sounds /b/ and /p/ are produced similarly, but they differ in that /b/ uses vocal fold vibration, while /p/ does not.

Other complex acoustic characteristics also make listening difficult for children with HL. For example, the *oo* and *ee* sounds have the same first formant (frequency) and differ primarily in their second formant. Because the second formant for *ee* is a high-frequency sound, children with hearing loss often confuse the *ee* and *oo* sounds; they may not be able to distinguish a word with the vowel sound *ee* from a word with *oo*. This vowel confusion may have played a part in Mary's vocabulary error.

As a practitioner, you will learn how to use tools such as the CASLLS to guide language assessments of children with HL. With practice and training, you will learn to determine a child's errors in relation to his or her overall listening and language-learning environment. The root cause of Mary's language problem likely relates to the inconsistent use of amplification, which causes her to miss important language cues.

Intervention

As a trained professional, you will play a vital role in the education and therapeutic intervention of children with HL. Parents need training and support to guide their child's language and literacy learning. As children enter school, both regular and special education teachers will require your help to meet the special educational and classroom needs of children with HL.

Below I will highlight intervention approaches for children with HL who are learning to listen and talk. Because you may also work with children who use sign language, Table 7.8 provides strategies for maximizing language and literacy development for manual communicators.

Intervention approaches for children who are hearing impaired often are intertwined with the mode of communication and age of identification. In the following section, I discuss LSL techniques. LSL techniques include "Learning to Listen" sounds, hand cues, acoustic highlighting, sound sandwich, sabotage, and language experience books. The last technique, language experience books, is discussed in a separate section below. LSL techniques are summarized in Table 7.9.

LEARNING TO LISTEN

When initial diagnosis and fitting of amplification devices have been addressed, an interventionist begins periodic family treatment sessions. Parents are coached to build communication through a natural developmental sequence using LSL techniques in meaningful daily experiences.

Table 7.8 **Facilitating Language Development for Children Who Use Sign Language**

Technique	Description
Letter calling	Present a word's sign, finger-spell the word, and then draw the child's attention to the printed version of the word.
Storybook reading	Expose the child to different book genres. Scaffold the reading interaction; activate the child's prior knowledge of story themes; support the child's story recall; and help the child identify the main theme, draw conclusions from the story, and provide story details.
Chaining	Explicitly link the finger-spelling, print, and sign versions of the word.
Sign placement	Sign words directly over text when reading, to make explicit links between signed and written word.

Table 7.9 **Auditory-Verbal Therapy Techniques**

Technique	Description
Learning to Listen (LTL) sounds	Sound–object associations used with young children as they learn new sounds and vocabulary. Commonly used LTL sounds are /ahhh/ with *airplane*, "moo" with *cow*, "quack quack" with *duck*, and /ssss/ with *snake*.
Acoustic highlighting	Strategies to improve audibility of spoken communication. Examples include slower rate, increased pitch, and providing greater contrast in sets (e.g., *airplane, cookie, dog* vs. the stimulus set *dog, hog, frog*).
Hand cue	A technique used to encourage a child to attend to spoken language. The hand is placed near or in front of the mouth to alert new listeners.
Sound sandwich	A way of emphasizing an auditory cue while providing a visual cue when necessary. A word or message is first spoken, and if not understood, it is then paired with a visual cue (e.g., object, lip reading, sign). The visual cue is followed by a second auditory cue (e.g., say "apple," show an apple [or the written word], and then say "apple" again).
Sabotage	A technique in which an adult makes a deliberate mistake to provide a child with an opportunity to recognize and try to repair the mistake.

In the Learning to Listen (LTL) technique, parents are instructed to play with their child using toys, paired with the LTL sounds. LTL sounds are associated with an object (e.g., a transportation vehicle, an animal) or a specific action. This type of activity is very similar to the auditory experiences parents use with children developing typically. For example, adults often say "uh-oh" to indicate that they have dropped a toy or make a motor sound when pushing a toy car. Children are repeatedly exposed to sounds connected to objects or actions in a deliberate and focused intervention program. During parent–child play interactions, parents use acoustic highlighting (i.e., strategies to improve sound audibility such as using a slower rate and increased pitch) and model hand cues (a technique that signals that the parent is speaking). Below is an example of an LTL interaction:

> The mother, father, and child with HL sit together on the floor with several toys. The mother makes the sound "ahhhh" in a melodic fashion; the father repeats the sound. A toy airplane is introduced, and the sound "ahhhh" is repeated as the airplane soars through the air. This is repeated. Finally, the mother produces an utterance paired with the LTL sound: "Mama has the airplane, ahhhh, airplane."

During similar interactions, parents learn how to encourage and then respond to their child's early communication attempts. During LTL activities, parents also learn to monitor and adjust the child's listening environment. Too much noise, visual distractions, and other factors affect early language-listening experiences.

As children begin to repeat the LTL sounds and eventually string together words, daily activities (e.g., cooking dinner, driving to school), interactive games, and book reading are used to expose children to important listening and language behaviors. Table 7.10 provides examples of how interweaving language training, listening exposure, and daily activities can be combined to develop foundational language skills. Activities used to teach foundational language concepts are sometimes called *extension activities*.

Table 7.10   **Literacy Ideas and Extension Activities across Different Book Genres**

Genre	Activities
Narrative storybooks	• Choose books that relate to or can be mimicked in daily events (e.g., falling asleep in *Goodnight Moon* [Brown, 2005]). • Role-play subtle nuances of story (e.g., emotions in *Bear Snores On* [Wilson & Chapman, 2001]). • Alter story text to fit child's interests or needs. • If working on specific vocabulary, extend the text into games around the house (e.g., focus on grammar or vocabulary with *Brown Bear, Brown Bear* [Martin & Carle, 2008]).
Manipulative storybooks	• Choose manipulative books that allow the child to touch and feel the book (e.g., *In the Ocean* [Wood & Pledger, 2001]). • Select a few favorite books and make movable features (e.g., add a window with a piece of tape and card stock or cutout characters). • Find corresponding characters from other toys or stuffed animals that can be used to relate elements from play and real life with the story line (e.g., *Little People Cars, Trucks, Planes, and Trains* [Fisher-Price, 2004]). • Rewrite the child's favorite recipes on cards that include pictures of the items and then allow your child to work "hands-on" with items, following the directions.
Role-playing	• Use props to correspond to a book and act out the story (e.g., for beginners, *Blue Hat, Green Hat* [Boyton, 1984]; for older or more sophisticated language users, *Jack and the Beanstalk* [Kellogg, 1997]). • Select books that detail an upcoming event (e.g., *Happy Birthday, Maisy!* [Cousins, 2008]). First read the book, then talk about what will happen at the child's party, then practice some aspects such as singing and blowing out candles. • Create or find books that allow you to include the child as a story character (e.g., *Picture Me with Jonah and the Whale* [MacKall, 1997]).
Experience books	• Encourage parents to create experience books and use them at home and in therapy. • Use photos and mementos (e.g., acorns, seashells, a wrapper) to enhance the meaning of an experience book page. Talk about an event with the child, and then decide how to caption it in a way that best represents the child's expressions. • Use the experience pages to talk about past and future, abstract concepts, and other language concepts that are difficult for the child to understand.

LANGUAGE EXPERIENCE BOOKS

The basis for the extension activities presented in Table 7.10 is a widely used tool: the language experience book. Associated with the language experience approach, events and teachable moments in a child's daily experiences are recorded with pictures or illustrations and narrated with varying levels of text. Parents and the interventionist help the child record experiences and use these books to promote language and literacy.

At the beginning stage of using the language experience book, the book's text usually is based on events in a child's life. For example, a child is shown a picture in which he is standing in front of the polar bears at the zoo. The adult writes a sentence or two below the picture: *Andrew went to the zoo for his birthday. The polar bears were eating fish.* Even before the time that the child can read the text, he is encouraged to "read" using emergent reading behaviors. (See Chapter 9 for more about emergent reading.) Integrating a language experience book into a child's intervention program provides complex language models and provides an opportunity for language expansion (Kaderavek & Pakulski, 2007).

As the child's language develops, the practitioner includes a theme-based language experience approach that combines storybook reading with extension activities. For example, after reading the book *Head to Toe* (Carle, 2000), the practitioner engages the child in singing "Hokey Pokey" and "Head, Shoulders, Knees, and Toes." Additional extension activities include discussions about body parts and related concepts. Examples of activities include (a) baking and decorating gingerbread boy/girl cookies, (b) tracing and coloring the child's body on large paper, (c) examining a skeleton or chicken bones left from dinner, (d) experimenting with muscles and movement, and (e) the child's growth record and changes in height and weight. Focus 7.7 and Focus 7.8 provide more ideas to consider regarding intervention for children with HL.

FOCUS 7.7 *Learning More*

There are dozens of useful websites that can provide ideas for therapy with preschoolers. Explore some of these websites and create extension activities based on one or more themes.

FOCUS 7.8 *Learning More*

Playgroup for Children with Hearing Loss

A playgroup is an excellent way to implement some of the early literacy and extension activities for preschoolers with HL. A playgroup may incorporate storybook reading, singing and dance/movement, and auditory and language-learning-based games and crafts. When young children are able to listen to stories and say or repeat certain story elements, reader's theater can be incorporated. Scholastic provides ideas on adapting reader's theater for young children (see www.scholastic.com/teachers/unit/readers-theater-everything-you-need).

Throughout a child's education, he or she will require monitoring and intervention. In some cases, as in Mary's example, audiological management may solve many of the child's language problems. Other children may require occasional support to develop new skills. For example, as a child's language and thought processes become more complex, he or she may have difficulty with new grammar or perhaps will demonstrate careless speech articulation. Other children, particularly those who did not get early or appropriate intervention, may require ongoing intervention.

Summary

- When a hearing loss occurs in the outer and middle ear, it is called a conductive loss and is typically the result of a medical problem such as a fluid-filled middle ear (otitis media) or damage such as a perforated eardrum.
- Sensorineural losses are caused by damage to the inner ear structures or auditory nerve, and they often result from genetic disorders or birth defects.
- When a child has both a sensorineural hearing impairment and a conductive disorder (e.g., permanent hearing loss due to genetic disorder co-occurring with a middle ear infection), the loss is called mixed.
- Auditory perceptual problems are generally caused by auditory processing disorder (APD) or auditory neuropathy/dys-synchrony (AN/AD). APD is caused by the malfunctioning of the auditory pathway to the brain or by small defects in the brain's auditory cortex and/or language processing centers. AN/AD is an auditory processing deficit that impedes the auditory signal as it travels from the cochlea to the brain. Like APD, AN/AD is not due to a malfunction in the outer, middle, or inner ear.
- Children with hearing loss who did not have early intense auditory training or who have other associated deficits are likely to have language impairments including morphologic and syntactic deficits, in addition to semantic, pragmatic, and speech production problems (i.e., articulation and phonological deficits).
- Due to developing understanding of the potential for auditory development in the brain and advances in amplification, current research demonstrates that when (a) environmental support is in place and (b) appropriate and high-quality amplification and early intensive intervention are provided, a child with HL who is identified and treated in the first few months of life has the potential of developing language commensurate with that of typically hearing peers when no other disorders exist. Children with HL who have co-occurring conditions may need to use sign language to become effective communicators.
- Factors that families of a child with HL need to consider include (a) early identification and audiological management, (b) choice of communication modality, and (c) family involvement in the remediation process.
- The MacArthur-Bates Communicative Development Inventory: Words, Gestures, and Sentences (Fenson et al., 2007) includes a questionnaire format and asks parents to identify various words that their child either says or signs. It includes vocabulary relating to home and people, action words, description words, pronouns, prepositions, and question words, and assesses the child's use of sentences and grammatical forms.
- The Cottage Acquisition Scales for Listening, Language, and Speech (CASLLS; Wilkes & Sunshine Cottage School for Deaf Children, 1999) includes a developmental checklist for assessment and planning for diagnostic therapy. The language section

includes steps from preverbal to complex sentences, including pragmatic development. The CASLLS was specifically designed for children with HL.

- The Ling Six Sound Test (Ling, 1989) is a procedure that can be used by anyone. The phonemes for the Ling Six Sound Test are *m, ah, oo, ee, sh,* and *s.* When a child is able to repeat each sound in response to an adult's request, the adult can be certain that the child has auditory access.
- In the Learning to Listen (LTL) technique, parents are instructed to play with their child using toys, paired with the LTL sounds. LTL sounds are associated with an object (e.g., a transportation vehicle, an animal) or a specific action. In combination with the LTL sounds, parents use acoustic highlighting (i.e., strategies to improve sound audibility, such as using a slower rate and increased pitch) and use model hand cues (e.g., a technique that signals that the parent is speaking) during parent–child play interactions.

Discussion and In-Class Activities

1. Before class, obtain a brief case description of a child with a communication impairment. Create a fictional character (mother, father, grandparent, etc.) who is coming to the clinic to discuss his or her child. During class time, in groups of three, take turns being the parent, the trained professional, and the observer. The observer's job is to keep track of open and closed questions, the duration of pause time before the professional responds, the use of appropriate body posture, and the professional's ability to reflect feelings. The professional uses client-centered counseling techniques to encourage the parent to talk. The parent stays "in character," expressing a range of emotions. For case histories and scoring forms that can be used for this activity, see Kaderavek, Laux, and Mills (2004).
2. In groups of three, discuss and practice LSL techniques. One student should demonstrate use of sabotage at the breakfast table, the second should demonstrate acoustic highlighting for a toddler while playing with play dough, and the third student should design an experience book that demonstrates reading the book *Curious George and the Pizza* (Rey & Rey, 1985) and engaging the child and family in a pizza-making activity.

Chapter 7 Case Study

Katie is a 6 year, 11-month-old female who has just started second grade. She was among the first children in her state to be referred from newborn hearing screening, completed in the hospital at birth. She was diagnosed with a profound bilateral sensorineural hearing loss and fitted with powerful digital hearing aids within the first few months of life. Katie's parents decided that they would work toward teaching Katie to listen and talk and were proactive in seeking the necessary information and appropriate services to reach this goal. Intervention focusing on speaking and

listening began when she was 3 months old; manual communication was not introduced. Katie received her first cochlear implant at 20 months of age and a second
implant at 5 years. She entered regular preschool at age 3 and has performed at grade
level academically. Although her academic performance meets or exceeds grade level,
she has difficulty following instructions in the classroom and must work diligently to
complete homework and prepare for spelling tests and other assignments.

The SLP administered three norm-referenced tests: the Peabody Picture Vocabulary
Test (PPVT; a receptive vocabulary test), the Clinical Evaluation of Language Function–
Preschool (CELF-P), and the Phonological Awareness Test (PAT).

Katie received the following standard scores (SS):

Test/Subtest	SS (M = 100)
PPVT	90
CELF-Preschool Total Language Score	85
Receptive CELF–Preschool score	90
Expressive language score	81
PAT	83
Rhyming	68
Syllable blend/segment	64/83
Phoneme isolation	92
Phoneme blend/segment	96/98
Phoneme grapheme	86
Decoding	90

Overall, Katie's normative assessment data indicate that her receptive-expressive
language, phonological awareness, and vocabulary knowledge are within normal
limits. However, the SLP noted that Katie showed frustration with some of the test
instructions and had difficulty with certain aspects of phonological awareness and
maintaining a typically paced conversation.

The SLP consulted with the educational audiologist, who completed a classroom-
based assessment followed by a home visit. The educational audiologist observed
that Katie struggles in note taking and following oral directions and that her slower
response time often interferes with her ability to take part in classroom discussions.
The educational audiologist concluded that Katie has been a high achiever primarily
through independent learning, despite the many obstacles she faces in the classroom
due to poor classroom acoustics.

The educational audiologist probed Katie's classroom listening skills using
criterion-referenced tests (e.g., Listening Inventories for Education [LIFE-R]; Anderson,
Smaldino, & Spanger, 2012; available from http://successforkidswithhearingloss.com
/tests/life-r).

Following the assessment, the SLP and the educational audiologist worked with
Katie's classroom teacher to develop a plan to improve classroom access to auditory/
oral instruction. The developed goals were (1) to provide Katie with preteaching notes

that she could use at home with her parents to prepare for new vocabulary and spelling words, (2) to teach Katie to advocate for herself and request that complex directions be restated or broken down when she is not able to synthesize the information quickly, and (3) to improve classroom acoustics by decreasing extraneous noise (e.g., put carpet squares under desks, stop shuffling of papers during important discussions), and encouraging the teacher and classmates to take turns when speaking.

Questions for Discussion

1. Explain why Katie could score reasonably well on standardized tests but find classroom learning so challenging.
2. Examine an audiogram of a child with a cochlear implant and explain how it is different from "normal hearing."
3. Compare language development of children with hearing loss across variables including age of identification, manual vs. spoken language use, and parental involvement.

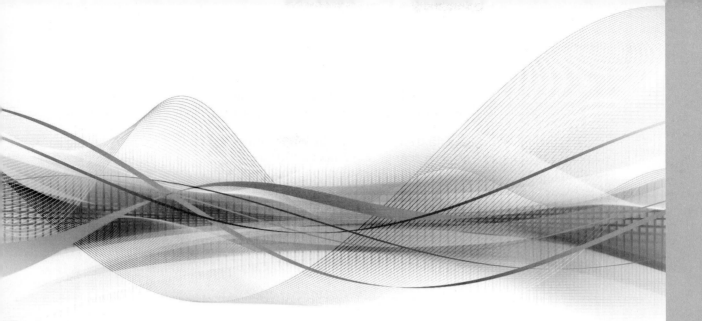

8 Children with Intellectual Disability

Chapter Overview Questions

1. What is the definition of *intellectual disability* (*ID*), and how has the definition changed since the 1960s?
2. What are primary causes and risk factors for ID?
3. How do knowledge-based and data-based processes impact how an individual learns and stores information? How does an interventionist modify stimuli and an intervention to account for processing differences?
4. Does ID represent a language delay or a language deficit? How are form, content, and use implicated in the various genetic syndromes of ID?
5. Why are criterion-referenced assessments important for individuals with ID? What criterion-referenced assessments should be completed?
6. What are the underlying theory and rationale for two intervention programs for individuals with ID?

This chapter describes issues, assessments, and interventions appropriate for children with intellectual disabilities. The term **intellectual disability (ID)** replaces the less-preferred terms *mental retardation, developmental disability,* and *cognitive impairment* (Executive Act on Intellectual Disabilities, 2003). In this chapter, the term *intellectual disability*

(*ID*) refers to individuals with core deficits encompassing both intellectual and social domains (Schalock & Luckasson, 2005). To clarify some issues regarding terminology, read Focus 8.1.

Along with changing terminology, there are other significant changes in the field of ID. Current perspectives move beyond identifying and focusing on intellectual deficits of persons with ID. Instead, practitioners evaluate and enhance functional skills, improve personal well-being, identify appropriate support systems within the family and community, and enhance competence through skill development and environmental modification (Schalock, 2004). This chapter will help you learn more about communication interventions that enhance an individual's quality of life in profound ways.

FOCUS 8.1 *Learning More*

Sometimes students are confused about the terminology used in the field of intellectual disabilities. Here are three common questions:

Is intellectual disability the same as developmental disability?

Developmental disability is an umbrella term that includes intellectual disability and also includes other disabilities that occur during early childhood. Some developmental disabilities are largely physical issues, such as cerebral palsy or epilepsy. Some individuals may have a condition that includes a physical and intellectual disability, such as Down syndrome or fetal alcohol syndrome (American Association of Intellectual and Developmental Disabilities [AAIDD], 2013).

Is intellectual disability the same as mental retardation? Why do some programs for individuals with intellectual disability still use the term *mental retardation*?

The term *intellectual disability* covers the same population of individuals who were diagnosed previously with mental retardation. Every individual who is or was eligible for a diagnosis of mental retardation is eligible for a diagnosis of intellectual disability. While *intellectual disability* is the preferred term, it takes time for language that is used in legislation, regulation, and even the names of organizations, to change (AAIDD, 2013).

How is the term *disability* used currently?

Disability is an umbrella term that covers impairments, activity limitations, and participation restrictions (World Health Organization [WHO], 2013). An *impairment* is a problem in body function or structure; an *activity limitation* is a difficulty encountered by an individual in executing a task or an action; a *participation restriction* is a problem experienced by an individual in involvement in life situations.

Sources: American Association of Intellectual and Developmental Disability (AAIDD, 2013). Retrieved at http://www.aaidd.org/content_104.cfm; World Health Organization (2013). Retrieved at http://www.who.int/topics/disabilities/en/

Description, Prevalence, Causation, and Major Characteristics

DESCRIPTION OF ID AND THE ECOLOGICAL MODEL

An individual is considered to have ID if the disability:

- Originates before age 18.
- Is characterized by significant limitations both in intellectual functioning and in adaptive behavior, as expressed in conceptual, social, and practical adaptive skills (AAIDD, 2012).

As this definition makes clear, to determine disability level, professionals must consider an individual's adaptive behavior as well as level of intellectual functioning.

Historically, professionals placed individuals with ID into one of four levels of impairment, based solely on IQ: mild (55–69 IQ), moderate (40–54 IQ), severe (25–39 IQ), or profound impairment (IQ below 25 or 20). The use of an IQ-based system was consistent with the general practice of institutional placement for individuals with ID—a practice common prior to 1960. Adaptive behaviors were not viewed as relevant to the diagnostic process because community placement was rarely considered. Although the American Psychiatric Association (APA) still includes the old severity grid in its *Diagnostic and Statistical Manual of Mental Disorders,* Fifth Edition (DSM-5; APA, 2013), the AAIDD recommends that the severity grid be eliminated as it does not reflect or represent best practices in the field of ID.

The current recommended classification system does not use the categories mild, moderate, severe, and profound based on IQ levels. The preferred model, visually presented in Figure 8.1, emphasizes the multidimensional aspects of ID (Dimensions I–V), and it also highlights interactions between an individual and his or her support system.

At present, most individuals with ID live and work in community settings; intervention is based on an ecological approach. The ecological approach considers an individual's functioning within the microsystem (i.e., family, caregivers), the mesosystem (i.e., school, neighborhood, community organizations, workplace), and the macrosystem (i.e., the sum of society's cultural views and practices regarding individuals with ID). The levels together influence individual functioning and quality of life; this is visually demonstrated in Figure 8.2.

Characteristics of each of the five dimensions within the ecological system include:

- *Dimension I:* **Intellectual ability** is represented by an IQ score two standard deviations below the mean: an IQ of approximately 70. Professionals typically use this dimension to determine eligibility for benefits and legal services.
- *Dimension II:* **Adaptive behavior** encompasses an individual's cognitive, communication, and academic skills, social skills, and independent living skills. A professional enhances adaptive behaviors by focusing on the social use of language, use of communication during daily living activities (e.g., making a phone call, buying groceries at the store), and reading and writing skills to facilitate independence, work, and community integration.
- *Dimension III:* Professionals directly observe an individual's participation, interactions, and social roles in everyday activities, because participation in a variety of

Figure 8.1 **Theoretical Model of Intellectual Disability**

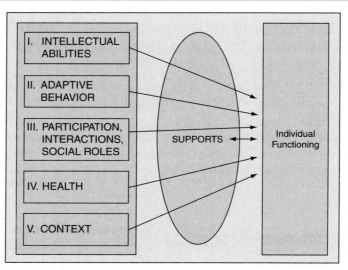

Source: From "American Association on Mental Retardation's Definition, Classification, and System of Supports and Its Relation to International Trends and Issues in the Field of Intellectual Disabilities," by R. L. Schalock and R. Luckasson, 2004, *Journal of Policy and Practice in Intellectual Disabilities, 1,* pp. 136–146. Used with permission.

Figure 8.2 **Three-Level Ecological Model of Intellectual Disability**

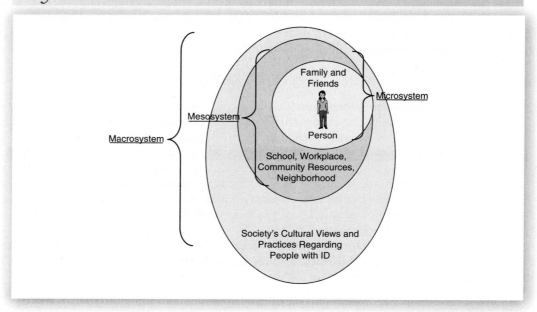

meaningful activities contributes to quality of life. Practitioners concentrate on the aspects of communication that are most likely to improve social interaction.

- *Dimension IV:* This dimension encompasses mental and physical health factors. There is variation in the degree to which health influences an individual's quality of life; some individuals have no significant health concerns, while others may be significantly affected (e.g., epilepsy, cerebral palsy). An individual's support system influences the impact of health concerns.
- *Dimension V:* Context describes an individual's family, the neighborhood, and community at all three levels of the environment (i.e., microsystem, mesosystem, macrosystem).
- *Supports:* The ecological model emphasizes the mediating effects of the support system on level of functioning. Support needs vary in intensity in relation to life activities and changes across the life span.

As an example of how the systems approach might work, imagine that you are working with an 8-year-old student with ID in a general education class. You communicate with the family and the teacher and discover that the student does not ask or answer questions in class. You collaborate closely with the classroom teacher, obtain lesson plans in advance of the class presentation and, along with the teacher, develop target questions and answers. You and the student practice asking and answering the questions; the teacher provides opportunities for the student to ask and answer target questions in class. This is an example of an ecological approach; you enhanced the student's participation in his community and facilitated communication skills used in everyday life. Think more about how practitioners use the ecological approach by discussing the questions in Focus 8.2.

FOCUS 8.2   *Clinical Skill Building*

With your classmates, discuss how you might use an ecological systems approach to facilitate the communication of (a) an adult who works at his local YMCA who communicates using simple sentences but is very difficult to understand, (b) a teenager who attends classes in general education classrooms at the local high school who would like to participate in an extracurricular activity, and (c) a 3-year-old child with one-word verbalization enrolled in an inclusive preschool classroom.

In your discussions, consider that ecological approaches differ from traditional approaches, particularly in assumptions about what is normal and abnormal. Ecological approaches acknowledge a wide variation in individual, family, community, and cultural modes for dealing with challenges. Family and community support systems can contribute to an individual's dysfunction or promote an individual's self-reliance and growth. As a result, ecological approaches consider the impact of an individual's communication impairment in relation to the functioning and relationships within the family and community. Intervention should focus on strengthening supports and minimizing barriers within the ecological system.

It is important to remember that the systems/ecological approach tends to focus on functional or life-skill goals that link aspects of language use, form, and function. For example, a systems/ecological communication goal might be stated as "John will use socially appropriate language when he greets and leaves his communication partners at his workplace" (e.g., "Hi," "How are you doing?" "See you later!").

PREVALENCE

The prevalence of ID (i.e., the number of persons identified at a given point in time) is 1 to 3% of the population; approximately 1.5 million people, ages 6 to 64, have been diagnosed with ID presently in the United States (Harris, 2006). ID occurs more frequently in males than females (WHO, 2001). Children with ID make up 15% of the caseloads of school-based SLPs; 9% of students ages 6 to 21 years of age receiving special education in U.S. schools are children with ID (CDC, 2007). The prevalence rates and the increasing levels of noninstitutionalization imply that most SLPs and educators will work with individuals with ID during their career.

CAUSATION AND RISK

The causes of ID vary in relation to two variables: the timing of the risk factor and the type of risk factor. In terms of timing, risk factors can occur before birth (prenatal), at the time of birth (perinatal), or after birth (postnatal). The types of ID risk factors include biomedical (i.e., physiological in nature), social, behavioral, and educational. Table 8.1 summarizes the various risk factors, organized along the dimensions of timing and type.

Table 8.1 **Risk Factors for Intellectual Disability**

Timing	Biomedical	Social	Behavioral	Educational
Prenatal	• Chromosomal disorders • Single-gene disorders • Metabolic disorders • Maternal illness • Parental age	• Poverty • Maternal malnutrition • Domestic violence • Lack of access to prenatal care	• Parental drug or alcohol abuse • Parental smoking • Parental immaturity	• Parental cognitive disability without support • Lack of preparation for parenthood
Perinatal	• Prematurity • Birth injury • Neonatal disorders	• Lack of access to birth care	• Parental rejection of caregiving role • Parental abandonment of child	• Lack of medical referral for intervention services at discharge
Postnatal	• Traumatic brain injury • Malnutrition • Meningoencephalitis • Seizure disorders • Degenerative disorders	• Impaired caregiver • Lack of adequate stimulation • Family poverty • Chronic illness in family • Institutionalization	• Child abuse and neglect • Domestic violence • Inadequate safety measures • Social deprivation • Difficult child behaviors	• Impaired parenting • Delayed diagnosis • Inadequate early intervention services • Inadequate special educational services • Inadequate family support

Source: From "American Association on Mental Retardation's Definition, Classification, and System of Supports and Its Relation to International Trends and Issues in the Field of Intellectual Disabilities," by R. L. Schalock and R. Luckasson, 2004, *Journal of Policy and Practice in Intellectual Disabilities, 1,* pp. 136–146. Used with permission.

A child's genetic makeup is a significant prenatal risk factor (Hodapp & Dykens, 2004). Experts have identified more than 750 genetic syndromes resulting in intellectual disabilities (Abbeduto, 2009). Genetic factors are a causative factor in 50% of cases of ID (WHO, 2001). Genetic syndromes can be inherited, but many genetic conditions are caused by genetic mutations. For example, **translocation** occurs when a broken piece of one chromosome attaches to another. In contrast, Down syndrome sometimes is caused by **gene duplication**. In this instance, chromosome 21 duplicates, resulting in three copies of the chromosome instead of two. Table 8.2 describes the genetic abnormalities that contribute to the most common syndromes resulting in ID.

Table 8.2   **Syndromes Associated with Genetic Causations of ID**

Syndrome and incidence	Behaviors noted as co-occurring	Genetic characteristics
Down syndrome • 1 in 750 births • 5–6% of all individuals with ID have Down syndrome (DS).	• Better performance on visual-spatial tasks than on verbal or auditory tasks. • Adaptive behavior strength relative to IQ. • Pleasant and sociable personality. • Pragmatic language and lexical skill strength relative to other language abilities.	Three separate chromosomal causes: • Trisomy 21 (child has 47 chromosomes instead of 46; chromosome 21 has 3 copies instead of 2). • An inherited translocation of chromosome pairs.[1] • Uneven division that creates cells varying in the number of chromosomes (some cells having 47 and some having 46).
Williams syndrome 1 in 25,000 births	• Strengths in language, auditory memory, and facial recognition. • Weaknesses in visual-spatial, perceptual, motor, and fine-motor skills. • Strength in understanding others' emotions and feelings (i.e., empathizing [see Chapter 9 for more about this term]). • Over-friendliness. • Pragmatic skills impaired in relation to other language abilities.	A deletion of a small piece of chromosome 7.
Prader-Willi syndrome 1 in 10,000–15,000 births.	• Food-seeking behavior and obesity. • Strength in visual processing. • Obsessive-compulsive disorders and poor impulse control are common. • Pragmatic difficulties; excessive talking on a narrow range of subjects.	A partial deletion of chromosome 15.
Klinefelter syndrome 1 in 1,000 births	• Learning disabilities. • Delayed expressive speech with phonological, lexical, and morphological skills more impaired relative to other language areas.	Males receive one, two, or three extra X chromosomes.

(continued)

Table 8.2 (*continued*)

Syndrome and incidence	Behaviors noted as co-occurring	Genetic characteristics
Angelman syndrome 1 in 20,000 births	• Absence or severe reduction in oral language. • Bouts of inappropriate laughter. • Generally happy disposition at all ages. • Hyperactivity and sleep disorders in younger children.	No active copies of a portion of chromosome 15.
Fragile X syndrome 1 in 4,000 males	• Verbal skills better than visual-spatial skills. • Relative strengths in daily living and self-help skills. • Can present with inattention, hyperactivity, and autistic-like behaviors. • Anxiety disorders common at all ages. • Lexical skills are strong relative to other language areas.	Sex-linked inheritance.[2] The disorder is mainly caused by the expansion of the CGG sequence located on the FMR1 gene on the X chromosome. The expansion of this triplet leads to "silencing" of the FMR1 gene.[3]

[1]Translocations are structural rearrangements of the chromosomes, including breakage and deletions.

[2]Sex-linked disorders: Males have an X and Y chromosome; females have two X chromosomes. Males (XY) are affected by a single recessive gene carried on the X chromosome; females (XX) are affected only if mother is a carrier and father has the disorder. Sex-linked genetic disorders are particularly significant for males.

[3]Penagarikano, Mulle, & Warren (2007).

Source: Based on information from "Intersyndrome and Intrasyndrome Language Differences," by J. A. Rondal, 2004. In J. A. Rondal, R. M. Hodapp, S. Soresi, E. M. Dykens, & L. Nota (Eds.), *Intellectual Disabilities: Genetics, Behavior, and Inclusion* (pp. 49–113). London: Whurr.

The development of chromosomal maps (**genotypes**) and the influence of genetics on an individual's **behavioral phenotype** (the connection between one's genetic endowment and observable outcome) is a rapidly expanding area of scientific research. Researchers are working to identify and compare language characteristics in relation to ID subtypes (Warren, Brady, & Fey, 2004). The genetic alterations result in a specific pattern of behavioral strengths and weaknesses; awareness of a syndrome's phenotype helps guide the assessment and intervention process. Table 8.2 provides a general description of behavioral characteristics associated with common syndromes. Remember, however, that whether a child has a genetic syndrome or is typically developing, an individual's functioning is due to a complex interaction of genes and environment (Abbeduto, 2009).

Despite our increasing understanding of genetics, in about 40 to 60% of cases, the exact cause of ID is unknown; cases of unknown etiology are called **idiopathic ID**. Experts believe that many cases of idiopathic ID are likely to have a genetic origin, but understanding the complex molecular mechanisms underlying idiopathic ID will continue to challenge scientists for years to come (Das Bhowmik & Mukhopadhyay, 2012). Individuals with idiopathic ID tend to be at the lower end of the IQ distribution (i.e., IQ of less than 50).

Genetics is a prenatal cause of ID. As demonstrated in Table 8.1, postnatal factors also impact the incidence of ID. A commonly occurring postnatal factor is **traumatic brain** injury (TBI). TBI is defined as an acquired injury to the brain caused by an external physical force, resulting in total or partial functional disability or psychosocial impairment adversely affecting an individual's educational or functional performance.

Unfortunately, the incidence of TBI is increasing in infants and preschoolers. Falling, car accidents, and physical abuse are common causes of childhood TBI. Approximately 8% of childhood brain injuries are caused by child abuse; the percentage is probably higher, but many cases of abuse go unreported. One of the primary forms of abuse is **shaken baby syndrome (SBS)**; SBS often is triggered when a caregiver loses control in response to an infant's crying. SBS is a term used to describe the constellation of signs and symptoms resulting from violent shaking or hitting the head of an infant or small child. You can learn more about the signs of potential SBS and find literature for families at www.dontshake.org.

The effects of childhood brain injury are profound because the human brain continues to make primary connections between motor and sensory areas throughout early infancy. Secondary brain development continues through age 5, primarily in the differentiation of verbal and nonverbal functions. Tertiary brain development continues up to age 8; temporal, occipital, and parietal lobes integrate functions resulting in coordinated movement, visual and auditory recognition, and sensory discrimination. The effects of brain injury may include motor, vision, and learning disabilities; communication impairments; and/or intellectual disabilities. Children with TBI sometimes have associated behavior problems including aggression or lethargy.

Although the occurrence of ID cannot always be prevented (as in the case of genetically based risk), professionals continually work to eliminate risk factors such as shaken baby syndrome. Other risk factors that can be prevented include the lack of access to birth care (a social risk factor), poor parenting and poverty (social, behavioral, and educational risk factors), and inadequate early intervention services (social and educational risk factors). You can learn more about the professional's role in the prevention of communication disorders and ID in Focus 8.3.

FOCUS 8.3   *Prevention*

A professional's role in intervention also encompasses the prevention of disabilities. The American Speech-Language-Hearing Association (2004) encourages SLPs to help prevent communication impairments, including those caused by intellectual disabilities. A document called *Preferred Practice Patterns for the Profession of Speech-Language Pathology* (available online, at www.asha.org/members/desk ref-journals/deskref/default) lists potential prevention activities:

- Identifying and contacting target groups
- Establishing professional relationships with target groups

- Providing consultation and educational strategies to groups:
  - Consultation may be provided to natural support systems, such as the family, or to direct service personnel, organizations, or policy-making groups.
  - Education may provide general information about communication disorders and intervention.
- Identifying and/or eliminating risk factors for the onset, development, or maintenance of a communication disorder as well as improving the target groups' ability to cope with communication disorders

CHARACTERISTICS OF ID AND THE IMPLICATIONS FOR REMEDIATION

Knowledge-Based and Data-Based Processing. Individuals learn and make decisions using previous knowledge and also by processing information from the immediate environment. **Knowledge-based processing** is processing that is based on an individual's previous experience or knowledge; it is sometimes called *top-down processing*. **Data-based processing** is processing that is based on incoming data; it is sometimes called *bottom-up processing* (Goldstein, 2012). An individual's response to a particular situation is influenced by both previous knowledge and incoming data. For example, in a difficult listening situation (e.g., a noisy restaurant), if you know the topic being discussed, it is easier to process the speech of your dining companions. If you don't know the topic (i.e., no previous knowledge), you will have more difficulty understanding the muffled speech (i.e., incoming data). A professional considers an individual's previous knowledge and the individual's ability to process incoming data when working with an individual with ID. Experts believe that neurological differences impact how an individual with ID stores and accesses previous knowledge and incoming data (Drew & Hardman, 2004). Consequently, it is important to consider how an individual with ID attends to stimuli, discriminates between different stimuli, and organizes, transfers, and stores information.

The section below lists important processing skills to consider when working with a person with ID. Figure 8.3 is a visual representation of these skills, and Figure 8.4 provides suggestions for strategies to accommodate individual differences.

Skills for Processing and Storing Information. **Attention** is the ability to orient and react to a specific stimulus. Individuals with ID typically have a delayed reaction time in response to stimuli. Therefore, caregivers should increase wait time so that individuals with ID have time to respond.

Discrimination is the ability to attend to specific stimuli in a field of similar stimuli. A disturbance of discrimination noted in individuals with ID is **stimulus overselectivity** (selective response to a limited number of stimuli cues). For example, a student may recognize his name, John, only by attending to the initial letter, *J*. Overselectivity accounts for the fact he selects any name starting with *J* (e.g., Jack, Jill) like his own name (Dube et al., 2003). Stimulus overselectivity also occurs during assessment, as when a student continually responds to an item because of its position (e.g., the upper-left corner of a page of pictures) rather than attend to all stimulus features before responding. When overselectivity occurs, the practitioner manipulates the task. For example, if a student looks only at the first letter, *J*, before selecting his name, the practitioner requires the student to point and say the letters (*J-O-H-N*) before making his selection. If the student consistently points to one picture without looking at all stimuli, the practitioner and student point and look at all four pictures together before the practitioner asks the student to point to a specific picture. Students are also trained to self-monitor a better visual scanning strategy (e.g., *Did I look at all my choices?*) to minimize overselectivity.

Organization refers to the ability to systematize incoming information to speed processing and facilitate retrieval. One organizational strategy, **chunking**, refers to organizing items into familiar manageable units. Individuals with ID have limitations in their ability to organize incoming information (Oross & Woods, 2003). For example, typical learners often use chunking to connect information within similar categories. You may associate words such as *sad, morose, pensive,* and *melancholy* as having similar meanings. An individual with ID may learn each new word as a completely new semantic concept—without

Figure 8.3 **Processes that Impact Learning**

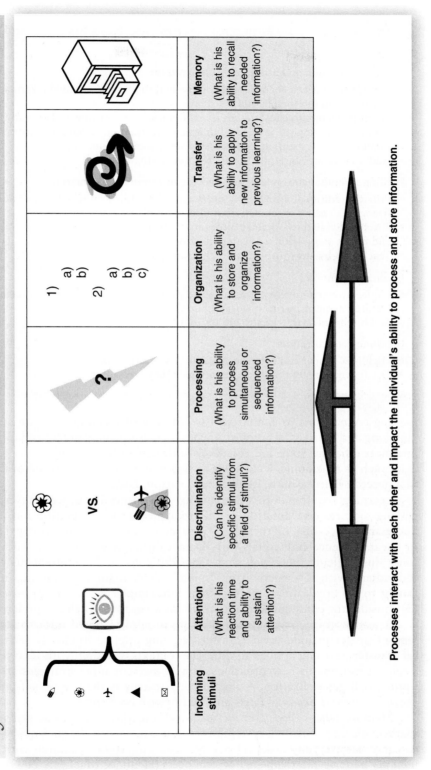

Processes interact with each other and impact the individual's ability to process and store information.

Figure 8.4   Strategies for Accommodating Processing Differences

Facilitate attention and accurate discrimination:
- Manipulate task to encourage the individual to attend to needed information (e.g., point to letters and say them aloud).
- Teach metacognitive techniques to facilitate self-monitoring and attending strategies.
- Give cues alerting the individual that new information is being presented.
- Limit extraneous stimuli to decrease stimuli competition.
- Add new stimuli carefully, with attention to stimulus load.

Facilitate simultaneous processing and organization of information:
- Provide additional visual or auditory cues (depending on which sensory avenue is a strength) to assist organization of information.
- Teach individual to organize information into meaningful components (e.g., chunking) and to use association and categorization strategies.
- Teach step-by-step problem-solving strategies.

Facilitate memory:
- Explicitly teach memory strategies and provide increased cues to aid retention (e.g., pictures, symbols, written words, charts).
- Teach rehearsal strategies to aid recall.

Facilitate generalization:
- Highlight similarities between old and new information.
- Teach behaviors in the situation in which they will occur.

making connections to similar words. The use of metaorganization strategies (such as chunking and word association strategies) makes learning and information retrieval faster and more efficient. Some individuals with ID benefit from training in organizational strategies such as mnemonic devices (e.g., using letters to remind oneself of the different steps in a process; Beirne-Smith, Ittenbach, & Patton, 2002).

Learning requires both simultaneous and successive processing. **Simultaneous processing** requires coordination of different pieces of information into a linked system. **Successive processing,** on the other hand, requires stimuli to be arranged in a step-by-step, or linear, sequence. Individuals with ID have difficulty with tasks requiring logic and planning; this difficulty may well stem from difficulty with simultaneous processing. Some individuals with ID benefit from "meta" problem-solving training, in which they are taught to (1) break down the problems into simpler elements, (2) generate alternatives, (3) consider the consequences of each alternative, and (4) select a preferred alternative.

Transfer of information is the ability to apply learned information to novel problems. Transfer includes **near transfer,** learning applied to closely related contexts, and **far transfer,** learning applied to different contexts. Children with ID often have difficulty applying learning to new situations. Simple metacognitive strategies are useful for facilitating skill generalization. A simple metastrategy is the use of self-questioning (*What should I do first? Second? Last?* and *Did I finish each step?*).

Memory (also called *working memory*) underlies many basic skills such as reading, mathematics, and vocabulary development; it is defined as the current information retained to carry out everyday tasks (Henry & MacLean, 2003). Children with ID use different memory patterns than same-age typical peers (Henry & MacLean, 2003), and the memory skills of people with ID lag behind mental age (Numminen et al., 2000). Researchers have studied the memory patterns of individuals with ID and have found deficits in nearly every aspect of memory storage and processing (Detterman, Gabriel, & Ruthsatz, 2000).

Rehearsal, or repetition of information, is an effective metaskill to aid memory; however, individuals with ID do not spontaneously rehearse information (Detterman et al., 2000). Rehearsal strategies include **verbal rehearsal**, in which the individual self-instructs and uses verbal labels to stimulate recall, and **image rehearsal**, in which the individual aids recall by associating task components with pictures. Chunking (described above) also facilitates memory. For example, a practitioner teaches a student with ID to remember to do three things after arriving at school: (1) *store materials* (hang up coat, put away books, turn in homework), (2) *get ready to work* (sign up for lunch, sit at desk, get out daily schedule), and (3) *start daily work* (begin first daily assignment, don't bother others while they are working). Chunking the information helps with information retention; the individual with ID remembers three categories instead of eight separate items.

Knowledge-based processing is facilitated when a practitioner engages the individual with ID in naturalistic and familiar contexts rather than isolated therapeutic tasks (Katims, 2000). Familiar environmental cues make it easier for the individual to access his or her knowledge base. Focusing on the communication events that occur during daily activities is called **functional communication**. Functional communication focuses the student's ability to express needs, wants, feelings, and preferences that others can understand.

There are many ways in which a professional enhances and takes advantage of an individual's knowledge base. For example, to improve writing skills, a practitioner targets familiar writing tasks such as writing a shopping list, filling out forms, and taking phone messages. Other strategies include:

- Selecting tasks likely to occur in daily life
- Linking new information to familiar activities and tasks
- Providing familiar cues to elicit behaviors
- Using social reinforcement rather than tangible rewards
- Building on an individual's strengths and interests

To summarize, professionals recognize that an individual's learning is influenced by both knowledge- and data-based processing abilities. An individual's ability to process incoming data influences his or her ability to complete a complex skill, while overall task familiarity and meaningful context similarly enhances performance and knowledge retention.

Motivation. **Motivation**, sometimes called *mastery motivation*, is the psychological capacity that leads people to demonstrate goal-directed behaviors to achieve the positive feelings associated with task competency. Children with ID demonstrate similar goal-oriented behaviors as children developing typically (Niccols, Atkinson, & Pepler, 2003). However, children with ID sometimes have reduced task mastery motivation in response to difficult tasks. Motivation increases when practitioners modify the tasks to match an individual's ability level (Harris, 2006). High motivation increases children's task persistence and positively correlates with competency in daily activities (Niccols et al., 2003). Professionals should consider motivational issues when developing intervention for people with ID. Later in this chapter, I present an intervention approach specifically designed to motivate school-age children with ID, called the IT's Fun program (Rosin, 2006). The IT's Fun program uses performance activities (i.e., role-playing, storytelling) to motivate students with ID to focus on effective communication strategies. Figure 8.5 illustrates motivated students participating in a performance.

Figure 8.5   **Intervention Activities Should Create Motivating Opportunities for Students to Focus on Improving Their Communication Skills**

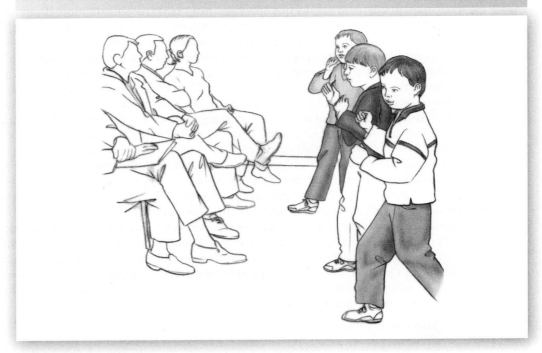

Connections

In this section, I present information that links important concepts discussed previously in this text to their application with ID. I revisit two topics introduced in Chapter 1: (1) a discussion of language delay vs. language disorder and (2) the application of Bloom and Lahey's classification system that divides language into the three domains of *form, content* (i.e., semantics), and *use* (i.e., pragmatics). Both topics represent important reoccurring concepts discussed in the ID literature. By the end of this section, you should be able to explain the two topics and understand the implications for clinical decision making.

LANGUAGE DELAY VS. LANGUAGE DISORDER

Is language development delayed or is it fundamentally disordered or deviant in individuals with ID? If one takes the perspective of language delay in ID, the communication behaviors of children with ID mirror the developmental sequence seen in children developing typically—but at a slower rate of acquisition. Ultimately, an individual with ID has the language abilities of a younger person.

Professionals believe that the language delay perspective accurately characterizes individuals with ID during childhood. Before age 10, language output of individuals with ID generally follows the expected developmental sequence except that there is a reduction in the quantity of language. The result is language output with shorter sentences, less grammar sophistication, and reduced vocabulary diversity (Rondal, 2004).

However, after age 10, there often are qualitative communication behaviors that suggest a language disorder. A professional defending the language disorder perspective might give an example of an adolescent with ID who asks the same questions repeatedly ("How old are you?" "What car you drive?") in spite of significant efforts to extinguish this behavior. Alternatively, the professional might describe a student who whispers continually under her breath, much to the annoyance of family and coworkers. It is unlikely that individuals developing typically would persist in such behaviors.

What would you say during this discussion? I hope that you would introduce several important points. First, you might point out that the population with ID is very heterogeneous. It is impossible to make a single generalization about a population that varies so widely and consists of individuals with very different etiologies (i.e., varying underlying causations).

After making this important point, you might explain (you are sounding quite wise at this point!) that a skilled professional does not see the language delay and language disorder perspectives as mutually exclusive. You explain that one can use a general developmental framework, particularly with young children, but continually examine the functional use of the communication skills that are the focus of intervention. A broad-based ecological perspective allows the professional to continually consider how an individual's communication differences affect his or her everyday life.

A clinical example demonstrates this decision-making process. You are working with a 10-year-old female child with Down syndrome (DS). You have been working on her production of four- to five-word sentences; you consider introducing the use of prepositional phrases in conjunction with the basic noun + verb combination (e.g., "The dog is eating food *under the table*"). However, this child's speech intelligibility is reduced when she attempts to produce longer sentences because she has difficulty producing rapidly sequenced motor movements. This is a communication disorder; her oral-motor problems often make her speech unintelligible (i.e., difficult to understand). Rather than introduce longer and more complex sentence structure, you decide to incorporate prepositional phrases within short sentences (e.g., "The dog is eating. He is *under the table.*"). You also decide to focus on overall intelligibility as a primary goal of intervention. During this decision-making process, you follow developmental guidelines when choosing your syntax target of prepositional phrases but adapt goals in response to the child's communication disorder.

FORM, CONTENT, AND USE WITHIN SUBTYPES OF ID

How does an individual's nonverbal cognitive ability (i.e., IQ) affect the form, content, and use domains? This is a second topic in the ID literature prompted by recent explorations of ID genotypes. Specifically, research demonstrates that within ID subtypes, language domains vary in relation to cognitive ability (Armstrong, 2010). In some cases, people with ID have language competencies surpassing expectations, given their nonverbal IQ. In other cases, language skills are less than expected. To learn more about nonverbal IQ, see Focus 8.4.

I explore the relationship between cognitive ability and language competencies in the section below in relation to three ID subtypes: Down syndrome, fragile X syndrome, and Williams syndrome. Within each syndrome, I compare language abilities to nonverbal IQ and discuss aspects of form, content, and use. Following this discussion, I return to the major topic—how IQ affects language ability—and reflect on the clinical implications.

Down Syndrome. Although overall language acquisition in DS is below expected levels in relation to an individual's nonverbal cognitive ability, there are relative strengths within language domains (Chapman & Hesketh, 2000). Specifically, vocabulary development

---

FOCUS 8.4 *Learning More*

Nonverbal intelligence, sometimes called *nonverbal* or *performance IQ,* is a measure that indicates a person's ability to carry out motor tasks or analyze and solve problems using visual reasoning. Nonverbal IQ is used to measure general ability for persons with language deficits. Tasks used in nonverbal IQ tests include the following:

- Recognizing and remembering visual sequences
- Understanding the meaning of pictures and recognizing relationships between visual concepts
- Completing visual analogies
- Recognizing causal relationships in pictured situations

It is unfortunate that nonverbal IQ sometimes is used to qualify or deny services to individuals with ID. In many states, SLPs and special educators cannot provide services to a student when his or her language ability and nonverbal IQ are equivalent, a practice called *cognitive referencing* (Goldstein, 2006). The assumption is that language skills cannot improve beyond one's language ability. Cognitive referencing oversimplifies the relationship between language and cognition and is a poor indicator of the potential benefit of communication intervention (Greenspan, 2006).

---

generally is equivalent to or above nonverbal cognitive levels, while morphosyntax (i.e., sentence length and grammar) skills are more impaired given the individual's nonverbal cognitive ability. It is thought that deficits in short-term memory negatively impact language learning in individuals with DS (Ypsilanti & Grouios, 2008). Sentences typically lack articles, propositions, pronouns, conjunctions, auxiliary verbs, morphological markings (e.g., verb tense, plural forms), and subordinate clauses (Rondal, 2004). Individuals with DS rarely progress beyond the simple sentence structures exhibited by a typically developing 2-year-old.

From an early age, children with DS evidence communication delay, including slowly developing turn-taking behaviors, delayed babbling, reduced imitation, and delayed use of gestures. Many children with DS do not produce their first words before 2 or 3 years of age (Rondal, 2004).

Children with DS typically have significant phonological deficits (Chapman & Hesketh, 2000). Speech difficulty is due to physiological differences of the articulators and vocal tract, motor programming deficits (Kumin, 2001), and frequent middle ear infections (Rice, Warren, & Betz, 2005). People with DS often have reduced respiratory control, resulting in shorter sentences and reduced intelligibility (Miller, 2006).

As mentioned above, individuals with DS have a relative strength in vocabulary development compared to their more significantly impaired morphosyntactic abilities (Ypsilanti & Grouios, 2008). Figure 8.6 visually demonstrates this relationship. Once word production begins, children with DS learn new vocabulary, although the rate of acquisition is not equivalent to that of peers developing typically. You might be surprised to know that many children with DS learn to read at functional levels. I highlight some research on reading ability of individuals with DS in Focus 8.5.

Figure 8.6   **Language Ability and Nonverbal IQ for Three Subtypes of Intellectual Disability**

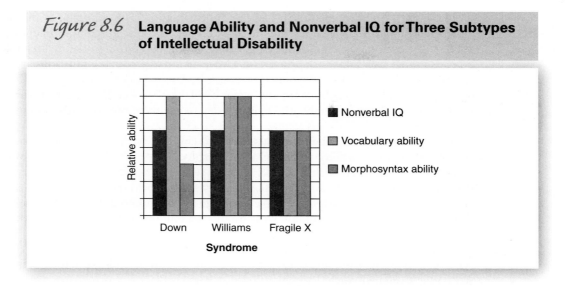

FOCUS 8.5   *Research*

Research demonstrates that individuals with Down syndrome are reading "overachievers." In a meta-analysis, Naess and colleagues (2012) examined high-quality studies evaluating the reading performance of individuals with DS. It is well documented that individuals with DS have vocabulary deficits and less-developed phonological awareness (i.e., sound awareness) than their typically developing peers. Given these deficits, one might suspect that individuals with DS would have trouble decoding, or "sounding out," unfamiliar words. Surprisingly, however, the researchers found that individuals with DS showed equivalent ability to decode unfamiliar words when compared to a group of children developing typically matched for word recognition level. This relative strength of nonword decoding was unexpected. If typically developing children were reading at a level higher than predicted, they would be

classified as overachievers; parents, teachers, and the students themselves would be amazed and thrilled (Oelwein, 2002)! These results—along with results of other recent studies—suggest that practitioners should make literacy a priority for children with DS. Suggestions for literacy interventions include (a) working on phonological awareness and the alphabetic principle by focusing on short words that do not place excessive demands on the student's short-term memory; (b) focusing on vocabulary development, particularly focusing on words that are useful in everyday life, and combining vocabulary and decoding practice to increase the meaningfulness of the text; and (c) focusing on the reading process, including the direction and names of the letters to help students learn what reading is about. You will learn about a model of reading (the interactive-to-independent model) for individuals with significant cognitive disabilities in Chapter 10.

Pragmatic abilities are variable in the DS population. For example, at the one-word level, children with DS demonstrate an appropriate range of pragmatic function, using a variety of speech acts, such as requesting, commanding, and question asking. In adolescence, conversational turn taking is appropriate. However, some pragmatic functions are impaired due to difficulty with morphosyntax. For example, children developing typically learn to use an indirect request (e.g., "Is there any paper available?" rather than a direct form (e.g., "I want paper!"). An individual with DS is unlikely to use the more complex indirect request.

Fragile X Syndrome. The language ability of children with fragile X is consistent with nonverbal cognitive ability (Abbeduto & Murphy, 2004). This is visually demonstrated in Figure 8.6. Children with fragile X develop receptive skills at one-half the rate of children developing typically and expressive ability at one-third the rate (Roberts, Mirrett, & Burchinal, 2001). As a result, receptive language is less impaired than expressive language. At the sentence level, individuals with fragile X demonstrate morphosyntax deficiencies and reduced sentence length.

Children with fragile X have persistent phonological impairments and difficulties with prosody (e.g., rate, inflection) and voice quality. Some children with fragile X speak with a high-pitched voice (Rondal, 2004).

Content (i.e., semantic or lexical development) is a comparative area of strength, with receptive vocabulary being relatively intact. Expressively, however, individuals with fragile X demonstrate word-finding problems (McDuffie et al., 2012).

The pragmatic skills of individuals with fragile X vary. Sometimes there are pragmatic deficits in conversational turn taking and topic maintenance (Abbeduto & Murphy, 2004). Off-topic and stereotypical language production sometimes is present (Belser & Sudhalter, 2001).

Williams Syndrome. Children with Williams syndrome have better-than-expected verbal abilities given their nonverbal cognitive skills; this pattern is very different from what is seen in most cases of ID (Landau & Zukowski, 2003; Rice et al., 2005). Figure 8.6 demonstrates this relationship.

Children with Williams syndrome have delayed verbal skills in early childhood; in fact, early vocabulary development is similar to that seen in children with DS. By adolescence, however, language abilities are equivalent to mental age, and some abilities, such as morphosyntax and lexical skills, surpass mental age (Rondal, 2004).

Individuals with Williams syndrome often have a hoarse voice, but it generally does not interfere with intelligibility (Rice et al., 2005). Articulation and prosody are usually good (Rondal, 2004).

Children with Williams syndrome are described as being "overly friendly." Despite their gregarious verbal style, they often have pragmatic weaknesses, including inappropriate eye contact, difficulty with topic introduction, poor topic maintenance, and inadequate conversational turn taking. Individuals with Williams syndrome frequently repeat topics and ask excessive questions (Rondal, 2004).

I hope you noted that language impairment varies in relation to nonverbal IQ. For some individuals, language is a relative area of strength compared to nonverbal intellectual ability. This is the case with individuals with Williams syndrome. In a second pattern, such as that shown in individuals with fragile X syndrome, language ability is generally equivalent to IQ. In yet a third pattern, seen in individuals with DS, there is a reduced morphosyntactical language ability compared to IQ, but there is a specific strength in lexical learning.

This information underscores the complexity of the relationship between cognition and language. I hope this discussion has persuaded you to take a multidimensional—rather than one-dimensional—view of language ability. As a practitioner, you need to develop the skills to consider independent aspects of form, content, and use in order to appreciate an individual's communication strengths. This perspective will positively impact communication intervention for people with ID.

Assessment

Practitioners typically assess communication skills with a combination of standardized normative tests and criterion-referenced protocols. The role of criterion-referenced assessment is important with people who have ID because particular problems arise in interpreting normative data with this population. In the following sections, I describe the limitations of norm-referenced assessments for individuals with ID, discuss one form of naturalistic assessment called functional assessment, and give an example of an established assessment tool for individuals with ID.

LIMITATIONS OF NORM-REFERENCED ASSESSMENTS FOR INDIVIDUALS WITH ID

Cascella (2006) reviewed 49 language tests published between 1994 and 2004. Students with mild ID were included in the normative sample for only 23 of the tests. When students with ID were included in the normative sample, typically only a few students were tested. For example, the Goldman-Fristoe Test of Articulation, Second Edition (Goldman & Fristoe, 2000), included only 23 students with ID; the Preschool Language Scale, Fourth Edition (Zimmerman et al., 2002), included only 1 student with ID. None of the 15 tests met the suggested requirements of at least 100 students in the ID normative sample group. Individuals with moderate to severe levels of impairment were not included for any tests.

Only 15 of the tests had separate normative samples for children with mild levels of ID. Separate norms allow comparison of student performance with other children with ID. The majority of the tests evaluated receptive and expressive vocabulary, syntax, and grammar; no recent test evaluated pragmatic ability. The lack of a pragmatic assessment is of particular concern because pragmatic ability often is weak in individuals with ID.

As these data demonstrate, there are obvious limitations with norm-referenced testing for individuals with ID. As a result, skilled professionals always include criterion-referenced protocols during the assessment process. Criterion-referenced protocols should include the following:

- A spontaneous language sample analysis to determine the individual's language skills as compared to typical language development patterns
- A discourse analysis to identify social communication abilities
- A classroom-based or workplace assessment to determine needed vocabulary and communication strategies
- An interview with the individual with ID, family, caregivers, and teachers to identify appropriate communication targets
- Evaluation of augmentative/alternative communication (AAC) devices, if appropriate (See Chapter 11 for more about AAC.)
- Evaluation of reading and writing abilities, as appropriate

FUNCTIONAL ASSESSMENT

During **functional assessment** (sometimes called *functional analysis*), a professional gathers information about a student's behavior in order to identify the function or purpose of an aversive behavior. This information is used to develop behavioral-change interventions. Functional assessment typically is used with students with ID who have challenging behaviors.

Challenging behaviors are usually classified in one of three areas: They are used (a) to gain attention or obtain a desired item (e.g., tantrums to obtain candy), (b) to avoid or escape an undesired event or demonstrate frustration (e.g., pulling own hair when asked to come to the table), or (c) as a sensory stimulus (e.g., rocking, self-biting). The characteristics of the challenging behavior are defined through interviews, rating scales, and direct and systematic observation. After defining the challenging behavior, a practitioner makes a hypothesis regarding the communicative purpose of the aversive behavior and substitutes a more appropriate behavior. I will provide more information on the intervention process in the section on intervention in this chapter.

Functional assessment takes specialized training; often a **transdisciplinary** team completes the assessment process. During a transdisciplinary assessment, families and practitioners from different disciplines work together and make collaborative decisions; members share roles and systematically cross discipline boundaries. Functional assessment draws from behaviorist as well as social/environmental theory. The advantages of functional assessment are that it is an ecological approach (i.e., considers the individual's environment) and that it incorporates all of the stakeholders into the intervention plan. The disadvantages include the level of expertise that is required to provide this type of assessment and the time needed to complete the process.

ACHIEVING COMMUNICATION INDEPENDENCE: A COMPREHENSIVE GUIDE TO ASSESSMENT AND INTERVENTION

Gillete (2012) designed *Achieving Communication Competence: Three Steps to Effective Intervention* as an assessment tool for AAC users and persons with severe communication disorders. It has several components, including the Communication Opportunities Inventory and the Communication Skill Inventory. The Communication Opportunities Inventory provides a list of 68 opportunities (e.g., eating at a restaurant, following directions, talking on the phone) that might potentially occur during daily activities. The assessor uses this list to evaluate the communication opportunities for a particular individual.

The Communication Skill Inventory allows the assessor to rate the individual in 11 communicative skill areas (categorized into four major domains). The four domains allow the assessor to consider whether the person with ID (aided or unaided) can (1) interact (e.g., Can he or she initiate an interaction? Are the interactions socially acceptable?), (2) communicate (e.g., Does he or she use symbolic communication such as words or signs, or nonsymbolic communication such as gestures or sounds?), (3) express (e.g., Does he or she vary message functions in relation to the communicative context? Is communication intelligible?), and (4) receive (e.g., Does he or she attend to others' communication?). Skills within the four domains are rated on a 7-point scale: A score of 1–2 represents no independence in using the skill, 3–5 indicates emerging independence, and 6–7 indicates that the skill is established.

Again, the Communication Skill Inventory measures an individual's independence in interacting, communicating, expressing information, and receiving information (see Figure 8.7). The goal of the Communication Skill Inventory is to collect information

Figure 8.7 **Communication Skill Inventory**

Inventory of 11 Essential Communication Skills

Directions: To complete the inventory, review the components of each skill and then provide a 1–7 score for each of the 11 skills on the inventory.

INTERACT	1	2	3	4	5	6	7	N/O
Participate	☐	☐	☐	☐	☐	☐	☐	☐
Indicate	☐	☐	☐	☐	☐	☐	☐	☐
Social Acceptability	☐	☐	☐	☐	☐	☐	☐	☐
Emotional Control	☐	☐	☐	☐	☐	☐	☐	☐

Comments:

COMMUNICATE	1	2	3	4	5	6	7	N/O
Unaided	☐	☐	☐	☐	☐	☐	☐	☐
Aided	☐	☐	☐	☐	☐	☐	☐	☐

Comments:

EXPRESS	1	2	3	4	5	6	7	N/O
Vary Message Functions	☐	☐	☐	☐	☐	☐	☐	☐
Intelligibility	☐	☐	☐	☐	☐	☐	☐	☐

Comments:

RECEIVE	1	2	3	4	5	6	7	N/O
Attention Skills	☐	☐	☐	☐	☐	☐	☐	☐
Behavioral Response Skills	☐	☐	☐	☐	☐	☐	☐	☐
Contextual Response Skills	☐	☐	☐	☐	☐	☐	☐	☐

Comments:

Communication Competence Rating Scale:

7 Established Independent

6 Established Independent with certain partners or in certain opportunities

5 Emerging Prompts or interpretations on 2/10 attempts (minimal assistance)

4 Emerging Prompts or interpretations on 4/10 attempts (moderate assistance)

3 Emerging Prompts or interpretations on 6/10 attempts (moderate/maximal assistance)

2 Potential Prompts or interpretations on 8/10 attempts (maximal assistance)

1 Potential Total prompting and interpreting required

N/O No Opportunity

Source: Courtesy of the Attainment Company, Inc.

about the individual's current communication skills and help identify realistic outcomes for intervention. Each skill is rated based on direct observation, information provided by informants, or information from a client interview. The structure of the entire *Achieving Communication Competence* battery allows the assessor to assess opportunities for communication across domains and develop a strategy to highlight communication strengths and weakness. The *Achieving Communication Competence* manual suggests ecological intervention goals and provides examples of intervention strategies.

Other assessment tools are appropriate for individuals with ID. Many instruments are complex and require specific training. One important new tool is called the *Supports Intensity Scale* (SIS; Thompson et al., 2004). The purpose of this tool is to evaluate a potential mismatch between an individual's repertoire of skills and the demands of the environment. The scale assists a practitioner in obtaining information from a wide variety of family members, friends, acquaintances, and paid support staff. After completing the scale, information is used to help the individual with ID engage in chronologically age-appropriate activities in community settings in a way that is consistent with his or her personal goals and preferences. The SIS and other newer assessment tools for individuals with ID underscore the need to consider both the student and his environment when developing an intervention program. Assessment should guide an SLP to ask and answer the following questions: "What support does this person need?" and "What skills does this individual need to learn?" and "How can the environment be modified to better accommodate this person's abilities and needs?" If you find yourself working with individuals with ID in your professional career, you will undoubtedly learn more about assessment tools, like the SIS, that are framed within an ecological approach to ID.

Intervention

A number of basic principles guide intervention for individuals with ID:

- Provide intervention from the prelinguistic stage through adulthood. Early and intense intervention is critical to ensure the highest possible functioning. Research demonstrates that intervention continues to facilitate communication change into adulthood (Chapman, 2000, 2003; Mattie, 2001).
- Follow a three-pronged approach to intervention programming that considers (1) typical language development patterns, (2) life span needs (i.e., What skills and concepts are required at different age levels?) and (3) modifications in response to an individual's communication strengths and weaknesses.
- Approach intervention from an ecological viewpoint by considering the individual's interests and motivation and also by soliciting input from family, teachers, and employers. Develop intervention approaches that maximize generalization and transfer of communication skills to daily life.

There are a number of good approaches for children with ID consistent with the above-mentioned principles: Research-tested approaches include milieu teaching (Yoder & Warren, 2002) and peer-training models (Schmidt & Stichter, 2012; Hughett, Kohler, & Raschke, 2013). Both approaches are discussed in other chapters in this book; consider how milieu teaching and peer-training models might be adapted for individuals with ID (see Focus 8.6).

In the following section, I introduce two additional interventions: functional communication training and an intervention called IT's Fun (Integrated Treatment Is Fun: A Program for Children with DS; Rosin, 2006; Rosin & Miolo, 2005). These two

---

FOCUS 8.6   *Intervention*

- Review the milieu teaching and peer-training approaches discussed in Chapter 6. What adaptations might be needed for children with ID?
- Make up a case example that describes a student who could benefit from peer

training. What intervention steps would be appropriate? How would you evaluate the impact of the intervention?

---

approaches are illustrative of different approaches appropriate for individuals with ID. At the end of this chapter, I present information on how an SLP can support an older student with ID as he or she transitions into the workplace.

Finally, it also is important to consider how individuals from different cultural groups may react to intervention planning for a family member with communication impairment. Individuals from different ethnic backgrounds can have very different communication styles, resulting in ethnic mismatch. **Ethnic mismatch** refers to a situation in which a student's home culture and the service provider hold conflicting expectations for the student's communication or behavior. An **ethnic group** is a group of individuals who share a common language, heritage, religion, or geography/nationality (Smedley & Smedley, 2005). To increase your cultural awareness and avoid potential ethnic mismatch, learn more about one ethnic group, Asian Americans, in Focus 8.7.

INTERVENTION APPROACH: FUNCTIONAL COMMUNICATION APPROACH

The functional communication training (FCT) approach is a behavioral intervention used to replace an individual's maladaptive or problem behaviors (e.g., tantrums, hitting, self-injury) with more socially acceptable communication options. It is built on the concept of

---

FOCUS 8.7   *Multicultural Issues*

Asia is the largest continent that includes East Asia (China, Hong Kong, Japan, Macau, Mongolia, Korea, and Taiwan), South Asia (Brunei, Burma, Cambodia, East Timor, Indonesia, Laos, Malaysia, Philippines, Singapore, Thailand, and Vietnam), and the Pacific Islands (Samoa, Hawaii, and Guam). Each country has its own language and unique culture. However, given that the cultures are broadly similar (i.e., there are more cultural similarities than differences), some generalizations are possible.

The cultural differences between an Asian family and an SLP could result in ethnic mismatch during intervention planning for an individual with developmental disorders. Seung (2013) discusses four major considerations in Asian culture to avoid ethnic mismatch: (a) the collectivist culture of Asian countries and the need to save face, (b) the high value placed on academics as contrasted to functional daily skills, (c) the authoritarian nature of Asia culture, and (d) the implications of a high-context culture.

(continued)

Asian culture is more collectivistic than many Western cultures. In a collectivist culture, members are very sensitive to the perceptions of others. The need to consider how others perceive the family or an individual is referred to as *face*; face is an abstract perception of each individual's "social self-worth." In Asian culture, someone losing face results in shame to the family (Parette, Chung, & Huer, 2004). Having a child with a developmental disability may cause a family to lose face. To maintain face, some Asian or Asian American parents of a child with a developmental disability disconnect from family members, either to hide the fact that the child has a disability or to cope with parental stress and shame.

Individuals from Asian cultures historically place a very high value on academics. Typically, a child's academic performance is seen as much more important than focusing on functional daily living skills. This viewpoint potentially impacts clinical decisions for children with disabilities; parents who are Asian American may be dissatisfied when nonacademic skills are suggested as intervention goals. SLPs should be sensitive to this perception when they counsel families about program planning.

Asian cultures tend to be authoritarian. Parents are seen as the authorities when making decisions about their child; it is likely that they will also rely on the professional's perspective, because professionals are perceived as having knowledge. Parents may not question a professional's suggestions because doing so would seem an affront to the professional's authority.

Communication styles are sometimes classified as either high-context or low-context communication. High-context styles are indirect, infer meanings from the context, have interpersonal sensitivity, and use silence and emotions to guide one's behavior. Low-context styles are direct, dominant, dramatic, animated, and open. Typically, Asian Americans follow a high-context style and European Americans follow a low-context communication style. If an SLP is not sensitive to a high-context communication style, there could be misunderstandings. For example, one SLP reported that prior to an Individualized Education Program meeting, she used small talk to put the family at ease. A few Asian mothers indicated that their perception of the small talk at the meeting was that the SLP was "not taking the meeting as seriously as the mothers did." This clearly was not the intention of the SLP; it was an example of miscommunication resulting from communication style differences.

Source: Seung, H. (2013). Cultural considerations in serving children with ASD and their families: Asian American perspective. *Perspectives on Language Learning and Education, 20,* 14–19.

---

functional assessment described above. The underlying assumption is that an individual with ID uses maladaptive behaviors to influence his or her environment, and communicative responses can replace inappropriate behaviors.

The FCT approach was developed in the 1980s. The steps for implementation of FCT include the following:

1. Identify the antecedent stimuli (i.e., time of day, settings, people, activities) that trigger maladaptive behavior.
2. Determine the purpose of the maladaptive behavior and the reinforcement that is sustaining inappropriate behaviors via a functional analysis that includes (1) manipulating task demands by altering the discriminative stimuli, such as making the task

easier or more difficult; and (2) changing the reinforcement schedule by presenting and withdrawing the reinforcement while documenting behavior changes.

3. Identify a communicative behavior equivalent to the maladaptive behavior (e.g., use of a sign, gesture, pointing response, verbalization) that will permit the individual to obtain the desired reinforcement (e.g., attention, task avoidance). The communication response needs to be as easy as, or easier than, the maladaptive behavior.

4. Monitor the generalization and use of the communication skill across situations (Bailey et al., 2002; Carr et al., 2004).

The process just described is similar to an experimental design implemented in highly controlled or laboratory-like conditions; this approach represents an outgrowth of Skinner's behaviorist theories. In Focus 8.8, consider the different ways Skinner's theories impact the FCT model.

To clarify the FCT model, imagine that you are a practitioner working with an individual with maladaptive behavior. First, as the trainer, you present two tasks. In the first task, you ask the individual with ID (the trainee) to point to pictures of easy vocabulary items; in the second task, you ask the trainee to point to pictures of difficult vocabulary items. The reinforcement schedule is systematically varied. At times, you provide 100% reinforcement (e.g., praise, shoulder pats); in other training sets, you reinforce the trainee after every third response. The occurrence of maladaptive behaviors is noted and interpreted. If, for example, the trainee demonstrates maladaptive behaviors during the more difficult tasks, the maladaptive behavior communicates *This task is too hard*. On the other hand, if the trainee produces more maladaptive behaviors during reduced reinforcement, you interpret the maladaptive behavior to communicate *I want more attention*. Subsequently, you introduce socially acceptable responses fulfilling the same function, such as coaching the trainee to say "This is too hard; help me" in the first case and "Look what I did!" in the second (Carr et al., 2004).

The use of FCT has changed since its introduction. Originally, FCT was used with nonverbal individuals, and the communicative replacement behaviors typically were signed, gestured, or implemented via augmentative communication. At present, individuals with autism, people with varying levels of ID, and individuals who are verbal are considered viable FCT candidates (Halle, Ostrosky, & Hemmeter, 2006).

The functional assessment process also has changed. Whereas professionals originally completed FCT within a controlled setting, now it is desirable to consider the person with ID within his or her daily routines (Dunlap, & Fox, 2011; McLaren, & Nelson, 2009). As a result, functional assessment now employs interviews and checklists along with descriptive behavioral observations of everyday interactions. An antecedent–behavior–consequence (A-B-C) chart (see Table 8.3) is a format that helps practitioners capture

---

FOCUS 8.8   *Learning More*

- Describe how Skinner's principles of behavior modification are demonstrated within the functional communication training (FCT) approach.

- Describe strengths and weaknesses of Skinnerian-based intervention. How has FCT been modified over the years to account for these weaknesses?

Table 8.3   **Example of an Antecedent–Behavior–Consequence (A-B-C) Analysis**

Questions	Occurred	Did not occur
Who	When working with peers she does not know well	When working with familiar peers
What	When asked to elaborate her response (e.g., say more than a few words)	When a minimal response is required
Where	During academic classes	Art class, playground, lunchtime
When	At the end of the day	Early in the day
Why	Student uses maladaptive behaviors when (a) working with unfamiliar listeners, (b) the task is more difficult (e.g., longer utterances, more complex work is required), (c) when she is fatigued.	

important environmental components triggering inappropriate behaviors. In the example provided in Table 8.3, the A-B-C analysis revealed that a student acted out with inappropriate behavior when she was with unfamiliar peers, when she was asked to produce more complex communication, during more difficult academic tasks, or when she was fatigued.

The professional uses the A-B-C chart to examine the *what, when, why,* and *where* associated with the occurrence of maladaptive behaviors. Typically, once the problem situation is identified, the professional completes a behavioral baseline. For example, the trainer records off-task vs. on-task behavior at 10-second intervals during an activity evoking the maladaptive behavior (time sampling) or counts the number of occurrences of a problem behavior within a specific block of time (frequency counts).

Following the baseline data collection, the FCT training begins. Figure 8.8 provides an example of a treatment interaction, and Figure 8.9 provides examples of intervention goals. The examples demonstrate how the practitioner uses FCT within ecologically valid situations as they occur during classroom, home, or work environments. During intervention, the practitioner remembers to:

- Provide frequent opportunities for the individual to practice the replacement communicative form in context. If needed, the practitioner additionally provides **massed trials,** which are intensive one-on-one training of the targeted behavior.
- Use behavioral modification techniques, including prompting, prompt fading, and reinforcement of successive approximations to teach the replacement communicative behavior (Halle et al., 2006).
- Teach tolerance to reinforcement delay so that the trainee does not always require immediate reinforcement. For example, if a child uses tantrums to obtain a favorite toy, the first step is to teach him to sign *I want toy!* as an alternative response and establish this behavior in everyday situations. As a second step, following the child's request, the practitioner shows a picture of the item and says, "John, hold on to this picture of the toy. You will get the toy in just seconds." Initially the delay is very brief, but gradually the delay is increased.
- Monitor the use of the replacement behavior in everyday interactions. If the maladaptive behavior occasionally emerges, the behavior may need to be extinguished by withdrawing reinforcement (e.g., time-out) or giving mild punishment (e.g., frowning

Figure 8.8   **Example of a Functional Communication Treatment (FCT) Sequence**

- *Maladapative behaviors:* Mark, a 14-year-old nonverbal boy with ID, engaged in stereotypical arm-flicking behavior and self-injurious fingernail picking. Functional analysis determined that maladaptive behaviors increased under low-stimulation conditions and decreased when Mark had access to his radio and other leisure items (e.g., photo album).
- The therapist taught Mark to request access to preferred leisure items by selecting a pictured item from a communication book. For example, if Mark handed the therapist a picture of a radio, he gained access to that item for 2 minutes.
- To demonstrate experimental control, the low-stimulation condition was reintroduced, and Mark's problem behaviors resumed at high rates. This reversal procedure was conducted several times, demonstrating that the reduction in maladaptive behaviors was a result of treatment.
- Mark was later taught to use his communication book at home and school. Also, he was taught to tolerate delays to reinforcement when an adult was unable to immediately provide an activity.

Source: Based on information from "Assessment and Treatment of Automatically Reinforced Self-Injurious and Stereotypic Behavior," by D. M. Gadaire, 2000, *Journal of Undergraduate Research, 1*. Retrieved December 7, 2006, from www.clas.ufl.edu/jur/200002/papers/paper_gadaire.html.

or reprimands). Alternatively, positive reinforcement of the communicative form may need to be increased.

Evidence Supporting the Functional Communication Approach (FCT). Published results of FCT interventions demonstrating intervention effectiveness at Level II appear in peer-reviewed journals. Much of this research uses single-subject designs. A single-subject design is an experimental design that focuses on the behavior of an individual subject

Figure 8.9   **Examples of Goals for Functional Communication Training (FCT)**

- Sasha will produce a signed "take a break" request with a subsequent reduction of off-task behavior. Requesting a break after 15 seconds of completing a demanding task such as stacking blocks will result in a high-quality break (1 minute of interaction with a favorite toy with adult attention); requesting a break without completing the demanding task results in 15 seconds of a low-quality break (no toy, no adult attention).
- Kallie will visually attend and sit through a 1-minute book reading after requesting and being given a favorite toy ("koosh" ball, silly putty), with subsequent elimination of self-stimulating behavior for 7 out of 8 consecutive days.
- Raini will shake her head *no* when given food she does not like for 7 out of 8 consecutive days, with subsequent reduction of tantrums. She will request and receive favorite food items using picture cards after finishing a meal without tantrums.

rather than comparing behaviors of subject groups; an example was completed by Wacker and his colleagues (2005). Wacker's study included 25 children with developmental disabilities between the ages of 1 and 6 years and consisted of five phases:

1. Functional analysis
2. Observation probes to collect baselines of problem behaviors combined into a category called *total problem behaviors* (i.e., behaviors included destructive behaviors such as aggression and self-injury as well as disruptive behaviors such as crying, task refusal, tantrums, and noncompliance)
3. FCT treatment phase during which parents modeled and reinforced a word, sign, or gesture such as *help, done,* or *play* to replace the maladaptive behavior
4. Evaluation of the occurrence of the replacement behavior in situations other than the training environment
5. Training on a second task (if needed)

The combined data indicated a decrease in total problem behaviors for 24 of the 25 children. The decrease for a child demonstrated via a single-case study design is visually presented in Figure 8.10.

INTERVENTION APPROACH: IT'S FUN PROGRAM

The IT's Fun program (Rosin, 2006; Rosin & Miolo, 2005) is a performance-based intervention designed to emphasize the communicative strengths (i.e., social skills, visual processing, receptive language) of school-age students with DS and to facilitate improvement in areas of deficit (i.e., intelligibility, respiratory control, prosody, increased verbal output). During a 3-week "speech camp" intervention format, participants complete theme-based activities including shared book readings, story reenactments, mime and improvisation,

Figure 8.10 **Example of Data from a Single-Case Study Design: Problem Behaviors Are Documented under Conditions of Free Play, Demand, and Attention**

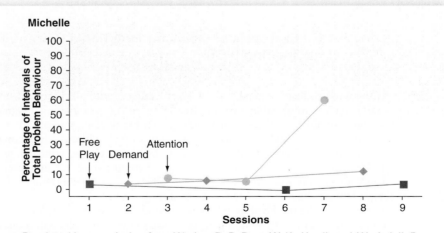

Source: Reprinted by permission from Wacker, D. P., Berg, W. K., Harding, J. W., Anjali, B., Rankin, B., & Ganzer, J. (2005). *Treatment effectiveness, stimulus generalization, and acceptability to parents of functional communication training.* Educational Psychology, 25, 233–256. Copyright © 2005 by Taylor & Francis Informa UK Ltd

vocal and physical warm-ups, singing and dancing, and play rehearsals, as well as presentation of their skills in a culminating end-of-the-week performance.

Professionals use specific strategies to increase participants' verbal output, vocabulary development, and literacy skills. For example, language facilitators (1) incorporate visual supports (words, pictures, and symbols) to help participants learn song lyrics and lines for the plays, (2) prompt participants to use metacognitive strategies to improve verbal production and organize information (e.g., using pictures, symbols, or a few words as a reminder), and (3) use scripts and routines to increase fluency and verbal output. The participants also are trained to use strategies such as body movement, gestures, and signing to facilitate verbalizations. Some "rules and tools" guiding their performances include (1) talking slowly, (2) saying all the sounds in words, (3) projecting their voices, and (4) formulating messages before speaking. Participants are given individual daily practice time to speak in front of the group. Dance and movement activities are used to increase and vary vocal quality and enhance the participants' fun and motivation. Figure 8.11

Figure 8.11   **Example of IT's Fun Treatment Sequence**

Description of student: Samuel is interested in sports and likes to discuss football. His speech is rapid and often difficult to understand. His communication goal is to increase meta-awareness to improve intelligibility. His talking rules include (1) slow down when talking, (2) stick to one idea at a time, and (3) say all the sounds in the words. He is in front of his peer group during the "In the Spotlight" time and is preparing to discuss Saturday's football game.

Adult: OK everyone, Samuel is going to tell us about the football game last week!
Samuel, what are you going to remember to do when you tell us your story?
Samuel: Talk slow!
Adult: Good! And what else?
Samuel: Say my words.
Adult: Right, you are going to say every sound in all your words. Anything else?
Samuel: (shrugs)
Adult: Look at your talking chart. What is your other talking rule?
Samuel: Say one idea at time.
Adult: That's right! Just tell us one idea before you tell us something new. Watch our faces to make sure we understand.

Samuel proceeds to tell his story with feedback from the adult and his peers. He evaluates his performance by assigning a face to his performance. He keeps his evaluations in his "talking diary."

Faces for Self-Evaluation

provides an example of a therapeutic interaction, and Figure 8.12 provides an example of communication goals.

Evidence Supporting the IT's Fun Program. The IT's Fun program has a documented Level III efficacy because intervention results are presented via case study examples (Rosin & Miolo, 2005). Experts indicate that the principles underlying the approach are theoretically sound (Miller, 2006).

Rosin and Miolo (2005) report pre- and post-intervention data for seven children with DS between the ages of 5 and 12 years. During the IT's Fun program, practitioners developed communication goals for each participant and used a performance rating measure (sometimes called goal attainment scaling) to rate the participants' abilities as follows: -2 = significant deficit, -1 = mild deficit, 0 = desired level of functioning, $+1$ = better than expected ability, $+2$ = much better than expected performance. Clinical researchers frequently use rating systems to document changes in overall daily functioning in individuals with ID (Jones et al., 2006; Schlosser, 2004).

The seven participants demonstrated improved communication and social skills and showed improved attitudes about talking following the 3-week intervention. Consistent with the Level III levels of evidence rating, the pilot study did not compare the focus intervention to alternative interventions. The authors indicate the intervention approach will continue to be examined with more sophisticated designs (Rosin & Miolo, 2005).

INTERVENTION: SUPPORTING THE STUDENT'S TRANSITION TO THE WORKPLACE

By the time most students with ID are 18, they have finished the coursework their school system has to offer, yet they are not prepared to enter the workforce (Hartman, 2009). Only 52% of postgraduates with ID obtain employment or receive employment training (Wagner et al., 2005). Core skills required for employment center around the individual's communication, social, and collaboration abilities. An SLP plays an important role in

---

Figure 8.12 **Examples of Goals for IT's Fun Approach**

- Tabitha will tell a story in front of a group using written cues. The story will have a beginning (initiating event), middle (exciting event), and conclusion. Tabitha will achieve a rating of 4–5 on intelligibility (sentences evaluated by interventionist using 5-point scale) for 4 of 5 consecutive days during storytelling.

  Rating scale: 5 = ≥ 90% of sentences intelligible, 4 = 80% of sentences intelligible, 3 = 70–60% of sentences intelligible, 2 = 50–70% unintelligible, 1 = ≥ 80% unintelligible.

- Michael will respond with a complete sentence (noun + verb + noun) on a related topic at least 5 times in a 5-minute group discussion 4 out of 5 consecutive days at a level of 5. Participation will be prompted initially with a nonverbal signal; prompt will be progressively faded.

  Rating scale: 5 = 5 interactions with no prompting, 4 = at least 3 responses with no prompting, 3 = produces 4–5 appropriate responses with nonverbal prompt, 2 = produces less than 3 responses with nonverbal prompt, 1 = produces less than 2 responses with nonverbal prompt or responses are off-topic.

facilitating the transition process; **transition** refers to the life changes that occur in the lives of young adults as well as the formal planning process that assists students with disabilities as they move from school environments to work environments (Wehman, 2013). Student involvement in the Individualized Education Program (IEP) process facilitates the transition process because student participation translates to goals that relate to the student's interests or personal motivation. However, in reality, most students with ID are not involved in their IEP process (Grigal & Deschamps, 2012).

The extent to which students learn, use, and generalize social and communication skills directly impacts a student's success in school, work, and community settings (Carter & Hughes, 2013). For example, employers consistently indicate that an employee's ability to communicate effectively, work well with others, and respond well to feedback are critical skills that impact hiring, promotion, and retention. Most models of transition place social and interpersonal skills as a foundational skill for successful transition to the community.

Many students with ID, as well as students with other significant disabilities, have social and communication challenges that limit their involvement and success in workplace and community activities. Fortunately, however, a number of strategies hold promise for increasing students' interactions and social ability (Carter & Hughes, 2013). The four major categories of educational practice facilitating student transition are (a) student-focused strategies, (b) peer-focused strategies, (c) support-focused strategies, and (d) compensatory strategies.

The primary student-focused strategy is social skills training. This approach involves explicit instruction targeting specific communication skills. A practitioner works with students with disabilities to facilitate their ability to initiate conversation or take conversational turns. The practitioner may also work on fostering more general social skills, including cooperation and assertiveness. Additional student-focused strategies include working with students on skills such as game playing or computer use to increase recreational or workplace access. Recommended practice is to focus on building a student's social skills in meaningful activities, such as eating lunch with peers, participating in a recreational activity, or working in a cooperative learning group.

Peer-focused strategies target working with a student's peer group. Sometimes classmates, coworkers, and employers are hesitant or unsure of how to support the communication and social skills of a student with a disability; or they may be willing to interact but hesitate to initiate conversation on their own. Peer-focused strategies focus on equipping typical communicators with opportunities and confidence to interact with individuals with disabilities. There are many strategies that facilitate peer-to-peer interactions. Typical communicators may need more information about a particular kind of disability and the communication and social challenges associated with the disability type. At times, it is useful to provide specific information about how a particular individual with a disability communicates his needs and preferences. Finally, an important component of peer-focused training is teaching specific strategies that facilitate daily communication. Helpful strategies include calling the student's name and waiting for eye contact before initiating a conversation, phrasing questions in ways that foster communication participation, and teaching peers how they can provide constructive feedback to facilitate improved interactions.

The third set of educational practice focuses on support-focused strategies. Support-based strategies aim to modify the environment so that a student with a disability has more opportunity to practice communication and social skills. Examples of support-based strategy include programs in which students with disabilities interact with peers who are typically developing. At present, approximately 40% of U.S. high schools offer social or activity clubs under a variety of names, such as peer buddy program, peer partner club, peer mentoring program, and Best Buddies (Hughes & Carter, 2012). The configuration of these programs varies greatly, but one successful option is offering course credit to students (both typically developing and disabled) as an elective course option and/or integrating regular peer interactions into an already existing course. Course assignments often include maintaining a journal and an end-of-semester project. In contrast, some high schools have developed extracurricular programs focusing on social or sports activities. Finally, some schools take an individualized approach and arrange for a peer buddy to regularly interact with the student with disabilities at lunch period, after school, or during class time.

The final set of educational practice focuses on compensatory strategies. An exciting application of technology is the ability to use iPad and iPhone apps to foster independence and job performance. For students with significant communication challenges, there are now apps that support communication (e.g., text-to-speech, photos that when touched respond with speech output). I discuss the use of communication apps in more detail later in this book, in Chapter 11.

In addition to communication apps, there are other apps that facilitate student performance within a community context. Other app types include daily living apps (e.g., task sequences are listed, tasks are "checked off " when completed, and/or the app records students' progress toward a reward), organizational apps (e.g., scheduled text or voice output is sent out to remind the student to complete a task), workplace support apps (e.g., a timer is set that shows the student how much time has elapsed and how much time is left to complete an activity), social skills apps (e.g., an app supplies conversational scripts in a variety of contexts), and medical apps (e.g., a prescription reminder alerts the student to take medication). If you want to learn more about transition planning and the use of apps, you can research the topic at www.ocali.org/center/transitions (type "apps" in the search box to find more about app technology and the transition process).

Summary

- The American Association of Intellectual and Developmental Disabilities (2012) defines *intellectual disability* (ID) as originating before age 18 and characterized by significant limitations both in intellectual functioning and in adaptive behavior, as expressed in conceptual, social, and practical adaptive skills.
- The ecological model of ID considers an individual's functioning in relation to his or her microsystem (i.e., family, caregivers), mesosystem (i.e., school, neighborhood, community), and macrosystem (i.e., society's views and practices regarding individuals with ID). Professionals use this model when developing intervention programs for individuals with ID.
- Five dimensions are considered in the ecological model: (1) intellectual ability, represented by an IQ two standard deviations below the mean, (2) adaptive behavior, (3) an individual's social interaction in everyday activities, (4) mental and physical health, and (5) an individual's environmental context including all three levels of system support (e.g., micro, meso, macro). The ecological model also emphasizes the mediating effects of an individual's social support system influencing his or her functioning.

- The prevalence of ID is 1 to 3% of the population; ID occurs more frequently in males than females. The causes of ID vary in terms of timing and type of risk factors.
- There are different ID subtypes; each subtype differs with regard to genotype and phenotype. An individual's cognitive processing and language characteristics also vary with respect to genotype. Cognitive processes include attention, discrimination, organization, transfer, and memory. Interventions should accommodate an individual's strengths and weaknesses.
- Prominent debates have focused on several topics, including (1) a discussion of individuals with ID as evidencing language delay vs. disorder and (2) the relationship of nonverbal IQ and language ability. Practitioners consider individual aspects of language form, content, and use with respect to ID genotype.
- Assessment should consider an individual's ecological system. Norm-referenced assessment has limitations for individuals with ID; criterion-referenced assessments are preferred as they describe an individual's functioning. Language sample analysis and functional communication strategy analysis are two important criterion-referenced assessments. Two intervention approaches, functional communication training and the IT's Fun program, offer valuable approaches for working with individuals with ID. An SLP also should consider how to help students with ID transition to the workplace.

Discussion and In-Class Activities

1. Compare the *Achieving Communication Competence* assessment tool (Gillette, 2012) with the observational assessment protocol for children with autism in Chapter 9. How are the assessments similar? How are they different? How is the *Achieving Communication Competence* similar to or different from an assessment protocol for a preschooler with specific language impairment?
2. Look at the data from a single-case study design (Figure 8.10). Examine and describe what might have taken place at different phases of the study and show how they are visually represented in this figure. Complete a literature search and find another communication study using a single-case study design. Describe the phases of the study (e.g., preintervention, intervention), and show how these phases of the study are visually represented in the data presentation.
3. Make a presentation on shaken baby syndrome (SBS). What are the signs that a family may be under stress and prone to SBS? What happens to the infant brain when a baby is violently shaken? Call the local Red Cross and obtain literature on its SBS prevention program and present the information in class. What are other possible causes of traumatic brain injury (TBI) in childhood, and what can professionals do to help raise community awareness to prevent childhood TBI?
4. Performance rating systems such as the one described in this chapter are viable tools for demonstrating behavior change. In a small group, describe a behavior or goal that is appropriate for an individual with ID and develop a rating system to describe behavior change relative to that goal. Complete a literature search and find other articles on similar rating systems. (Note: Search for goal attainment scaling, functional

communication measures, or performance evaluation.) Discuss the pros and cons of performance rating systems.

5. List aspects of the IT's Fun approach that make it an appropriate program for school-age students with ID. In small groups, identify aspects of the program that could be incorporated into other intervention programs. For example, how could aspects of the IT's Fun approach be incorporated into individual therapy sessions for a 12-year-old student with Down syndrome who has difficulty with the /s/ and /l/ phonemes and incorrectly uses pronoun forms (e.g., substitutes *he* for *his* and *she* for *her*)?

6. Find information regarding the communication styles likely to be used by members of different ethnic groups. Determine whether communication patterns reflect a high- or low-context communication style. You can begin to find information by looking at the website www.pbs.org/ampu/crosscult.html.

Chapter 8 Case Study

Jonah, a 3-year-old male, has Down syndrome. His father is an engineer, and his mother is a kindergarten teacher. Jonah has two older sisters, ages 13 and 11. Jonah's hearing has been checked, and it is within normal limits. He wears glasses. His health is good.

Since birth, Jonah's parents have been reading to him and using simple sign language along with spoken language. A developmental specialist has been visiting Jonah at his home once a month since birth. Jonah will attend an inclusive preschool program in the fall; it is a program with six children who are typically developing and six children with special educational needs.

At present, Jonah has about 20 words; some are spoken, and others are approximations of manual signs. Jonah has difficulty producing words with varying syllables. So, for example, he pronounces *Daddy* as *Da-Da, pudding* (a favorite food) as *puh, baby* as *ba-ba,* and so forth. Jonah likes music and rhythm games (e.g., clapping, pounding a drum, shaking a tambourine). He is more vocal and varies his sound production more during rhythm activities than at other times.

Jonah has some expressions, such as "What is that?" and "Give me that!" The expressions are always said in the same combination and are primarily prosodic units (i.e., inflection patterns) with poor intelligibility. The individual words (i.e., *what, is,* and *that*) are never used in any other combinations or in isolation.

Jonah often points at what he wants, and his sisters (who dote on their brother) are eager to figure out what he wants. Jonah's mother has been teaching Jonah to sign *please.* He now uses the sign *please* for almost all his requests throughout the day rather than labeling items directly.

You have been asked to work with Jonah. Your plan is to have Jonah, his parents, and his sisters (when they are available) come to your office twice a month and develop a home program.

Questions for Discussion

1. Jonah's parents want to start working on two- and three-word combinations because of his use of three-word phrases such as "What is that?" You feel that Jonah is at the

one-word stage and would like to see him begin to use some action words, words for appearance/disappearance, and modifiers (*big, pretty*). Review the developmental information in Chapter 2 (early word learning stage) and develop an explanation for why Jonah needs to continue to emphasize a variety of word types into his corpus.

2. What environmental factors might be limiting Jonah's word/sign production? With members of your class, develop a mock counseling session in which you make suggestions to the family on how they can help Jonah increase his use of meaningful words and signs. Role-play your intervention session.

3. What do you think might be going on with Jonah's use of phrases? You might want to consider the implication of something called "giant words." **Giant words** are two- or three-word combinations that the child hears frequently. When the child says one of these, he or she really is treating the phrase as a polysyllabic single word. At this stage of development, the child typically does not use the words separately or in novel combinations with other words. Explain the role of giant words in terms of Jonah's language development.

4. How might you take advantage of Jonah's love of music and rhythm to facilitate his production of two-syllable words with varying sounds (e.g., *doggie, bunny, mommy*)? With your classmates, write an intervention goal to improve Jonah's production of CVCV (consonant–vowel:consonant–vowel [e.g., *Daddy, baby, cookie*) words with varying sound patterns.

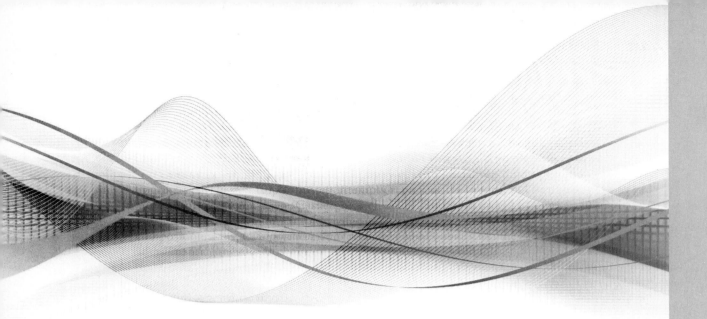

9 Children on the Autism Spectrum

Chapter Overview Questions

1. What characteristics are common to all students with autism spectrum disorder (ASD)? What behaviors are associated with low-functioning autism? What behaviors are associated with high-functioning autism?
2. What evidence indicates that ASD is likely to have multiple etiologies?
3. How do fundamental skills related to cognitive constructivist theory impact the intervention of children with ASD?

4. What is the difference between communicative functions and communicative means? What differences in communication functions and means might a practitioner expect to see in a child with ASD?
5. What theoretical underpinnings form the basis of the applied behavior analysis (ABA) and *SCERTS*™ intervention approaches? What are some examples of intervention goals that reflect the two different interventions?

This chapter describes individuals diagnosed with autism. It is designed to help you understand how children with autism are likely to communicate and behave and how practitioners assess and intervene with children in this population. Children on the autism spectrum are some of the most challenging and interesting individuals to work with. Ninety percent of school-based speech-language pathologists (SLPs) (ASHA, 2012) report that they work with children with autism; this area of intervention is the second most common intervention on their caseload—preceded only by articulation and phonological disorders!

One challenging aspect of working with children with autism is their contradictory pattern of ability vs. disability. For example, I know of a child with autism who was unable to meaningfully communicate with others but read verbatim from a telephone book. This child demonstrated **hyperlexia**, a precocious reading ability inconsistent with overall ability. He read the words aloud but did not comprehend what he was reading. An ability discrepancy such as hyperlexia is frustrating to families and may prompt them to seek novel treatments without proven treatment efficacy. The information in this chapter will help you consider and evaluate assessment and treatment options for children with autism. This set of skills will guide your intervention when you are responsible for helping families make important decisions.

Description of the Disorder

Dr. Leo Kanner, an Australian pediatrician, first described children with autism in 1943. Kanner provided case descriptions of children demonstrating a unique combination of symptoms. One case, Donald T., was noted to "hum and sing many tunes accurately," have an "unusual memory for faces and names," know an "inordinate number of pictures in a set of Compton's encyclopedia," and recite the alphabet "backward as well as forward." However, along with his precocious abilities, Donald T. "almost never cried to go with his mother, did not notice when family or playmates came or went, and was happiest when left alone" (Kanner, 1943, pp. 217–218).

As you learned in Chapter 6, the *Diagnostic and Statistical Manual of Mental Disorders,* Fifth Edition (DSM-5; American Psychiatric Association, 2013) is the manual clinicians and researchers use to diagnose and classify mental disorders. DSM-5 uses the term **autism spectrum disorder (ASD)** to categorize individuals who (a) have deficits in social communication and social interaction *and* also (b) demonstrate restricted repetitive behaviors, interests, and activities (RRBs). RRBs include a very broad category of behaviors, such as preoccupation with restricted patterns of interest (e.g., having very specific knowledge about clocks and time); adherence to specific, nonfunctional routines (e.g., insisting on walking on specific parts of the sidewalk); repetitive motor manners (e.g., hand flapping); and preoccupation with parts of objects (e.g., peering at the wheels of toy cars while spinning them). The symptoms of people with ASD fall on a continuum, with some individuals showing mild symptoms and others having much more severe symptoms. Use of the term ASD allows clinicians to account for the variations and severity of symptoms and behaviors from person to person. The ASD category now is an umbrella term that applies to individuals who were previously classified as having either autistic disorder, Asperger's disorder, childhood disintegrative disorder, or the catchall diagnosis of pervasive developmental disorder not otherwise specified. Researchers found that these separate diagnoses were not consistently applied across different clinics and treatment centers, which resulted in the now all-encompassing category of ASD. Under the DSM-5 criteria, individuals with ASD must show symptoms from early childhood, even if those symptoms are not recognized until later. You can review the specific criteria for diagnosis of ASD in Table 9.1.

Under the DSM-5 criteria, there is a new category called "social (pragmatic) communication disorder"; this diagnosis is used to identify individuals who have difficulties with social skills but do not show restricted or repetitive patterns of behavior. SLPs play an important role in helping to make this differential diagnosis. ASD must be ruled out before a diagnosis of social (pragmatic) communication disorder is made.

Table 9.1 DSM-5 Criteria for Autism Spectrum Disorder

Currently, or by history, must meet criteria A, B, C, and D

A. Persistent deficits in social communication and social interaction across contexts, not accounted for by general developmental delays, and manifests *all three* of the following:
   1. Deficits in social-emotional reciprocity
   2. Deficits in nonverbal communicative behaviors used for social interaction*
   3. Deficits in developing and maintaining relationships
B. Restricted, repetitive patterns of behaviors, interests, or activities as manifested by *at least two* of the following:
   1. Stereotyped or repetitive speech, motor movements, and use of objects
   2. Excessive adherence to routines, ritualized patterns of verbal or nonverbal behavior, or excessive resistance to change
   3. Highly restricted, fixated interests that are abnormal in intensity or focus
   4. Hyper- or hypo-reactivity to sensory input or unusual interest in sensory aspects of environment
C. Symptoms must be present in early childhood (but may not become fully manifest until social demands exceed limited capacities)
D. Symptoms together limit and impair everyday functioning

*It is important to note that in relation to ASD, DSM-5 omits criteria related to delay in or lack of development of spoken language. Rather, as part of the DSM-5 diagnostic process, an evaluator is to specify whether the ASD occurs "with or without accompanying language impairment." Because the language component is downplayed in the new ASD criteria, SLPs must (a) ensure that individuals with ASD who have a language impairment receive a diagnosis of *both* language disorder *and* autism spectrum disorder and (b) strongly advocate for language goals to be included in ASD intervention plans (Paul, 2013).

CHARACTERISTIC DEFICITS OF ASD

ASD is now viewed as a single disorder that presents with significant individual variety. Every individual with ASD will have significant problems with the social/communication domain, but there will be significant variation in the severity of the symptoms. For example, students with severe autism (referred to as low-functioning autism [LFA]) may be nonverbal or have extremely limited verbal communication. Students with LFA need individualized, specialized, and intensive levels of intervention. On the other hand, students with high-functioning autism (HFA; formerly referred to as Asperger's syndrome) often can be educated in general education settings. However, students who are diagnosed as having HFA also need intervention provided by special educators and an SLP because even though they communicate verbally, they are likely to have communication patterns that include (a) odd prosody and intonation, including a too-rapid rate, "jerky" phasing, and too-loud volume; (b) differences in nonverbal communication, including limited use of gestures and facial expressions; (c) use of unusual phrases and vocabulary; and (d) one-sided and disorganized conversational style lacking a give-and-take with the listener. The current use of a more general classification of ASD encompassing the full range of the autism spectrum (LFA vs. HFA) requires clinicians to carefully describe (a) the details of the severity of the ASD symptoms, (b) when the symptoms were first noticed and whether the symptoms have gotten more severe over time, (c) the individual's intellectual ability (i.e., IQ), and (d) any associated conditions (e.g., gastrointestinal dysfunction, sleep disturbances, attention-deficit/hyperactivity disorder [ADHD], epilepsy, motor problems). In the sections below I highlight behaviors likely be observed in LFA and HFA.

COMMUNICATION AND SOCIAL DIFFERENCES

A child with more severe forms of autism will display differences in social and communication abilities from a very early age and will experience communication challenges associated with Communication Subdomain 1 (refer to Chapter 2); recall that Subdomain 1 focuses on early-developing pragmatics (i.e., communication "use"). Typical early indicators of ASD include:

- Child does not respond when a family member calls his or her name.
- Child does not point at objects spontaneously or in response to adult questions.
- Child uses presymbolic techniques to gain adult attention, such as pulling on a parent's sleeve or hand instead of making eye contact and pointing.
- Child does not imitate motor movements such as playing patty-cake or "so big!"
- Child does not engage in pretend or imaginative play (Baranek, Parham, & Bodfish, 2005; Rogers, Cook, & Meryl, 2005).

To see examples of these indicators, view the video clip www.youtube.com/watch?v=YtvP5A5OHpU&feature=youtube called *Bringing the Early Signs of Autism Spectrum Disorders into Focus* (Kennedy Krieger Institute and American Academy of Pediatrics, 2013). In the video, what behavioral indicators listed above do you see in the children with ASD? What communication deficits are associated with Communication Subdomain 1? What Subdomain 1 skills might be targeted for intervention?

As noted in the DSM-5 criteria, social interaction and communication impairments are the central deficit of ASD. Parents may describe children with ASD as stiff and unresponsive in infancy, saying they are not "cuddly." In infancy and early preschool, there are nonverbal signs of ASD: Compared to their typically developing peers, children who are on the autism spectrum use fewer gaze shifts (e.g., lack of alternating gaze between an object and the communication partner), have less positive emotional affect (e.g., less smiling or laughing with communication partner), and demonstrate less frequent use of conventional gestural interactions. Children with more severe autism sometimes demonstrate hand leading, which is using another's body to communicate (e.g., moving the mother's hand toward an object); hand leading often replaces pointing. Also, children with autism may have fewer intentional vocalizations and show limited responsiveness to the interaction and communication attempts of others.

In contrast to the significant early communication deficits noted in children who have been identified with LFA, children with HFA often achieve normal language milestones during the preschool years. For example, they are often reported to talk using single words by age 2, use phrases by age 3, and demonstrate many typical self-help and adaptive behaviors during the preschool years. However, after age 3, children later diagnosed with HFA begin to demonstrate communication differences. Children with HFA typically demonstrate deficits associated with Communication Subdomain 5 (i.e., later-developing discourse skills [higher-level pragmatic deficits]) as well as potential deficits with sophisticated vocabulary use associated with Communication Subdomain 3.

As you would expect, all children diagnosed with ASD have difficulty with peer relationships, which poses a particular challenge in the later elementary school and teenage years. Even students with HFA demonstrate challenges interacting with peers, but their deficits are often more subtle (e.g., not understanding sarcasm/humor, not perceiving a situation from a peer's point of view). An individual with HFA has difficulty making friends and often is socially isolated, bullied, and teased. The situation is compounded because children with HFA sometimes have conduct problems such as aggressive and disruptive behaviors, negativity, noncompliance, and anxiety (Klin, McPartland, & Volkemar, 2005). To work on peer relationships, peers are sometimes incorporated into interventions for students with ASD. Learn more about peer intervention in Focus 9.1. Also review the information on peer social communication interventions in Chapter 6.

About 75% of children with ASD evidence echolalia (Bishop & Mogford, 1997). **Echolalia** represents either immediate or delayed imitation. In immediate echolalia, the child imitates the communication partner's utterance; in delayed echolalia, the child produces a previously heard sentence or phrase. Sometimes the child imitates radio or television jingles. Echolalia is more likely to be seen in children diagnosed with LFA. Traditionally, experts thought that all echolalia should be eliminated as an aberrant behavior. However, children may use echolalia to communicate. For example, a child may say "Do the Dew" repetitively (from the Mountain Dew commercial) to indicate his need to change activities. Intervention approaches for echolalia now focus on substituting appropriate verbalizations or gestures (Paul & Sutherland, 2005).

Behavioral Differences. The sensory impact of taste, smell, and touch are very meaningful for all infants and toddlers. However, with maturity, the senses of sight and sound overshadow olfactory (smell) and tactile (touch) stimulation. A potential explanation for the sensory behaviors exhibited by children with ASD is that the early-developing senses of taste, smell, and touch are neurologically immature or suppressed (Bregman, 2005). Accordingly, children with ASD often are hypersensitive to sensory stimulation and demonstrate discomfort in response to noise, touch, smell, or visual stimulation; this hypersensitivity can make children with ASD anxious in new situations, potentially resulting in an increase in stereotypic behaviors such as rocking or hand flapping—behaviors typically associated with LFA. Sometimes these unusual sensitivities may contribute to behavioral symptoms such as resistance to being cuddled or touched.

Children with ASD often have narrow and rigid interests related to physical objects or external stimuli. This interest can become a fixation that limits their ability to interact

---

FOCUS 9.1   *Issues for School-Age Students*

Interventions that incorporate a child's peer group can positively impact social abilities in school-age children with ASD. In fact, a recent randomized, control-group study (Level I level of evidence) demonstrated the effectiveness of peer training. Researchers compared the social behaviors of students with ASD who received one-on-one social skills training with a comparison group in which peers were trained to interact with individuals with ASD (Kasari et al., 2012). Social skills improved more when peers were trained—even compared to one-on-one coaching! Peers developing

typically can learn facilitative strategies such as (a) making sure you have your friend's attention, (b) waiting for your friend to talk, (c) saying something nice (e.g., compliment), (d) continuing to talk, and (e) answering questions. A meta-analysis of peer interventions with students with ASD also concluded that peer interventions are highly effective. Goldstein (2002) stated, "given that a problem relating to others is a core social deficit associated with autism, the effectiveness of these interventions in increasing social interaction with peers in particular is quite striking" (p. 390).

with others. For example, I worked with a child who was fascinated by clocks. In every interaction, the child would seek out, point to, and stare at clocks in the environment. Other children with ASD may focus on visual patterns or motion. For example, some children may like to spin or twist an object, while others fixate on light as it refracts through the window. The repetitive physical exploration of toys and objects is another barrier limiting social development and interaction.

A common pattern seen in individuals with HFA is an overwhelming interest in a very narrow subject area. Interests sometimes reflect topics that are fascinating to many children, such as an interest in dinosaurs, video games, or superheroes. However, an individual with HFA generally incessantly discusses the topic, to the exclusion of other subject areas, and lacks awareness of the listener's response to this preoccupation. Focus 9.2 prompts you to consider how a student with HFA might be classified using Fey's (1986) assertiveness–responsiveness communication rubric (see the discussion in Chapter 5).

Motor and Perceptual Differences. Many individuals with ASD have delayed motor development and look clumsy or awkward. They may have difficulty performing activities such as throwing a ball, opening a container, or climbing stairs. Some children with ASD, typically children with LFA, demonstrate a pattern of walking on their toes, a gait descriptively called toe walking. It is likely that some of the motor behavior and body placement difficulty arises because of the individual's limited body awareness with respect to the physical environment (Klin et al., 2005). The motor deficits also affect the development of self-help skills (e.g., dressing, feeding, toileting). As in the other domains, the motor deficits of individuals with HFA are likely to be subtle (e.g., difficulty with balance and difficulty making rapid, alternating movements such as flexing and extending a limb; Freitag et al., 2007).

Learning Differences. Children with ASD often have significant cognitive and learning differences. It has been estimated that 68% of children diagnosed with ASD have intellectual disability (ID); 20% have mild ID, 11% moderate ID, 7% severe ID, 3% profound ID, and 28% unspecified level of ID; Yeargin-Allsopp et al., 2003). Students identified as having LFA are more likely to have significant cognitive impairment (Fombonne, 2005).

Students with ASD often demonstrate memory impairments, with the result that they are likely to have significant difficulty remembering where objects are located or recalling daily events. However, tasks that require rote memory, such as simple visual or auditory patterns, may be relatively intact (Tsatsanis, 2005). Examples of simple memory tasks include asking a child with ASD to match line drawings or to remember a visual sequence

FOCUS 9.2   *Clinical Skill Building*

- How would you classify a child with high-functioning autism using Fey's (1986) assertiveness–responsiveness communication rubric? Why?

- Does a child with autism predominately have a deficit of form, content, or use? Give an example of a communication interaction that demonstrates your answer.

of objects or pictures. Studies have demonstrated that individuals with HFA use visual cues to recall letters during a memory task, whereas students developing typically use verbal strategies (Koshino et al., 2005). Consequently, children with ASD are more likely to recall event sequences when practitioners use visual stimuli as a memory cue than to use a verbal description or request.

A deficit in empathizing, a new term for the previously used terms *theory of mind* or *mindblindness,* is considered to occur for many individuals with ASD (Baron-Cohen et al., 2005). **Empathizing** describes the ability to perceive another's motives or thoughts as well as the ability to understand how another person might feel in a particular situation. Children with ASD often have difficulty taking another person's perspective and fail to understand others' emotions. A child with ASD assumes that if he knows something, then everyone knows what he knows. Lack of empathy is demonstrated when a student with HFA continues to talk even when others are bored or disinterested in the conversation.

Prevalence of Autism and Co-Occurrence of Other Disorders

In 2012, the Centers for Disease Control and Prevention (CDC, 2012) significantly revised its estimate of the prevalence of autism in the United States. We now know that ASD affects 1 out of every 88 children in the United States. This represents a 23% increase from the CDC's estimate of 1 in 110 children reported in 2009 and a 78% increase over the 2007 estimate of 1 in 150. The data still indicate that ASD affects males more than females (males: 1 in 54; females: 1 in 252).

The CDC reports a prevalence of 1 in 83 for European American children, 1 in 127 for Hispanic children, and 1 in 98 for African American children. However, the largest increases in the current survey were noted among Hispanic children, African American children, and children with ASD who have typical intellectual ability. Consequently, researchers believe that the lower prevalence noted in Hispanics (1 in 127) and African Americans (1 in 98) may be due to limited availability of community services and assessments rather than true differences in prevalence. The overall increase of the occurrence of ASD between 2009 and 2012 is thought to be at least partially attributable to the improvement in identification in nonmajority groups as well as better identification of ASD in older students, ages 14 to 17, who have mild ASD and may have been previously undiagnosed (Blumberg et al., 2013).

The reported numbers of children with ASD are alarmingly high; however, the true prevalence in the United States may be even higher than the 2012 CDC report! For example, a South Korean study (Kim et al., 2011) directly screened children for ASD rather than relying on medical or educational records (the method the CDC used). The South Korean study reported a prevalence of 1 in 38 among the screened schoolchildren; two-thirds of the children had been previously undiagnosed. So, with direct screening for ASD, experts suggest that the reported U.S. rate may also increase.

Several associated conditions occur relatively frequently in individuals with autism. I have already mentioned the increased incidence of intellectual disability; epilepsy also co-occurs. Specifically, epileptic seizures occur in 20 to 30% of individuals with ASD (Shea & Mesibov, 2005). A less frequent medical condition occurring at a higher-than-chance level is tuberous sclerosis, a genetic disease that causes benign tumors to grow in the brain and other vital organs.

Causation/Risk Factors

Autism is thought to have multiple etiologies (i.e., causes) that include both genetic and environmental factors. The most recent genetic research suggests that it is unlikely that there is a single major gene linked to ASD. Instead, research suggests that small gene mutations occur, increasing an embryo's susceptibility to developing ASD (Gilman et al., 2011; Neale et al., 2012). Researchers estimate that approximately 25% of all cases of ASD are caused by spontaneous mutations of genes that occur in the sperm, egg, or very early embryo development following conception. Importantly, these studies have found that these tiny mutations occur most frequently in children born to older parents—especially older fathers. It is thought that these gene mutations inhibit brain development and neural interconnectivity (Kong et al., 2012).

Research on environmental factors and ASD suggests that certain types of environmental exposures during pregnancy or infancy may increase or decrease autism risk. For example, Volk et al. (2013) found that exposure to high levels of air pollution during pregnancy resulted in a threefold incidence of ASD. In a second study, researchers reported that mothers taking folic acid (vitamin B9) in the weeks before and after conception significantly reduced the risk of autism in her child; children of mothers who took folic acid had a 39% reduced risk of developing ASD (Surén et al., 2013). Together, the emerging research suggests a genetic–environmental linkage in that a genetically at-risk embryo may be more susceptible to chemical or environmental factors. Fortunately for parents, however, research indicates that ASD is not caused by exposure to too many vaccines or thimerosal-containing vaccines, such as the measles, mumps, and rubella (MMR) vaccine (DeStefano, Price, & Weintraub, 2013). Learn more about recent ASD research at the websites www.autismspeaks.org and www.asatonline.org.

Connections

In this section, I examine aspects of ASD in relation to two important concepts introduced in the initial chapters of this book: (1) developmental issues and (2) family involvement.

DEVELOPMENTAL ISSUES

Sensorimotor Skills. As you recall from the discussion of cognitive constructivist theory in Chapter 2, cognitive growth in children developing typically progresses from sensorimotor stages to subsequent development of object permanence, means–end behavior (i.e., demonstration of cause and effect), imitation, and symbolic play. A child's imitation ability facilitates interpersonal relationships and reciprocal (e.g., person-to-person, back-and-forth) interactions.

This developmental sequence from sensorimotor awareness to symbolic play varies in children with ASD. While children with ASD are likely to develop sensorimotor skills related to objects (i.e., object permanence, means–end), they have difficulty with the sensorimotor skills linked to social interaction and awareness of others. For example, you might observe a child with ASD demonstrating means–end behavior when he turns the crank on a jack-in-the-box to make the lid pop open, yet you observe difficulty with a seemingly less-complex task such as imitating a simple motor act like waving "bye-bye." The child may also demonstrates little, if any, imaginative or symbolic play. Focus 9.3 prompts you to consider information on Piaget and how it applies to children with ASD.

FOCUS 9.3   *Learning More*

What does a child's ability to participate in symbolic play tell us about the child's cognitive development? (Clue: Go back to Chapter 2 and review the information on Piaget's cognitive constructivist concepts.)

Professionals accommodate children's learning differences within intervention programs. Imitation skills are taught through techniques such as reciprocal imitation training (RIT; Ingersoll & Schreibman, 2006). Using RIT, the practitioner facilitates imitation (1) by initially imitating the child's actions, gestures, and vocalization while simultaneously describing the behaviors (i.e., describing what the child is doing); (2) by initiating bids for child imitation of adult behavior using a duplicate toy (i.e., adult models actions slightly different from the child's and encourages the child to imitate; both the adult and child have the same object); and (3) by modeling play with different toys (i.e., generalizing the child's new imitative skills to different objects).

Joint Visual Attention. Children with ASD have more difficulty achieving joint visual attention than do other children with language delay; consider the children with ASD that you watched on the video *Bringing the Early Signs of Autism Spectrum Disorders into Focus*. As discussed in earlier chapters, and as you saw in the video, joint visual attention is the ability of a child to share a common focus of attention and to alternatively lead and follow others' focus. The ability to share others' referential cues precedes the child's ability to name objects and actions. In other words, joint visual attention precedes symbolic understanding and is a skill that typically develops within the first 18 months of life. Joint visual attention skills at older ages facilitate children staying in pretend and social play and to use more sophisticated and flexible interactive play routines.

Because children with ASD look at, point to, and respond less often to adults' communication bids than do their typically developing peers, it is important to target joint visual attention behaviors. To increase joint visual attention, an adult can watch a child's gaze and focus of attention; the adult joins the child at eye level and asks, "What do you want?" or "Look, cookie!" Waiting and eliciting a verbal or nonverbal response from the child before providing the item facilitates joint visual attention skills.

FAMILY INVOLVEMENT

Family-focused treatment is an important intervention component in a wide range of communication disorders. However, it is particularly important in the treatment of ASD because earlier and more intensive intervention predicts better treatment outcomes (Strock, 2004). Fifty years ago, medical professionals told parents that they had "caused" their child's autism. Professionals believed that autism developed in response to cold and rejecting mothers and absent fathers. Thankfully, research has clarified that parents do not cause their child's autism. Professionals know that rather than causing a child's autism, family support and involvement are key intervention components. Home intervention programs often train parents to:

- Implement behavior modification programs to reduce the child's negative behaviors.
- Involve the child in interactions to enhance the child's social-emotional and communication behaviors, such as facilitating attending skills, child participation during interactions, and the ability to follow commands.

- Facilitate the child's independence, self-monitoring, goal-setting, and self-evaluation abilities.

As I discussed in Chapter 4, federal laws such as IDEA 2004 mandate that children must be educated in the least restrictive educational environment. Families need to work closely with schools to ensure appropriate educational placement and identify effective interventions. Families often are overwhelmed by the amount of information and terminology involved in the educational process. Parents require support to become effective educational advocates for their child. As a child's SLP or special educator, you will be an important resource throughout the child's educational process.

As a child matures, the child's family may begin to focus on his or her peer relationships. Even a child with ASD who has normal intellectual ability requires family support and intervention to maximize social inclusion with typical peers. The school years are a challenging and difficult time for adolescents and families (Shea & Mesibov, 2005).

Assessment and Progress Monitoring: Autism

As an SLP working with a child diagnosed with ASD, your first task is to describe and quantify the child's communication and social behaviors. As I discussed at the beginning of this chapter, children with autism often demonstrate a broad range of deficits that vary in severity and frequency. The process begins with screening for ASD.

IDENTIFYING CHILDREN WITH POTENTIAL ASD: SCREENING

As you have learned, there are several stages in the assessment process: screening, diagnostic assessment, and progress monitoring. It is now recommended that all children receive autism screening at 18 and 24 months of age. One screening tool is called the Modified Checklist for Autism in Toddlers (M-CHAT). The M-CHAT (Robins et al., 2001) is a scientifically valid tool for screening children between 16 and 30 months of age, designed to assess a child's risk of having ASD; the American Academy of Pediatrics has approved this screening tool. You can view the M-CHAT online and even complete the M-CHAT for a child in your life (see www.autismspeaks.org/what-autism/diagnosis /screen-your-child).

Professionals carefully consider family concerns during the screening and assessment process; 69 to 88% of families of a child with ASD report sensing the problem prior to the child's third birthday (CDC, 2007; see Focus 9.4). Unfortunately, although parents often

FOCUS 9.4 *Family Issues*

What parental concerns might you hear that could indicate a potential for ASD in their children?

sense that something is wrong at an early age, the median age of identification of ASD is 5.7 years (Shattuck et al., 2009). The large gap between the first signs of ASD and identification underscores the critical need for improved community awareness, early screening, and professional training.

Once a child is screened, if the behaviors are consistent with potential ASD, the physician refers the child for a complete speech-language assessment battery. One of the first goals of assessment is to rule out other diagnoses, such as hearing impairment or behavioral issues. In some cases, an SLP may be the first professional to suspect that the child is on the autism spectrum. In this case, the SLP completes a speech-language evaluation and then refers the child to the family's physician. The physician, often in conjunction with a team of pediatric specialists, makes the ASD diagnosis.

The assessment protocol includes a variety of evaluative procedures. As in any other speech-language evaluation, an SLP obtains a full picture of the child's hearing, oral-motor skills, and speech production (if the child is verbal), including intelligibility, prosody, volume, and fluency. Typically, the language/communication assessment will include at least one norm-referenced test as well as observational assessments during a variety of activities. Information provided by the SLP will be added to information obtained by other members of a multidisciplinary team. A team member will assess the child to determine the presence of core features of ASD. Table 9.2 lists two examples of evaluation instruments used to assess core features of ASD; specialized training is required to use these assessment tools reliably.

ASSESSMENT OF VERBAL AND NONVERBAL COMMUNICATION FUNCTIONS

The assessor must consider a child's **communicative functions**. Communication functions describe what motivates a child to communicate. Communication functions include requesting, commenting, protesting, turn taking, imitating, and social greeting.

Table 9.2 **Assessment Tools for Children with ASD**

Tool	Description
Checklist for Autism Spectrum Disorders (Mayes et al., 2009)	• Completed by a practitioner based on a 15- to 20-minute structured interview with the parent, child's teacher, or child observations. • Developed to provide a comprehensive list of all core and associated symptoms of ASD. • Can be used to assess both low-functioning (LFA) and high-functioning autism (HFA). • Reliability coefficient for the checklist was highly significant ($r = .72$). Validity: All the children with LFA and 99% of those with HFA were correctly identified using the checklist; none of the children with ADHD were misdiagnosed with autism.
Childhood Autism Rating Scale (CARS; Schopler, Reichler, & Renner, 1988)	• Parent questionnaire and observation. • 15 items rated on a 7-point scale from normal to severely abnormal. • Appropriate for children of all ages, including preschoolers. • Reliability coefficients for CARS ($r = .78$) were highly significant. Validity: There is good psychometric support for CARS; however, CARS is better at detecting LFA than at detecting HFA.

Children developing typically demonstrate communication functions using a variety of communication means. **Communication means** (or communication forms) describe how the child communicates. Communication means can reflect either verbal behaviors (e.g., sounds, word approximations, words) or nonverbal behaviors (e.g., gestures, eye contact). As you would suspect, children with ASD typically have a reduced range of communication functions because they are less motivated to interact with others and often demonstrate limited or unusual communication means (e.g., taking a parent's hand rather than making eye contact, using echolalic verbalizations).

Observation of a Child in Play Interactions. During the assessment process, an assessor involves a child in a range of activities and observes the child's ability to participate and imitate during simple turn-taking games. Activities include involving the child in "baby games" such as patty-cake, peek-a-boo, and "so big!" The adult also solicits the child's turn taking during back-and-forth motor activities such as rolling a ball, pushing a car, or block building (i.e., the child and the adult take turns building a block tower). In addition to monitoring the child's ability to interact during simple motor-imitation games, the practitioner observes and models simple play routines to determine the child's level of symbolic play. The practitioner knows that a child developing typically begins to participate in simple symbolic play activities, such as rocking and feeding a doll, at around age 2. Throughout the assessment session, the practitioner observes the child's social and affective responses (i.e., his or her facial expression, eye gaze, smiling, laughing) during practitioner–child and parent–child interactions. The child's caregiver is included in the assessment because caregivers are an important information source about the child's abilities. Parents indicate whether the child's behavior during the assessment typifies his behavior at home.

The practitioner uses **communication temptations** to entice, surprise, or elicit a child's conversational attempts (Prizant et al., 2006). When using a communication temptation, the practitioner "sabotages" the situation, increasing the likelihood of communication (a form of pragmatic pressure!). For example, the child and the practitioner engage in a play dough activity. During the activity, the practitioner uses containers with tight-fitting lids. In order to participate, the child must request adult assistance. Other examples:

To determine whether the child can protest	• Give the child an undesired object. • Place the child's hands in something wet or sticky.
To determine whether the child can comment	• Have interesting objects or toys in a bag and pull them out one at a time. • Give the child some duplicate objects and then "surprise" him with a different object. • Complete a desired or surprising action (e.g., blowing bubbles, letting the air out of a balloon, playing with a wind-up toy) and watch for the child's response.
To determine whether the child can request	• Place a desired toy or object up high or in a jar with a tight lid. • Play a tickle game such as "I'm going to get you!" and wait for the child to request repetition of the action.

Figure 9.1 provides a simplified version of an assessment protocol suitable for children with ASD. Communication temptations are included in the assessment process.

Figure 9.1 **An Observational Tool for Assessing Communication and Interaction of Young Children with ASD**

Communication Means (i.e., How does the child communicate?)		Gazes at communication partner	Uses 3-point gaze (partner and objects)	Gestures (Conventional = C, Unconventional = UC)	Vocalizations (Conventional = C, Unconventional = UC)	Speech (E = Echolalic, S = Spontaneous)	Describe
Communication Functions (i.e., What is the child's motivation for communication?)	Comment						
	Request action						
	Request object						
	Social functions (e.g., "Hi," "Bye")						
	Share enjoyment, exclaim, tease						
	Other communication functions						
Response to Communication Temptations	Doing something silly	Describe child response:					
	Bubbles with too-tight lid	Describe child response:					
	Switching toys	Describe child response:					
	Pretending not to understand	Describe child response:					
	Withholding part of toy	Describe child response:					
	Other temptations	Describe child response:					
Receptive Ability							
Responses to Others' Communication	Response to name	Describe child response:					
	Response to yes/no question	Describe child response:					
	Response to *wh* question	Describe child response:					
	Identifies objects?	Describe child response:					

Source: Information from *The SCERTS Model: A Comprehensive Educational Approach for Children with Autism Spectrum Disorders. Vol. 1: Assessment,* by B. M. Prizant, A. M. Wetherby, E. Rubin, A. C. Laurent, and P. J. Rydell, 2006, Baltimore, MD: Brookes; and "Assessing Communication in Autism Spectrum Disorders," by R. Paul, 2005. In F. R. Volkmar, R. Paul, A. Klin, and D. Cohen (Eds.), *Handbook of Autism and Pervasive Developmental Disorders. Vol. 2: Assessment, Intervention, and Policy* (3rd ed., pp. 799–816). Hoboken, N J: Wiley & Sons.

Table 9.3 **Example of a Progress-Monitoring Tool**

Teacher verbal question	Teacher nonverbal cue (provided at the same time as question)	Child rating
"John, what do you want to drink today?"	Show two drink options.	3 2 1 0
"John, what do you want to eat today?"	Show two food options.	3 2 1 0
"John, after you finish your snack, what would you like to do next?" (Provide stimulus when snack is over.)	Show two pictures of desired activities.	3 2 1 0

Rating scale: 3 = child spontaneously points and verbalizes following teacher question; 2 = child spontaneously points following teacher question; 1 = child points following teacher prompt if child does not respond to initial question (teacher provides prompt "John, *point* to the one you want"); 0 = No response following prompt.

FOCUS 9.5 *Clinical Skill Building*

Develop a rating scale to document a child's use of (a) social greetings (a communication function), (b) protesting (a communication function), or (c) pointing (a communication means).

During an assessment, the assessor observes both expressive and receptive abilities. The receptive portion of the observational protocol allows observation of the child's ability to understand and respond to others' verbal communication.

ONGOING PROGRESS MONITORING

A final component of assessment is the ongoing evaluation of a child's social and communication progress. Progress monitoring documents a child's carryover of targeted skills to the natural environment and generalization of new skills to novel situations. One way to document both the quality and quantity of new behaviors is to use ratings scales. An example of a progress-monitoring tool is shown in Table 9.3. The assessor uses a self-developed tool, such as this one, to document the child's use of requests in a novel situation such as snack time. It is important for practitioners to be familiar with developing rating scales; develop your clinical skills by considering the questions in Focus 9.5.

Intervention

There are a number of viable intervention approaches for children with ASD; Table 9.4 lists examples of current approaches. Evidence from many more randomized ASD research studies are in progress and will be available in the years ahead. Below I present two currently used intervention approaches in more detail: applied behavior analysis (ABA; Lovaas, 2003) and the *SCERTS* model (Prizant & Wetherby 2006; Prizant, Wetherby, Rubin, Laurent, & Rydell, 2006). ABA is considered a focused intervention practice; it uses specific instructional

Table 9.4 **Examples of High-Quality Intervention Programs**

Program	Description
Early Start Denver model (Rogers & Dawson, 2010)	• Uses techniques from applied behavior analysis (ABA) for early intervention with toddlers; emphasizes relationship building and interactive play. • Data showed that the program improved social and communication skills and also improved brain activity related to social responsiveness (Dawson et al., 2012).
Pivotal response treatments (PRT; Koegel & Koegel, 2006)	• Based on ABA methods, PRT uses structured operant teaching techniques in the child's natural environment; adults follow a child's interests and communication attempts. • Focuses on communication, academic, social, self-help, and recreational domains. • Meta-analysis (Rogers & Vismara, 2008) indicated that, based on the number and type of published studies, PRT meets the criteria as a "probably efficacious intervention."
LEAP (Learning Experiences and Alternative Program for Preschoolers and Their Parents) program (Strain & Bovey, 2008)	• The Kennedy Krieger School LEAP program serves students on the severe end of the autism spectrum who struggle with behavioral challenges. • A variety of evidenced-based strategies are used; there is a focus on functional independence. • A randomized, control-group study found that children in LEAP intervention made significantly more progress than comparison children at the end of 2 years on measures of cognitive, language, autism symptoms, problem behavior, and social skills (Strain & Bovey, 2011).

approaches designed to promote skill acquisition for individual children. In contrast, the *SCERTS* program is an example of a comprehensive treatment model. Comprehensive treatment programs are multicomponent programs that implement a variety of intervention practices, organized around a conceptual framework and designed to facilitate multiple student outcomes (Odom et al., 2010). Understanding two different intervention models and the theoretical foundation supporting their use will help you thoughtfully consider new approaches in the future. I provide an informational link and discussion questions with regard to the LEAP approach—another high-quality ASD intervention—in Focus 9.6.

FOCUS 9.6   *Learning More*

The LEAP approach incorporates a variety of intervention practices (see Table 9.4). Like the *SCERTS* approach (discussed in detail later in this chapter), the LEAP approach is a *comprehensive treatment model.* Go to the LEAP website, www.kennedykrieger.org /special-education/educational-programs /leap-program, and consider some of the interventions used in this program (e.g., sensory integration, work-based learning, expressive therapy). Divide into groups and research these terms. Discuss with your classmates what you have learned. Do you believe the LEAP approach may be an appropriate approach for older students with ASD? Why or why not?

Clinical Skill Building

What is the theoretical foundation of ABA? What behavioral principles are likely to be part of ABA, given the theoretical roots?

What behaviors and language production are most likely to be facilitated with a highly structured ABA intervention?

INTERVENTION APPROACH: APPLIED BEHAVIOR ANALYSIS (ABA)

To understand the **applied behavior analysis (ABA)** approach, keep in mind the behavioral conditioning theories of the 1970s (i.e., links between an initial eliciting stimulus, child behavior, and contingent positive or negative stimuli). ABA developed from the work of Lovaas (2003) and his colleagues at the University of California, Los Angeles. ABA, sometimes also referred to as the Lovaas approach, is an early intensive behavioral intervention, discrete trial training, and intensive behavior treatment (IBT). I use the term ABA to refer to the general form of intervention, based on Lovaas's principles. ABA's operant, learning-based philosophy states that any behavior (even language) can be broken down into separate behaviors, measured in precise terms, and manipulated through principles of reinforcement. With regard to the ABA program, improve your clinical skill and ability to apply theoretical information by answering the questions in Focus 9.7.

Specific instructional techniques, or methods, emerged from the ABA approach. A primary method is discrete trial therapy (DTT), a method that uses behavioral techniques to facilitate child behaviors such as (1) receptive identification of objects, pictures, and actions; (2) early play and self-help skills; (3) verbal labeling; (4) early concept development (e.g., recognition and naming of color, shape, size); (5) use of prepositions; (6) use of emotion words; and (7) use of simple carrier phrases such as "I see " and "I want " (Lovaas, 2003). Behavioral techniques include the use of prompting, cuing, chaining, fading, and differential reinforcement.

Figure 9.2 is an example of a DTT teaching sequence. As Figure 9.2 illustrates, DTT intervention is primarily practitioner directed and skill rather than activity based. Typically,

Figure 9.2 **Example of Discrete Trial Therapy Teaching Sequence**

Steps to Teaching Naming of Actions

- Adult assembles three pictures (e.g., *waving, eating, sleeping*).
- Adult presents one picture and asks, "What is he (or she) doing?" Adult immediately prompts the word by saying "waving." Adult reinforces the child for each response. Adult continues until the child accurately names all three pictures with high accuracy without prompt.
    - Reinforcement at this stage is often social or includes the use of tokens that the child trades for privileges or prizes.
- Adult intermixes the pictures until the child is 90% accurate in unprompted attempts.
- Adult generalizes labels so that the child describes (a) actions the adult performs, (b) actions the child performs, and (c) actions in books.

parents and trained therapists implement DTT intervention in a child's home for 20 to 40 hours per week, on an individual basis. Later, after 1 to 3 years of intervention, the intervention takes place with a paraprofessional in an inclusive classroom (Smith, Groen, & Wynn, 2000). Figure 9.3 provides examples of DTT treatment goals.

Evidence Supporting the ABA Approach. In the past several years, a number of meta-analyses have examined the effectiveness of the ABA approach. Recall that meta-analyses contrast and combine results from different studies in order to identify patterns across study results. An indication of intervention effectiveness determined by meta-analyses is considered Level I evidence in the evidenced-based practice model. Prior to the current round of meta-analytic studies, ABA had been shown to be efficacious at Level II (i.e., nonrandomized but well-designed studies).

Several of the meta-analytic studies report that ABA is helpful for many, but not all, children with ASD (Howlin, Magiati, & Charman, 2009; Reichow & Wolery, 2009). For example, Rogers and Vismara (2008) concluded that the ABA approach met the criteria for "probably efficacious." Other research teams supported the general positive effects of ABA and state that, given the lack of strong evidence for other ASD interventions, ABA should be an intervention of choice for children with autism (Eldevik et al., 2009). However, the generally positive conclusions about ABA are not unanimous. Following their meta-analysis, Spreckley and Boyd (2009) stated in the *Journal of Pediatrics* that ABA did not result in "significant improvement in cognitive, language, or adaptive behavioral outcomes compared with standard care" (p. 342). However, looking across the entirety of meta-analyses, today's SLP can still recommend ABA—particularly in the case of intervention for preschool and kindergarten-age children. However, future research will determine whether ABA is the best approach for all students with ASD and whether it is effective for older, school-age students with ASD (Odom et al., 2010).

INTERVENTION APPROACH: *SCERTS*

The ultimate goal of communication intervention for children with ASD is to help the children interact with others in their natural environments. As an alternative to behaviorally based approaches, the *SCERTS* **approach** is based on social interaction, developmental,

Figure 9.3   **Examples of Goals for Discrete Trial Therapy***

- Without prompting, John will correctly imitate 20 different gross motor behaviors (e.g., waving bye-bye, touching ears) when asked "do this" within 2 seconds of request with 90% accuracy.
- John will correctly respond with 90% accuracy with the response "happy" or "sad" when the trainer presents a picture of a child either smiling or crying when pictures are randomly presented. (Note: Child previously demonstrated receptive knowledge of verbs *smiling* and *crying*.)
- John will produce with 90% accuracy without prompting the prepositions *on top*, *under*, or *beside* when asked, "Where are you?" while John sits on top of, under, or beside a table or chair.

*All goals in the DTT program require careful sequencing of task presentations; each of the listed goals is introduced as one part in a series of structured intervention steps (Lovaas, 2003).

FOCUS 9.8   *Intervention*

Refer to the continuum of naturalness in Chapter 5 to refresh your memory regarding clinician- vs. child-directed therapy. Describe how the ABA and *SCERTS* approaches reflect variations in terms of the continuum of naturalness. Can these approaches ever be combined for a particular child?

and family systems theories. The *SCERTS* approach emphasizes enhancing children's turn-taking, choice-making, emotional-regulation, and problem-solving abilities (Prizant, Wetherby, Rubin, Laurent, & Rydall, 2006). *SCERTS* stands for *Social Communication, Emotional Regulation, and Transaction Support*. The term **transaction support** refers to the interpersonal support provided by a child's adult and peer communication partners, the environmental modifications used to promote social communication and emotional regulation, and the enhancement of family support systems (Prizant, et al., 2006). Transactional goals support learning by reinforcing and motivating a child to use the targeted behavior and integrate new behavior into daily life. Consider how the *SCERTS* approach is different from the ABA intervention described above by reading Focus 9.8.

The *SCERTS* approach addresses a child's social communication abilities and social relationships as the primary focus of intervention. Figure 9.4 lists the challenges of children with autism at various stages of development. The listed challenges motivate the intervention strategies used in the *SCERTS* approach.

At the earliest levels, a child needs to establish joint visual attention and improve the frequency of communicative functions such as requesting, commenting/labeling, and negation. At advanced language levels, individuals with ASD need support to improve discourse abilities, repair communication breakdowns, and use language in less familiar social situations. The *SCERTS* approach uses a facilitative intervention style rather than the adult-directive techniques characteristic of ABA methodologies. The *SCERTS* approach uses the following methods:

- Following the child's lead
- Offering choices and alternatives within the child's daily routines and activities
- Responding to the child's intent and reinforcing communication attempts
- Modeling a variety of communication functions at the child's level
- Elaborating the child's verbal and nonverbal communication attempts (Prizant & Wetherby, 2006)

An example of a *SCERTS* treatment sequence is shown in Figure 9.5.

In the *SCERTS* approach, communication partners embed learning sequences within the child's everyday activities. Embedding instruction increases the generalization of the targeted behaviors and encourages the involvement of the child's parents, classroom teachers, siblings, and peers. Because intervention aims to improve both the quality and the quantity of interactions, the practitioner in a *SCERTS* intervention uses both frequency counts and behavioral rating systems to document child and communication partner objectives.

For example, if the intervention goal is to increase a student's ability to negotiate more effectively with peers, a professional might document how frequently a classroom peer uses

Figure 9.4   **Challenges for Students with ASD at Different Stages of Communication Development**

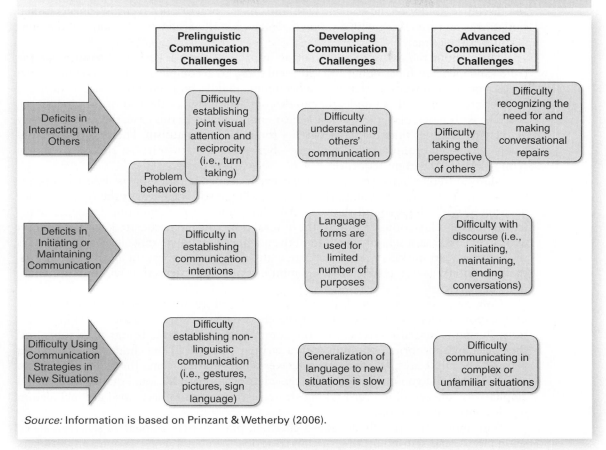

Source: Information is based on Prinzant & Wetherby (2006).

Figure 9.5   **Example of a *SCERTS* Treatment Sequence**

Communication challenge: Tabitha tends to engage in solitary play and does not typically make eye contact or verbal or nonverbal requests when interacting with others.

• During playtime, the communication partner modifies the toy selection to include toys that require adult assistance (e.g., wind-up toys, toys with tight lids) or by placing favorite toys in locations that require Tabitha to initiate a request.
• The communication partner captures Tabitha's interest in toys and then responds to any communicative attempt.
• With Tabitha's more frequent communication attempts, the communication partner delays responding to encourage vocalization or gestures.

Source: Information based on *The SCERTS Model: A Comprehensive Educational Approach for Children with Autism Spectrum Disorders; Vol. 1: Program Planning and Intervention,* by B. M. Prizant, A. M. Wetherby, E. Rubin, A. C. Laurent, & P. J. Rydell, 2006, Baltimore, MD: Brookes.

a wipe-off white board to map out negotiations and record compromises during a cooperative science project. In this case, the practitioner has taught the typically developing peer to use this negotiation strategy (Prizant et al., 2006). At the same time, the practitioner rates the discourse ability of the student with autism; the practitioner records conversational initiations and turn taking with a rating scale (i.e., 3 = all of the time, 2 = some of the time, 1 = none of the time).

Throughout the *SCERTS* intervention approach, there is an effort to increase the child's independent functioning and self-regulation. To accomplish this, intervention often focuses on natural routines that have a beginning, middle, and end. For example, during a shared interaction with a puzzle, the puzzle completion signals the end of the interaction, whereas with block play, there is not a clear ending point. In this case, the puzzle activity is likely to be easier than the block activity for a child with autism. The practitioner considers what social routines will challenge—but not overly frustrate—a child with autism with respect to the event sequence.

Many different activities have a clear event sequence that can be used to improve social functioning. A very young child in the prelinguistic stage learns the play sequence associated with ring-around-the-rosy. An older child in the emerging language stage learns during classroom free play the interaction routine associated with making a choice. In contrast, a school-age child in the advanced language stage learns in gym class the communication skills needed to participate in a group activity. In all three examples, the practitioner facilitates the child's communication and interaction within reoccurring daily activities.

Communication partners learn to use visual and auditory cues to signal the communication sequences. For example, if the child with autism is practicing asking questions during a shared conversation, the communication partner brings up a topic and then cues an appropriate question with a written sentence (if the child is a reader) or a picture. The adult says, "I had an exciting weekend!" and then cues the child with autism to ask, "What did you do?" Eventually, the adult promotes additional question types and emphasizes conversational turn-taking strategies; parents and peers also are included in the discourse intervention.

With more linguistically advanced children, practitioners emphasize self-regulation, self-analysis, and self-monitoring of conversational strategies. For example, practitioners videotape shared conversations between children and train a child with ASD to evaluate and modify conversational strategies (Scherer et al., 2001). As you see from the examples above and the goals listed in Figure 9.6, this approach is flexible. The practitioner constantly evaluates the child's current level of functioning and targets skills to improve the child's independence and daily interaction with others. Examples of *SCERTS* intervention goals are shown in Figure 9.6.

Evidence Supporting the *SCERTS* Approach. The *SCERTS* approach is based on evidence that children learn the most when (1) they are engaged in meaningful activities, (2) families are included as a central part of intervention, and (3) social interaction and functional communication are central intervention components (National Research Council, 2001; Strain, Schwartz, & Bovey, 2008).

Prizant and Wetherby and their colleagues describe children with ASD and the results of *SCERTS*-based interventions (e.g., Prizant et al., 2006). Published case studies and research supporting the underlying theory of *SCERTS* intervention places the *SCERTS* model at Level III in the scientific studies evidence hierarchy.

Figure 9.6 **Examples of *SCERTS* Communication Goals**

- **Child goal:** Child will independently modify communication strategy (use his picture symbols) to obtain desired item when communication partner does not understand vocalized communication attempt in 8 out of 10 consecutive attempts.
- **Partner goal:** Communication partner will present a series of prompts moving from least directive to more directed (i.e., looking at communication board, pointing to communication board, saying "Show me what you want") to cue child to use picture symbols.
- **Transactional goal:** Communication board is updated to reflect child's current interests and is available throughout the day to promote spontaneous use.

Source: Information based on *The SCERTS Model: A Comprehensive Educational Approach for Children with Autism Spectrum Disorders; Vol. 1: Program Planning and Intervention,* by B. M. Prizant, A. M. Wetherby, E. Rubin, A. C. Laurent, & P. J. Rydell, 2006, Baltimore, MD: Brookes.

Summary

- *Diagnostic and Statistical Manual of Mental Disorders,* Fifth Edition (DSM-5; American Psychiatric Association, 2013) uses the term *autism spectrum disorder* (*ASD*) to categorize individuals who have (a) deficits in social communication and social interaction *and* also demonstrate (b) restricted repetitive behaviors, interests, and activities (RRBs). There will be variations in how these behaviors are demonstrated when considering a student with HFA vs. LFA. DSM-5 also has a diagnostic category called "social (pragmatic) communication disorder" for an individual with social skill deficits who does not demonstrate restricted or repetitive patterns of behavior.
- ASD affects 1 out of every 88 European American children in the United States; it affects males more than females. The prevalence of ASD is increasing; this may be due to better identification of ASD in (a) nonmajority groups, (b) older students with high-functioning ASD, and/or (c) increased awareness of ASD. Intellectual disability and epilepsy are the most frequently occurring associated conditions.
- Current research points to a complex association between genetics and environmental factors that together cause increased risk for ASD.
- Deficits in sensorimotor skills, imitation abilities, and the development of joint visual attention are associated with ASD; families play a strong role in the intervention program of children with ASD.
- Intervention approaches vary on the continuum of naturalness; applied behavior analysis (ABA) and the *SCERTS* approach demonstrate this variation. ABA draws strongly from behaviorist theory, has Level I research data supporting its use, and seems particularly appropriate for preschool and kindergarten children. The *SCERTS* approach is based on development and social interactionist theory, emphasizing ecological validity; the *SCERTS* approach represents a comprehensive treatment model.

Discussion and In-Class Activities

1. Your instructor will divide the class into groups and assign each group either high- or low-functioning autism. Complete a same–different rubric for your assigned ASD category. In other words, decide how your ASD category is the same as or different from ASD on the other side of the spectrum. Write two intervention goals (refer to Chapter 5 for a review of good goal writing), one for your side of the spectrum and one for the other side. Explain whether your goal targets the language domain of form, content, or use. In what way does the goal target the indicated language domain? How will this goal improve the child's daily life?

2. View videotape clips of children with ASD at www.autismspeaks.org (in the video glossary). Discuss the communications functions and means that you see in the different video clips, using the observational tool in Figure 9.1 as a guide. Discuss the decision-making process used to classify the various communication patterns.

3. Develop a series of intervention steps that a professional could use in a behavioral intervention program (such as ABA) with the ultimate goal of improving the child's ability to (a) name objects and actions during an adult–child shared book reading, (b) choose a favorite toy during free play, or (c) follow one-step commands.

4. In a small group, choose one or more of the communication goals listed below:

   - Labeling objects
   - Requesting toys
   - Answering *wh-* questions (e.g., *what, when, where*)
   - Labeling actions
   - Asking a question
   - Following simple one- and two-step directions
   - Greeting people socially
   - Maintaining a conversation with a communication partner
   - Improving an individual's syntax and semantic skills

   Develop an intervention to improve an individual's communication functioning in the targeted area via (a) an adult-directed approach and (b) a social interaction intervention (similar to the *SCERTS* approach). List the pros and cons of each method for improving the specific communication goal.

5. The *SCERTS* approach focuses on helping children make real-life changes in their social and communication behaviors. In small groups, discuss how you could document a child's behavioral, social, and communication changes (a) at home during dinner hour, (b) during a family routine such as bath time or bedtime, (c) with peers during free play, (d) in the classroom during an academic activity, or (e) during a rule-based game with peers. Consider a variety of methods to document change, including rating scales, behavioral sampling, and transcription of child communication. Discuss the pros and cons of each method, and brainstorm how documentation could be adapted to make it work for a classroom teacher.

Chapter 9 Case Study

Vijay is a 12-year-old male diagnosed with high-functioning autism. He attends middle school with his typically developing peers. He is good at math and enjoys his computer class. He spends two periods a day in the resource room, where a special educator helps Vijay on his organizational strategies and coaches him in his more difficult subjects (e.g., language arts). You have been working with Vijay on his conversational skills; the focus of intervention has been initiating a conversational topic, staying on topic, and using appropriate discourse strategies to change topics.

Vijay would like to join the chess club. However, he demonstrates inappropriate behaviors (i.e., he "acts out") when he is unfamiliar with the routine or is experiencing new situations. He has difficulty with peer interactions when they involve humor, sarcasm, or kidding around.

Questions for Discussion

1. How can you assist Vijay to conversationally interact and handle chess club?
2. Will your goals more likely reflect an ABA or a *SCERTS* intervention approach?
3. In small groups, write some intervention goals for Vijay. Describe how you would document progress.
4. Could Vijay's peers be trained to incorporate some facilitating strategies? Describe some possible strategies and a plan for documenting the peers' use of strategies.
5. How could the scheduling or planning for the chess club be modified (or elaborated) to assist Vijay's adaptation to novel situations?

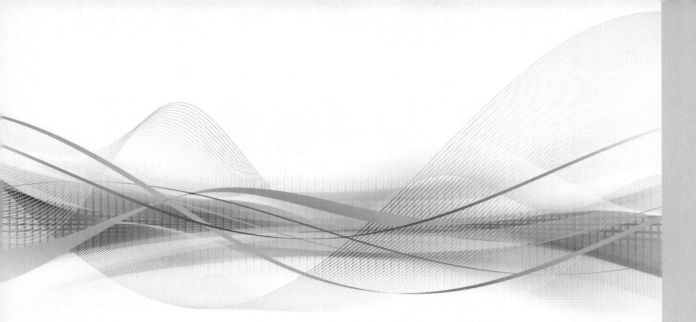

10

Early Literacy, Reading, and Writing for School-Age Children

Chapter Overview Questions

1. Why does a practitioner working with emergent literacy take a preventive approach? What are the primary emergent literacy targets?

2. What is the embedded-explicit model of emergent literacy intervention? Give examples of embedded and explicit intervention techniques.

3. How does a practitioner assess emergent literacy skills? How does a practitioner assess school-age reading and writing skills?

4. What skills are foundational for school-age readers?

5. What are some intervention strategies for advanced-level phonological awareness skills, narratives, reading comprehension, and writing?

6. What are some target skills within the five levels in the interactive-to-independent model of literacy?

7. What level of evidence exists regarding Gillon's Explicit Phonological Awareness program and Nelson's Writing Lab approach?

This chapter outlines important aspects of written language and literacy development. I discuss early literacy development as well as aspects of later reading and writing development pertaining to school-age children. I refer to the early stage of reading development as **emergent literacy**. Emergent literacy refers to the skills, knowledge, and attitudes that are precursors to conventional reading and writing (Sylva et al., 2011). **Conventional reading** refers to the ability of children to decode (i.e., sound out) unfamiliar words and draw meaning from written text. Children with spoken language impairments often have associated difficulties with written language development (Catts et al., 2002). The reasons should be obvious to you by now: Language development encompasses more than spoken language. A child who is language proficient can, for example, hear and differentiate phonemes, understand complex syntax, infer meaning from vocabulary, and move from less formal conversational-style discourse to more formal academic-sounding language. Skills in each domain—phonological, syntax, vocabulary, and discourse—are needed during reading and writing. Underlying language impairments in language domains have far-reaching effects that negatively impact children's reading and writing abilities throughout their school years (Bishop & Clarkson, 2003). In fact, approximately 50% of children with language impairment at age 5 will be diagnosed with reading disability (Catts et al., 2002).

The Role of the Speech-Language Pathologist in Reading and Writing

The American Speech-Language-Hearing Association (ASHA) strongly advocates that speech-language pathologists (SLPs) indirectly and directly incorporate reading and writing interventions into clinical practice (ASHA, 2001, 2007). Indirect involvement occurs in the early years, when SLPs collaborate with classroom teachers and special educators to include literacy-based objectives and activities in prekindergarten programs;

FOCUS 10.1　*School-Based Issues*

ASHA recommends that SLP school caseloads not exceed 40 students per week; however, the average SLP caseload is 53 students, and some SLPs have school caseloads as large as 110 (ASHA, 2002b). Because of large caseload demands, some SLPs question their ability to focus on children with reading and writing deficits.

To overcome the challenge of a large caseload, one approach is to use workload analysis. Rather than compute workload by counting the number of students served, workload analysis considers face-to-face contact time in addition to time needed for paperwork, classroom visits, collaboration with classroom teachers, and IEP development. This approach gives work credit for SLPs who provide classroom-based support to students with reading and writing deficits. For more information about workload analysis, go to the ASHA website, at www.asha.org/about/publications/leader-online/archives/2002/q3/020910c.htm.

it occurs in later school years when SLPs work with general education teachers to provide effective classroom interventions. SLPs are using new approaches to increase their ability to spend more time in classrooms, working with teachers (see Focus 10.1). SLPs work directly with students when early literacy, reading, and writing goals are included in language intervention programs.

However, despite the connections between oral language and reading development, some SLPs do not feel comfortable including reading and writing goals in their speech and language interventions. Consider the following excerpt, sent as a letter to the editor of an SLP journal.

> I am an SLP in the schools. I am concerned about stepping into the role of reading specialist/resource teacher when our plate is so full with working within the traditional role of an SLP in oral comprehension, oral expression, articulation, voice, and stuttering. (From Jan 22, 2008, Letters to the Editor, ASHA Leader. Copyright © 2008 by the American Speech Language Hearing Association.)

The above letter provoked a number of responses from other SLPs. The example below is representative:

> We must be cognizant that speech-language pathology is a fluid discipline and continue to keep pace with new perspectives and developments. It was only in the 1970s that we began to consider our role in treating children with language disorders! We need to embrace the range of disabilities that fall under our purview and applaud the fact that our profession allows SLPs to develop specializations across a wide range of communication disorders. (From May 6, 2008, Letters to the Editor, ASHA Leader. Copyright © 2008 by the American Speech Language Hearing Association.)

Needless to say, I agree with the second writer. I understand that it can be difficult to develop new areas of expertise. However, in this case, SLPs are compelled to become knowledgeable in written communication because of current educational policy and research evidence. For example, federal law (IDEA, 2004) mandates that SLPs report the academic risk factors for a student receiving school-based SLP services. Further, research evidence overwhelmingly demonstrates the higher-than-expected academic risk factors for students with language impairments (e.g., Catts et al., 2008).

A professional's role change is different when working with younger children than when working with older school-age students. With the earliest ages, an SLP may be the first to detect a child's language impairment. Research demonstrates that the presence of language impairment (LI) in preschool and kindergarten is an important indicator of a potential reading disability. Consequently, prior to school entry, an SLP is likely to be at the forefront in leading an early literacy and language intervention program. I talk more about the role of the professional in preventing reading disabilities in the section below.

At later ages (first grade and beyond), an SLP generally works alongside other educational professionals. The education team typically includes the classroom teacher, reading specialist, school psychologist, special education teacher, resource room teacher, and SLP. The general reading assessment program is typically administered on a schoolwide level, and the education team and school administration monitor the results. The SLP's role in assessment and intervention is typically domain specific, such as targeting the student's narrative ability, spelling abilities, or focusing on written language skills.

In this chapter, first I discuss the role of the SLP and special educator with regard to setting up a prevention program for young children who are at risk for reading disability. Then I describe the primary targets that should be the focus of an early literacy prevention program, including phonological awareness, print concepts, alphabetic awareness, and early writing. I provide information on assessment of early literacy skills. Finally,

I outline an intervention model: the embedded-explicit approach. Practitioners use the embedded-explicit approach to implement a literacy prevention program in preschool and kindergarten classrooms.

In the second major subsection, I provide information useful to SLPs and special educators who work with older, school-age children with reading or writing deficits. I describe specific language-focused areas, including narratives, spelling, reading comprehension, and writing. I also describe a literacy model for students with more significant levels of impairment (e.g., children with autism); this approach is called the interactive-to-independent model of literacy. In several subsections in this chapter, I describe cultural considerations related to children's literacy development.

In the final major section of this chapter, I present detailed information on two intervention approaches for children with reading impairments. There are dozens (if not hundreds) of intervention approaches for children with reading impairments. I have picked two approaches because (a) both were developed by SLPs, (b) both have peer-reviewed evidence documenting their effectiveness, and (c) the two approaches (one for younger children and one for older school-age children) demonstrate the connections between theoretical knowledge and clinical application.

Emergent Literacy

PREVENTION OF READING DISABILITY IN YOUNG CHILDREN AT RISK FOR READING FAILURE

When practitioners provide literacy interventions to preschoolers, they are participating in a preventive program. A preventive program is like a vaccination for a child. Doctors do not wait until a child has chicken pox to give a vaccination; instead, doctors give the vaccination to prevent chicken pox. Similarly, SLPs and educators participate in emergent literacy preventive interventions to reduce the chance of reading failure in later school years. The goal is to "catch children before they fall" (Torgenson, 1998, p. 1). In essence, this means that practitioners strive to identify children *before* they experience reading failure by monitoring children's reading development. Early identification of reading risk is paramount because reading interventions are much less successful once children reach third grade (Hanselman & Borman, 2012).

A number of fundamental language skills are required for early literacy development; these skills include a child's phonological awareness, print concepts, alphabetic knowledge, oral language development, and emergent writing. Consequently, much of early language and literacy intervention is focused on these critical domains. Assessment in a prevention program uses the response to intervention (RTI; Greenwood, et al., 2011) approach introduced in Chapter 4. RTI uses scientifically based research to guide intervention. In Focus 10.2, I describe how three different curriculum-based reading assessments are currently used to monitor students' reading growth and evaluate the effects of instructional programs from emergent to conventional reading levels and even into the later elementary grades. Curriculum-based assessments are used in the RTI model to continually make sure that children's reading skills are improving. In the following section, I describe the primary literacy targets included in a preventive literacy approach focusing on emergent readers.

FOCUS 10.2   *Clinical Skill Building*

Curriculum-Based Measurement

Curriculum-based measurement (CBM), as it pertains to reading, is a progress-monitoring assessment used to monitor students' growth in reading development. Just like the use of individual growth and development indicators (IGDIs) described in Chapter 4, CBM is another approach appropriate for educators who are using the response to intervention (RTI) approach. Using CBM, educators evaluate whether a student needs extra intervention or a change of approach to maximize reading development.

In a review of the literature, Wayman and her colleagues (2007) evaluated which CBM measures were most effective for monitoring children's reading development. Three approaches are most commonly used in CBM reading: reading aloud, maze selection, and word identification. To complete the reading aloud CBM, students read aloud from a passage for 1 minute, and the number of words read correctly is scored. Phoneme omissions, insertions, substitutions, hesitations, and mispronunciations are counted as errors. In maze selection, students read through a passage in which every seventh word has been deleted and replaced by three word choices—one correct choice and two distractors. Students

read the passage silently, usually for 1 to 3 minutes, making selections as they read. In word identification, students read aloud from a list of high-frequency words for 1 minute, and the number of words read correctly is scored.

Different CBM reading measures are suitable for children at different ages. Word identification is most appropriate for beginning readers and is appropriate for the RTI approach for early identification and prevention. In contrast, the reading-aloud CBM is the most appropriate for primary-grade students (grades 1–3); adding the maze selection task to the word identification CBM task is helpful when evaluating intermediate-grade students (grades 3–7). For older secondary students, maze selection is the best CBM assessment to monitor reading growth.

To learn more about CBM, you can access examples of reading passages at the University of Oregon–sponsored website: www.easycbm.com/info/demos.php.

Source: Based on information from Wayman, M. M., Wallace, T., Wiley, H. I., & Renáta, T., & Espin, C. A. (2007). Literature synthesis on curriculum-based measurement in reading. *Journal of Special Education, 41,* 85–120.

PRIMARY TARGETS OF EMERGENT LITERACY PREVENTION PROGRAMS

Primary Target: Phonological Awareness. Phonological awareness (PA) is the best predictor of a child's reading ability (Catts et al., 2002). **Phonological awareness (PA)** refers to the ability to reflect on and manipulate phonemic segments of speech. Phonological awareness develops from word and syllable awareness (e.g., rhyming and recognizing, identifying the number of syllables in words) to awareness of individual sounds in words. A child demonstrates awareness at the individual sound level by recognizing that /k/ /æ/ /t/ can be blended together to form the word *cat*. At the beginning stages of PA development, a child recognizes larger sound units; he or she learns that sentences are made up of words, and words are made up of syllables. At more sophisticated levels of PA development, a child demonstrates the ability to sound out and blend individual sounds. The ability to decode at the phoneme level is critically linked to reading development. The term **decoding** is used to describe the ability to read a printed word by relating the letters to corresponding speech sounds (Gillon, 2006). PA instruction should not be confused with **phonics instruction**, which entails teaching students how to use letter–sound relationships to read or spell words. You can read more about phonics instruction in Focus 10.3.

Many children begin to develop awareness at the word and syllable levels by age 2. Specifically, about one in four children at age 2 can complete a rhyming detection task in which they are asked to identify the word that does not rhyme (e.g., *hat, cat, bell*). Phoneme-level identification (i.e., identification of specific sounds) takes longer. Most children do not achieve mastery of phoneme-level awareness until age 5. Table 10.1 lists the different PA tasks and developmental age guidelines.

You might suspect that children with oral speech and language deficits have more difficulty with PA tasks and later reading development than children with typical language development (Catts et al., 2002; Puranik et al., 2008). You are correct in this assumption. However, you may be surprised to know that some children who do not have obvious oral language deficits sometimes have difficulty with phonological awareness tasks. "Hidden" PA deficits can significantly impede reading and writing development (Gillon, 2004). Consequently, knowledgeable professionals monitor PA skill development for all children during the early school years; they also support classroom teachers in providing high-quality PA instruction. With SLP assistance, general education teachers learn to provide more explicit and frequent exposure to PA concepts to children whose PA skills are developing more slowly.

Primary Target: Print Concepts and Alphabetic Awareness. The term **print concepts** is used to describe children's understanding of the use and function of print during reading and writing. **Alphabetic awareness** describes children's understanding of letter

---

FOCUS 10.3   *Learning More*

What is the difference between phonological awareness (PA) and phonics? *Phonological awareness* describes the broad range of understanding related to the sounds of speech. At beginning levels, PA includes awareness of words and word parts, and at more advanced levels, it includes phonemic awareness, or understanding of a word's individual sounds. To develop PA, a child learns to pay attention to the sounds in words in an abstract way, learning that sounds in and of themselves do not contain meaning.

Phonics is a form of instruction that focuses on improving a student's understanding and use of the alphabetic principle. Phonics instruction teaches that there is a predictable relationship between phonemes and graphemes (i.e., letters represent sounds in written language). For example, during phonics instruction, a student might be taught that the /el/ sound potentially is represented by different spelling patterns, as in *laid, late,* or *lay*.

Table 10.1 **Developmental Age Levels and Examples of Early Phonological Awareness Skill Areas**

Age at which a child is expected to have greater than 75% accuracy	Skills	Examples
Early to late preschool	Word awareness	• "Can you point to a word on this page?"
	Syllable awareness	• "Let's clap the syllables in your name."
	Rhyming	• "Can you make a big word from these two words? (*cow, boy*)"
		• "Let's play a rhyming game. You finish this sentence: The silly old *cat* wore a big *hat* and sat down on a _____."
Late preschool–early kindergarten	Beginning sound awareness	• "Do these words start with the same sound? (*boy, ball*) How about these two? (*dog, man*)"
	Sound blending	• "What word am I saying? /b/ /i/"
	Onset-rime	• "Look at these pictures. What word am I saying? ("b" [pause] "ubbles")"
Kindergarten	Phoneme identification	• "What sound do you hear at the beginning of the word *pig*?"
	Sound segmenting	• "How many sounds do you hear in the word *boot*? Show me with these blocks." (Child touches one block at a time as he or she says the word, phoneme by phoneme.)

Source: From "Embedded-Explicit Emergent Literacy Intervention I: Background and Description of Approach," by L. M. Justice and J. N. Kaderavek, 2004, *Language, Speech, and Hearing Services in Schools, 35,* pp. 201–211. Reprinted with permission.

names. Table 10.2 lists the different skills included within the print concepts and alphabetic awareness domains. Like phonological awareness, early awareness of print concepts and alphabetic awareness strongly predict later reading proficiency.

Primary Target: Oral Language Skills. The important skills of phonological awareness, print, and alphabetic concepts are learned within a stimulating oral language environment (Stanovich, 2000). A high-quality oral language environment is fostered when adults frequently engage children in extended conversations. Although this seems obvious, research in preschool classrooms demonstrates that the majority of teacher talk is "management talk." Management talk includes giving directions and gaining children's attention. Surprisingly, as little as 10% of teacher–child conversation in early childhood classrooms relates to reading and writing (Rosemary & Roskos, 2002).

For many children, opportunities for high-quality oral language discourse are not much better at home. While children in high-income families hear approximately 2100 vocabulary words per hour, children in families who are struggling economically hear only 600 words per hour; home literacy environments can foster or limit language development (Hoff, 2006). Consequently, practitioners promote the importance of an

Table 10.2 **Print Concepts and Alphabetic Awareness Terms, Descriptions, and Teaching Examples**

Term	Description	Teaching examples
Environmental print awareness	Children recognize familiar symbols and demonstrate knowledge that print carries meaning.	• Point out signs (e.g., McDonald's sign) and letters in children's daily life. • Ask children to sort items (e.g., put all the similar candy wrappers in one pile).
Concepts of print	Children demonstrate accepted standards of practice for interacting with print.	• Demonstrate left-to-right directionality in reading and writing. • Ask children, "Where do I start reading?" (front-to-back directionality of books). • Ask children, "Show me the big long word on this page!" Children learn the meaning of *word*, *letter*, *sentence*, *author*, and *title* and recognize that words are set off by the surrounding space. • Involve children and demonstrate the different functions of print (e.g., a newspaper, a letter, a shopping list). • Demonstrate the use of punctuation and ask children to point out different punctuation marks (e.g., "What do we do when we see a ? ?").
Alphabetic letter knowledge	Children recognize printed letters and understand the letter–sound relationship.	• Play games using letters in children's names; sort and identify letters using blocks, draw and paint letters, play games with magnetic and foam letters. • Help children sort pictures and objects that start with the same letter. • Ask children to find words that have the same first letter as their name. • Sing the alphabet song and have children hold up a letter. • Play "find the hidden letter" or bury plastic letters in a sandbox and have the children find and identify the letters.

Source: From "Embedded-Explicit Emergent Literacy Intervention I: Background and Description of Approach," by L. M. Justice and J. N. Kaderavek, 2004, *Language, Speech, and Hearing Services in Schools, 35*, pp. 201–211. Reprinted with permission.

enriched oral language environment during the preschool years, including opportunities to learn sophisticated vocabulary.

Primary Target: Emergent Writing. Children's writing skills, such as name writing and invented spelling, are strong predictors of later reading proficiency (Puranik & Lonigan, 2012). Early writing puts a child in an active role; children consider how to use a written symbol to communicate meaning. As students' phonics skills develop, they learn to represent sounds with letter combinations. Unfortunately, only 27% of U.S. fourth-grade students exhibit proficient writing abilities; 15% have writing abilities at "below basic" levels (U.S. Department of Education, 2002). To improve this poor outcome, practitioners work with early childhood teachers to foster emergent writing (e.g., Kaderavek & Justice, 2004).

Children's writing development begins with early scribbles and what look like random marks. These unsophisticated attempts represent children's exploration of writing as a means of communication (Casbergue & Plauché, 2005). In order to compose written language, children draw on their knowledge of the alphabetic principle as well as their language **composition skills**. *Composition skills* refer to a child's ability to integrate pragmatic, syntax, and semantic language domains to formulate and express thought (Berninger et al., 2006).

Children move from making scribbles and marks to making letterlike shapes. The formation of letterlike shapes is followed by children's beginning attempts to represent the sounds they hear in words. Table 10.3 demonstrates the stages of writing development and describes the important concepts learned at each stage.

Table 10.3 **Writing Development**

Level	Writing	Concepts	Child learns to:
Preschool	Scribble with or without drawing; letterlike forms; random letter strings	• Writing differs from drawing • Print carries meaning • Concept of *letter*	• Pay attention to print • Control a writing implement • "Write" across the page from left to right • Produce some letterlike shapes
Late preschool to mid-kindergarten	Syllabic writing; writing that the child can "read" (including some conventional letters)	• Chooses own words to make a written text • Concept of word in text • Recognizes own name • Recognizes others' names	• Recognize most letter names • Form and orient many letters • Control letter size • Use letters to make words • Leave spaces between words • Know some letter sounds
Mid-kindergarten to mid-first grade	Simple texts that can be partially read by others; writing is labored	• Produces messages that others can read • Concept of *sentence* and *story*	• Write name fluently • Organize words into sentences • Use punctuation • Recognize all letter names • Know most letter sounds • Distinguish between upper- and lowercase letters in writing
Late first grade to second grade	Writing in phrases with greater fluency	• Writes extended and coherent text • Learns vowel patterns in single-syllable words	• Link sentences • Monitor and correct text • Write phrases with fluency • Write simple paragraphs • Apply writing process (brainstorm, compose, proof, revise)

Sources: Based on information from *Words Their Way: Word Study for Phonics, Vocabulary, and Spelling Instruction* (4th ed.), by D. R. Bear, M. Invernizzi, S. Templeton, and F. Johnston, 2007, Upper Saddle River, NJ: Pearson; "Early Writing and Spelling Development," by J. N. Kaderavek, S. Q. Cabell, and L. M. Justice, 2009. In P. M. Rhyner (Ed.), *Emergent Literacy and Early Language Acquisition: Making the Connection.* New York: Guilford; and *Literacy Development in the Early Years* (5th ed.) by L. M. Morrow, 2005, Boston: Allyn & Bacon.

Although most children follow a general development in the early stages of writing, children's writing development does not follow a step-by-step path. Children sometimes use less-sophisticated writing (e.g., scribbling) when they attempt a difficult task. In contrast, they may produce a sophisticated writing attempt at other times. For example, a 3-year-old child may painstakingly write her name accurately, but in a dramatic play situation, while pretending to write a shopping list, she may scribble and say, "This is my shopping list!" Both efforts are appropriate and demonstrate important aspects of writing development. The name-writing task represents a child's understanding that writing demands the use of specific letters and that certain letter combinations represent a unique word. On the other hand, a child's scribbled shopping list demonstrates awareness of the function of print in everyday life.

ASSESSMENT OF CHILDREN'S EARLY LITERACY SKILLS

In the section above, I described the early literacy domains most frequently targeted within preschool programs. However, it is important to remember that early literacy development begins in infancy in a child's home (Morrow, 2007). Consequently, professionals monitor children's early literacy development from an early age and carefully consider the quality and quantity of home literacy experiences. If a child is not demonstrating enjoyment of shared parent–child book reading, the professional works to improve home book-reading practices and monitors the child's literacy growth.

Early literacy assessment tools are typically criterion-referenced rather than norm-referenced assessments (Justice, Invernizzi, & Meier, 2002). This reflects a prevention approach consistent with the response to intervention (RTI) model. Consistent with RTI, practitioners do not wait until a child has a literacy delay before implementing a high-quality language-literacy program. Instead, practitioners monitor literacy development for all children and implement intense literacy interventions as needed. As you can see in Figure 10.1, practitioners monitor a broad range of early literacy domains in young children. Along with the literacy features described above, practitioners also consider children's social literacy and literacy orientation.

Social literacy considers children's affective (i.e., emotional) response to shared literacy experiences. In Figure 10.1, a child's social literacy is documented in items 1–8, as well as items 12, 13, 15, and 24. Parent–child shared book reading is a critically important early learning context for building children's social literacy. Children who are frequently read to and participate in warm, engaging storybook interactions more frequently become successful readers and writers. Further, children's ability to demonstrate joint visual attention and back-and-forth discourse during shared storybook reading supports oral language and literacy development. Much of what children learn about print and the alphabet they learn through literacy socialization (Battle, 2009). More information about literacy socialization is provided in Focus 10.4.

Frequent, positive social literacy interactions lead to high literacy orientation. **Literacy orientation** includes aspects of children's temperament, motivation, and attention in response to book reading; literacy orientation is an important component of social literacy (Chang & Burns, 2005; Kaderavek & Sulzby, 2000). Most children enjoy shared storybook reading. Some children do not. It is hypothesized that children with language impairments are more likely to have a negative orientation to literacy than are children developing typically (Kaderavek & Sulzby, 2000). Literacy orientation impacts the success of literacy interventions because children with high orientation show more improvement in response to treatment in comparison to children with low orientation (Justice et al.,

Figure 10.1 An Early Literacy Observational Checklist

Child's name: _____ Birth date: _____ Chronological age: _____ Observer: _____

Emergent Literacy Accomplishments	Typically Mastered By	Emergent Literacy Component					Child's Accomplishments		Notes/ Comments
		S	O	L	P	PA	Occasionally	Frequently	
(1) Content to stay in lap	Before 12 months								
(2) Asks for books/indicates books are to be repeated	Before 12 months								
(3) Gestures and laughs during book reading	Before 12 months								
(4) Indicates wants favorite book	Before 12 months								
(5) Focuses on picture	Before 12 months								
(6) Makes spontaneous sounds/words/gestures during book reading	Before 12 months								
(7) Independently manipulates, looks at books	Before 18 months								
(8) Enjoys many different stories	Before 18 months								
(9) Handles book properly (pages left to right, etc.)	18–36 months								
(10) Names actions of characters (running, etc.)	19–22 months								
(11) Points to pictures when asked	Before 36 months								
(12) Joins in, repeats phrases during book reading	Before 36 months								
(13) Tells stories from books	24–60 months								
(14) Writes, attempting to make letters	30–40 months								
(15) Dramatic play (acts out stories)	36–48 months								
(16) Predicts plots (what happens next)	36–48 months								
(17) Points to print/knows print is read	36–60 months								
(18) Reads environmental print (cereal boxes, etc.)	36–48 months								
(19) Plays with words (rhymes, etc.)	36 months								
(20) Claps out syllables in words	36–48 months								
(21) Scribbles	36–48 months								
(22) Says scribbles are "writing"	48–60 months								
(23) Recognizes the first sound in words	60–66 months								
(24) Retells story (beginning, middle, end)	60–72 months								
(25) Recognizes 12–21 uppercase letters	60 months								
(26) Recognizes 9–17 lowercase letters	60 months								
(27) Writes some real words, including first name	60 months								
(28) Names 4–8 letter sounds ("that says /m/")	60 months								
(29) Blends and segments sounds in words	2nd semester kindergarten								
SUMMARY		_/12	_/12	_/11	_/11	_/5			

S = Social literacy; O = Orientation/interest in literacy; L = Language development; P = Print and alphabetic awareness; PA = Phonological awareness

FOCUS 10.4 *Clinical Skill Building*

Aspects of social literacy can be compared to the description of language *use* (see Chapter 1). Discuss how book-reading interactions lend themselves to development of language use. Specifically, how does literacy socialization provide a vehicle for parents to share their viewpoints about the value of reading and writing? How might literacy socialization vary, depending on a families' culture or ethnicity? Finally, how does literacy socialization allow children to experience different patterns of communication use?

If literacy socialization can be considered a component of language use, what other aspects of form and content also are impacted in literacy learning? In the form–content–use model, which language component is involved if a student has lexical deficits contributing to his or her reading problem? What component is involved if a student has difficulty with structural knowledge?

2003). In the observational checklist (Figure 10.1), children's orientation to literacy is documented in items 1–8, 12, 13, 15, and 22.

In addition to informal observational tools, there are other published early literacy assessment tools. A frequently used prekindergarten assessment is the Phonological Awareness and Literacy Screening–Pre-Kindergarten (PALS-PreK; Invernizzi et al., 2004). The PALS-PreK evaluates a range of early literacy skills, including rhyme, beginning sound awareness, name writing, upper- and lowercase letter identification, letter–sound knowledge, and print concepts. The assessor calculates a raw score by summing the points obtained on each subtest and comparing the child's scores with those of other children the same age. The comparison scores reflect a child's ability in the spring prior to kindergarten enrollment. Total administration time of the PALS-PreK is 20 to 25 minutes. The PALS-PreK documents a broad spectrum of emergent literacy skills but particularly focuses on a child's phonological awareness skills. The SLP plays an important role in the assessment of PA because PA deficits are a primary risk factor for reading development and because of SLP's knowledge of phonetics and phonological disorders (Hogan, Catts, & Little, 2005).

EARLY LITERACY INTERVENTIONS: THE EMBEDDED-EXPLICIT APPROACH

The embedded-explicit approach describes a two-faceted intervention model practitioners use to foster children's early literacy development (Justice & Kaderavek, 2004; Kaderavek & Justice, 2004). Through **embedded interventions**, practitioners work to enhance children's oral language, phonological awareness, print and alphabetic concepts, and emergent writing in meaningful activities and classroom interactions. Potential interactions include storybook reading, dramatic play, center-time activities, and even transitional routines (e.g., "signing in" at the beginning of the school day). Teachers learn to take advantage of naturalistic opportunities to target emergent literacy skills.

For example, imagine that you are at a sandbox and children are digging for objects in the sand; prior to the children's arrival, you placed objects in the sandbox with the letter *B* in the initial position (e.g., *bucket, ball, bat, book, basket, bone*). You also buried several plastic letters *B* and *M*. As the children find objects, you say, "That's a bucket.

What sound do you hear at the beginning of *bucket*? /b/. Good, I hear a /b/ sound, too!" When a child finds a letter *B* or *M* you ask, "What letter is that?" Oh, yes, that's a letter B. It makes the /b/ sound, doesn't it? Is that the sound you heard at the beginning of *bucket*?"

As you can see from the example above, during embedded interventions, an adult often primes the activity to foster literacy discussions. However, the adult follows the children's focus of attention, and the context is highly engaging and child centered. Embedded learning opportunities occur throughout the school day and should be fostered across interactions.

In contrast to embedded approaches, **explicit intervention** emphasizes the importance of structured, sequenced adult-directed instruction. In explicit interventions, the adult selects a particular literacy target and carefully sequences the child's exposure; here the adult takes a more direct route to enhancing literacy. Explicit approaches are less naturalistic because the adult selects the goals and specifies the teaching sequence and materials. In explicit intervention, the adult typically uses modeling, demonstration, prompts for child response, and regular guided practice. Explicit interventions typically occur in individual or small-group sessions for relatively short (e.g., 5- to 15-minute) periods; sessions are presented intermittently throughout the school day or week.

Children need exposure to both embedded and explicit literacy instruction. Figure 10.2 demonstrates the kinds of embedded and explicit learning that occur in a literacy-rich

Figure 10.2 **Embedded and Explicit Language and Literacy Activities in the Preschool Classroom**

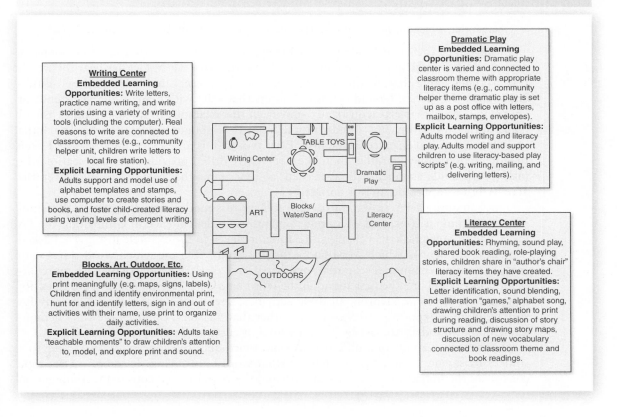

Writing Center
Embedded Learning Opportunities: Write letters, practice name writing, and write stories using a variety of writing tools (including the computer). Real reasons to write are connected to classroom themes (e.g., community helper unit, children write letters to local fire station).
Explicit Learning Opportunities: Adults support and model use of alphabet templates and stamps, use computer to create stories and books, and foster child-created literacy using varying levels of emergent writing.

Dramatic Play
Embedded Learning Opportunities: Dramatic play center is varied and connected to classroom theme with appropriate literacy items (e.g., community helper theme dramatic play is set up as a post office with letters, mailbox, stamps, envelopes).
Explicit Learning Opportunities: Adults model writing and literacy play. Adults model and support children to use literacy-based play "scripts" (e.g. writing, mailing, and delivering letters).

Blocks, Art, Outdoor, Etc.
Embedded Learning Opportunities: Using print meaningfully (e.g. maps, signs, labels). Children find and identify environmental print, hunt for and identify letters, sign in and out of activities with their name, use print to organize daily activities.
Explicit Learning Opportunities: Adults take "teachable moments" to draw children's attention to, model, and explore print and sound.

Literacy Center
Embedded Learning Opportunities: Rhyming, sound play, shared book reading, role-playing stories, children share in "author's chair" literacy items they have created.
Explicit Learning Opportunities: Letter identification, sound blending, and alliteration "games," alphabet song, drawing children's attention to print during reading, discussion of story structure and drawing story maps, discussion of new vocabulary connected to classroom theme and book readings.

classroom. As you can see from the activities listed in Figure 10.2, both embedded and explicit early literacy experiences actively engage children as learners; worksheets and drill activities are avoided.

Early Intervention: Phonological Awareness (PA). The sandbox example above demonstrates an embedded PA learning opportunity. Adults also provide embedded PA instruction when they incorporate rhymes and chants into the classroom or read storybooks such as *The Cat in the Hat* and draw attention to rhyming words. Research demonstrates, however, that explicit exposure to PA should also be included in the early childhood classroom; many children will not grasp PA concepts without explicit instruction (Bradley, Danielson, & Hallahan, 2013). I describe several explicit PA learning opportunities below.

One of the easiest PA tasks is syllable recognition. **Syllable recognition** is a child's awareness that a word is made up of syllable subunits. Syllable recognition is considered a word-level task; a child does not need to recognize individual phonemes to recognize syllables. When I engage a child in a syllable recognition task, I ask him or her to clap or tap out word syllables. For example, following a book reading about zoo animals, I may suggest:

> Let's clap out el-e-phant. Now let's clap out ti-ger. Which word has more syllables? Let's clap it again. That's right, el-e-phant has three claps, doesn't it? *Elephant* has three syllables! *Tiger* has two claps. *Tiger* has two syllables!

Children should also be exposed to phoneme-level tasks such as activities to build initial sound awareness. In the following example, Samantha and I take turns pulling objects out of a "treasure chest":

> Samantha, which of these words starts with the /b/ sound? *Snake, boat, sandwich, ball.*

I introduce each word individually. I exaggerate and emphasize the initial sound in each word. I go back and let Samantha say the words with me and let her hear the words several times. Note that, at this stage, I only include objects that start with two different sounds (/b/ vs. /s/); I avoid choosing objects that start with many different sounds or choosing sounds that are acoustically similar. In this example, to make the task easier, I contrast the stop-plosive /b/ sound with the fricative /s/ sound. I make sure that Samantha stays interested and engaged in the task. Even though it is an explicit intervention, I keep the interaction gamelike rather than like a repetitive drill. I provide clues and scaffold the task (i.e., provide as much help as needed) so that Samantha feels successful. I keep the activity brief—approximately 5 minutes.

As Samantha's PA skills improve, I add more sounds, include acoustically similar sound comparisons, and encourage Samantha's independence in completing the PA tasks. Modifying a task also changes the difficulty level. In the example just given, I asked Samantha to identify which word had a target sound ("Tell me which word starts with /b/."). This is a beginning-level initial sound awareness task. I can make the task more difficult if I say, "Tell me the first sound in the word boat" or "Tell me which word does not belong: *bus, bun, hat.*" During all these activities, I remember that the goal of early PA skill building is exposure to PA concepts rather than mastery. Children typically demonstrate initial sound awareness by late preschool or early kindergarten.

In another example of a different PA skill, I introduce the concept of *onset-rime* to a student by saying, "Sean, can you tell me what word I am saying? l – amp." Onset-rime consists of the initial sound (in this case /l/) and the vowel + final consonant combination

/æmp/. The ability to recognize onset-rime is connected to rhyming because a child must have awareness that words "sound the same at the end" in order to rhyme words. After onset-rime skills, children generally learn sound blending and sound segmentation: "What funny word is the puppet trying to say? /s/ /I/ /t/" (Answer: *sit*). Sound segmentation is a skill generally demonstrated during kindergarten or first grade. It is important to note that recent research suggests that a shorter but more intensive intervention (e.g., 20 hours over a 10-week period) focusing on phoneme-level (e.g., initial sound awareness, sound segmentation) vs. syllable-level skills (e.g., syllable identification, rhyming) is the most time-effective intervention, resulting in improved reading outcomes for at-risk children. An SLP should consider this information when developing a PA intervention program (Carson, Gillon, & Boustead, 2012).

Practitioners often seek out effective preschool curricula to guide their early literacy interventions. Find out how specific preschool curricula are ranked for effectiveness by using the information provided in Focus 10.5.

Early Intervention: Print Concepts and Alphabetic Knowledge. Children are exposed to print concepts and alphabetic knowledge through both embedded and explicit learning opportunities. Adults use an embedded approach when they point out that print can be seen in traffic and store signs. During a discussion of environmental print, a child is likely to learn (a) the meanings of *word, letter,* and *sentence*; (b) that readers read the print and not the illustration; (c) that readers read from left to right and top to bottom; (d) that there are different letters and letters have different names; and (e) that letters make sounds and sounds make up words.

Print referencing is an explicit teaching technique that exposes children to print and alphabetic concepts (Justice & Ezell, 2002). For example, during book reading, an adult reader includes comments to draw the child's attention to specific print and alphabetic concepts. Below I list several examples of print referencing:

- "This is the *title* of the book. Can anyone show me where the *author's* name is on this front cover? That's right, the *author* writes the book." (Concepts of print)
- "Where should I start reading—here or here?" (Adult points to illustration and then text; concepts of print)

FOCUS 10.5   *Clinical Skill Building*

Currently, many early childhood literacy curricula have been evaluated in randomized control studies. You can research information about the effectiveness of specific literacy programs via the *What Works Clearinghouse* (*WWC*). The WWC is sponsored by the U.S. Department of Education; it is a review process that evaluates the effectiveness of different programs, products, practices, and policies. The stated goal of WWC is to provide educators with the information they need to make evidence-based decisions. To research early childhood curricula at WWC, go to http://ies.ed.gov/ncee/wwc/findwhatworks .aspx; and then click on "Early Childhood Education and Literacy" in the "Find what works for" menu.

- "What does this sign say in this picture? That's right, it says STOP!" (Awareness of environmental print)
- "Can anyone find the uppercase *T* on this page?" (Alphabetic awareness)

Early Intervention: Oral Language. One of the best opportunities for embedded oral language learning is through repeated exposure to shared storybook reading. Children who are frequently read to are more likely to demonstrate literate language. **Literate language** refers to the frequently occurring syntax and morphological features that occur in books and written text (Greenhalgh & Strong, 2001). Through repeated readings, children become familiar with the way written language sounds; they internalize word usage, grammatical forms, and idiosyncratic features of written language. Consider the following example:

> "Oh, my!" the small, furry teddy bear exclaimed. "I think I have misplaced my favorite honey jar. Where could I possibly have placed it?" Because the bear could not find his cherished honey jar, he sat down glumly on the closest tree stump.

In this example, do you think I was talking to you in a conversational style, or do you think I was reading to you from a book? I imagine that you said "reading from a book." What features in the example led you to this decision? There are several clues.

First, I used **dialogic speech**, which is the use of quotation or spoken language by a character in the story. In this example, I used the dialogic marker *exclaimed,* but I also could have used a word such as *complained, whined,* or *said.* Dialogic language is rarely used during informal discourse (i.e., conversation) but occurs often in written language. Children learn to understand dialogic speech when they hear written text.

A second indicator is the use of descriptive vocabulary, such as *small, furry* (teddy bear), *my favorite* (honey pot), *cherished* (honey pot), and *closest* (tree stump). A descriptive adjective before a noun makes a noun phrase (NP). A verb and its modifiers and/or associated auxiliary verbs make a verb phrase (VP). Literate language typically demonstrates more NP and VP elaboration. Children with language impairments have difficulty with descriptive words, and they fail to use elaborated NP and VP combinations (Ukrainetz et al., 2005). Written language also uses Tier 2 vocabulary. (See Chapter 5 for a discussion of Tier 1, 2, and 3 vocabulary.) In the example above, I used the verb *misplaced,* the adjective *cherished,* and the adverb *glumly.* These words are relatively rare and may be unfamiliar to children. When children listen to storybooks, they are exposed to Tier 2 vocabulary.

Literate language also includes more sophisticated verb forms. In the example above, I used past tense verbs. Written text often includes past tense verbs; in contrast, in face-to-face conversations, verb use often reflects present tense. In the example above, I used the past tense verbs *exclaimed, misplaced, could,* and *sat.*

Cognitive verbs, sometimes called mental verbs, are another advanced verb form. **Cognitive verbs** include words such as *thought, knew, remembered, decided, imagined, forgot, asked, told, explained, called,* or *yelled.* We use cognitive verbs to describe the actions and thoughts of characters in text. Oral language uses cognitive verbs less frequently; written text offers more opportunities for exposure to cognitive verbs.

Literate language requires decontextualization and cohesive language devices. **Decontextualized language** allows the listener to understand what is spoken or written, without background information or environmental cues. This contrasts with conversational speech. During a conversation, both the speaker and the listener share the same context (i.e., the same environmental stimuli and shared experience), and the listener has the ability to ask questions if there is a need for more information. When one reads a book, it is not possible to ask the author questions; consequently, literate language must be decontextualized.

The use of **cohesive language** devices requires the speaker or writer to use words that link information from one sentence to another. In the example above, after I introduced the main character (the teddy bear), I referred to the bear as *he* in the fourth sentence. This represents a linkage between an introduced referent and the pronoun referring back to the referent. Another cohesive device in the example is the use of the subordinating conjunction *because*. Subordinating conjunctions such as *because, so, then,* and *therefore* make cause-and-effect story connections and highlight the temporal (i.e., time) sequencing of story events (Curenton & Justice, 2004).

Practitioners use embedded opportunities during storybook reading to enhance children's use of literate language features. Practitioners also explicitly increase children's oral language and literate language during story role-plays, storytelling with felt board or puppets, and with child-dictated stories (Justice et al., 2003; Stanovich, 2000).

Early Intervention: Emergent Writing. Children have embedded opportunities to practice writing during classroom routines and dramatic play. A classroom routine may include children signing out books from the classroom library to take home. Children incorporate writing into dramatic play when literacy objects (e.g., doctor's prescription pad, clipboard, pens, magazines) are included in a play area centering on a specific theme—in this case, the doctor's office. During dramatic play, the practitioner uses adult-mediated writing to foster children's emergent writing skills. An example of adult-mediated writing is the adult modeling and demonstrating writing a letter, addressing an envelope, stamping a letter, taking a letter to the post office, and receiving and "reading" a letter. Children's experiences with literacy-rich dramatic play centers (e.g., library, veterinarian's office, grocery store, restaurant) dramatically increase the quality and quantity of children's reading and writing activities (Morrow, 2005).

Professionals also use the explicit approach of **story dictation** to foster early writing skills. Story dictation provides children the opportunity to learn that writing is speech written down. Using the language experience approach, the adult writes down a story as the child dictates his or her experiences. The child illustrates the story or supplements the story with photographs. The adult reads the story back to the child and points to each word as he or she reads it aloud.

CULTURAL CONSIDERATIONS IN EMERGENT LITERACY DEVELOPMENT

Young children who must learn English as a second language and children who use African American English face additional challenges in learning to read and write. In the past, sometimes teachers, SLPs, and researchers failed to recognize the learning challenges faced by minority students. Other times, preconceived notions of "what it takes to be academically successful" are just plain wrong! I will describe two recent studies illustrating both points.

The first example demonstrates the complexity of early language and literacy learning for children who speak Spanish at home and English at school. Cardenas-Hagan, Carlson, and Pollard-Durodola (2007) evaluated the acquisition of early literacy skills for children who are in **dual language programs**.

In dual language programs, the goal is for students to maintain the first language (L1) while learning English as a second language (L2; Cloud, Genessee, & Hamayan, 2000). Teachers use both L1 and L2 at different times of the day; in many programs, English is used 50% of the day and Spanish the remaining 50%. Sometimes the ratio of English/Spanish represents a ratio as high as 90%/10%.

Researchers concluded that instructional decisions for L2 learners must include (a) assessment of children's knowledge of letters and letter sounds in both English and Spanish at the beginning of the school year and (b) careful consideration of instructional time in L1 vs. L2. Children with low literacy skills at the beginning of the school year may benefit from increased instructional time in Spanish. For other children—children with higher literacy skills in either Spanish or English—the amount of instructional time in L1 vs. L2 may not significantly impact literacy development.

The second example demonstrates how preconceived notions of academic readiness are sometimes incorrect. Specifically, I point to findings indicating that preschoolers who use many features of African American English (AAE) are *not* necessarily at greater risk for reading failure. This finding contrasts with other reports indicating frequent AAE use in older school-age children is a reading risk factor (Connor & Craig, 2006). What is going on here?

It appears that many young children who enter school with AAE dialect as a primary speaking pattern learn to use General American English (GAE) at school. The movement from primary AAE dialect to GAE is evidence of code switching. As you recall from Chapter 2, code switching refers to an individual's ability to alternate between formal and informal language or between dialectal language patterns and GAE.

Research has revealed some interesting results about code switching in young urban preschool children (Connor & Craig, 2006). At the beginning of formal schooling, urban preschoolers may have minimal exposure to GAE. As a result, at the beginning of the school year, preschoolers may demonstrate high use of AAE features. However, with exposure to GAE, Craig and her colleagues (Connor & Craig, 2006; Craig & Washington, 2004) report that many students learn to code switch with a subsequent decrease in AAE features. The ability to code switch is a sophisticated metalinguistic skill. Children who code switch demonstrate a level of linguistic ability that bodes well for later academic success.

Now, back to the issue I raised earlier. I stated that preschoolers who use many features of AAE are not necessarily at greater risk for reading failure. The lack of relationship between high AAE use and early literacy weakness centers on the ability of children to code switch. Young children who are able to code switch and adapt their linguistic patterns once they are exposed to GAE are likely to have good underlying linguistic skills. On the other hand, children who fail to code switch, even though they have exposure to GAE, may have underlying linguistic deficits. In sum, it is not AAE use that limits academic development but rather underlying language abilities.

School-Age Children with Language Impairment

Increasingly, because of the 2001 No Child Left Behind (NCLB) legislation (see Focus 10.6 for more information about NCLB) and our increasing understanding of the connections between oral and written language, practitioners assess and provide intervention for school-age students in reading and writing domains. Research summarized by the

FOCUS 10.6   *School-Based Issues*

No Child Left Behind Act of 2001

The No Child Left Behind Act of 2001 (Public Law 107-110), often abbreviated as NCLB, is a U.S. federal law proposed by President George W. Bush. NCLB establishes standards-based education reform based on the belief that setting high standards and establishing measurable goals improves students' educational outcomes. The effectiveness of NCLB has been debated. Specifically, critics argue that NCLB-mandated testing is not appropriate for all students (e.g., students with disabilities, students with limited English proficiency) and/or that teachers "teach to the test" and are less likely to provide best instructional practices to meet students' needs (Forum on Educational Accountability, 2007).

National Reading Panel (NRP) in 2000 (NICHD, 2000) identified specific skills that—in the opinion of the panel reviewers—are necessary foundations for reading development in school-age children (see Figure 10.3). Important identified component skills included phonological awareness, the ability to match letters and sounds (i.e., phonics), and the development of reading fluency, vocabulary, and text comprehension.

The American Speech-Language-Hearing Association (ASHA, 2001, 2002a) supported the NRP recommendations. However, some experts suggest that the NRP description of reading development is limited because reading is broken down into a series of isolated component skills. Critics of the NRP report argue that a skills-based approach does not account for the underlying mental structures required to become a successful reader and writer (Damico & Nelson, 2010; Strauss, 2003). As an alternative to the skills-based view of reading development, another approach has been forwarded, sometimes referred to as the meaning-based approach to reading (Damico & Nelson, 2010).

Advocates of a meaning-based approach suggest that children should (a) first be exposed to literacy during adult–child reading- and writing-aloud activities, (b) progress to guided reading and writing activities in naturalistic settings, and (c) gradually move to independent reading and writing. As an SLP, you will want to provide balanced reading interventions fostering both component-reading skills and meaning-based literacy activities. In this chapter, I have emphasized the importance of both naturalistic, meaning-based literacy activities and interventions focusing on literacy skill development.

In the section below, I describe information on the literacy domains frequently targeted by practitioners who work with school-age students. I provide an overview of advanced levels of phonological awareness in addition to a discussion of narrative production, spelling, reading comprehension, and writing. At the end of this section on school-age students, I discuss issues related to working with classroom teachers and multicultural considerations.

SCHOOL-AGE STUDENTS: PHONOLOGICAL AWARENESS

Many school-age students with language impairments or learning disabilities continue to struggle with PA skills. Consequently, practitioners frequently assess and provide PA intervention for school-age children. Assessment and intervention for older students typically emphasizes sound blending and segmenting.

Figure 10.3 National Reading Panel: Background and Recommendations

In 1997, Congress asked the director of the National Institute of Child Health and Human Development (NICHD), in consultation with the secretary of education, to convene a national panel to evaluate the research-based knowledge focused on the best methods to help children become skilled readers. The recommendation was to approach reading development from a skills-based perspective. While this approach has not been universally accepted, the reading domains described below are targeted in U.S. public school reading curricula. The panel evaluated the literature, focusing on three areas[1] of reading research:

Domain: Phonological Awareness

Definition and rationale for inclusion: Phonological awareness (PA) involves teaching children to focus on and manipulate phonemes in spoken syllables and words. Correlation studies have identified PA as one of the best school-entry predictors of how well children will learn to read during the first 2 years of instruction.

Findings: Teaching children to manipulate phonemes in words is highly effective under a variety of teaching conditions and with a variety of learners across a range of grade and age levels.

Domain: Fluency

Definition and rationale for inclusion: Fluent readers are able to read orally with speed, accuracy, and proper expression. Fluency is one of several critical factors necessary for reading comprehension.

Findings: Guided repeated oral reading procedures have a significant and positive impact on word recognition, fluency, and comprehension. Steps to guided oral reading include: (a) adult or peer reads a passage aloud while modeling fluent reading at the student's independent reading level,[2] (b) student rereads the text quietly by himself or herself several times, (c) student reads aloud with adult encouragement and feedback, and (d) sequence is repeated (typically 3–4 times) until the student can read the passage fluently.

Domain: Reading Comprehension

Definition and rationale for inclusion: Reading comprehension is a student's ability to gain meaning from text and repair misunderstandings when they occur. Deficits in reading comprehension limit children's long-term academic performance.

Findings: Reading comprehension is a complex cognitive process requiring (a) vocabulary development and vocabulary instruction and (b) use of metaskills during reading such as semantic organizers,[3] question answering (i.e., readers answer questions posed by the teacher and receive feedback), question generation (i.e., readers ask themselves questions about various aspects of the story), or summarization (readers learn to integrate ideas and generalize from text information).

[1]The panel also looked at the domains of (a) teacher education and (b) computer-based reading instruction but concluded that there was not enough research available to draw strong conclusions.

[2]A student's independent reading level is the level at which he can read with 95% word accuracy; it should be "relatively easy" for the student.

[3]Readers make graphic representations (i.e., story maps) to assist comprehension.

Source: Based on information from *Report of the National Reading Panel. Teaching Children to Read: An Evidence-Based Assessment of the Scientific Research Literature on Reading and Its Implications for Reading Instruction: Reports of the Subgroups* (NIH Publication No. 00-4754), National Institute of Child Health and Human Development, 2000, Washington, DC: U.S. Government Printing Office.

School-Age Students: Phonological Awareness Assessment. With young children, an assessor is likely to use informal tests or a screening assessment such as the PALS-PreK to assess PA skills. However, for a student of school age, an assessor is more likely to use a norm-referenced assessment (for examples of norm-referenced PA tests, see Table 10.4). Whether the assessment is criterion based or norm referenced, PA skills are assessed in the order of developmental sequence and difficulty (see Table 10.1). The practitioner remembers that PA skills can be assessed with a variety of tasks and that some tasks are easier than others. For example, it is easier to identify sounds at the beginning of words (e.g., "What is the first sound you hear in the word *duck*?") than to identify the final sounds in words. A practitioner also knows that matching tasks (e.g., "Which words have the same sound at the beginning? *top, man, tin*") and same–different tasks (e.g., "Do these words start with the same sound? *pin, fin*") are easier for children than production tasks ("Give me a word that rhymes with *cat*").

Table 10.4   **Examples of Norm-Referenced Assessments for Older Students for Identification of Reading and Writing Deficits**

Language domain	Test	Age/grade range
Narrative development	Test of Narrative Language (TNL; Gillam & Pearson, 2004)	5–11:11 years
Phonological awareness	Lindamood Auditory Conceptualization Test–3rd (Lindamood & Lindamood, 2004)	5–18:11 years
	Test of Phonological Awareness—Second Edition: PLUS (TOPA-2+; Torgesen & Bryant, 2004)	K–3rd grade
	Comprehensive Test of Phonological Processing—Second Edition (CTOPP-2; Wagner et al., 2013)	4:0–24:11 years
Writing	Test of Written Language—4 (TOWL-4; Hammill & Larsen, 2009)	9–17:11 years
	Oral and Written Language Scales—II (OWLS: Written Expression [WE] Scale—Second Edition; Carrow-Woolfolk, 2011)	3–21:11 years
Reading	Woodcock Reading Mastery Tests—Third Edition (WRMT-III; Woodcock, 2011)	4:6–79:11 years
	Test of Reading Comprehension Skills (TORC-4; Brown, Wiederholt, & Hammill, 2006).	7–17:11 years
	Gray Oral Reading Tests–Fifth Edition (GORT-5; Wiederholt & Bryant, 2012)	6:0–23:11 years
Spelling	Test of Written Spelling, 4th Edition (Larsen, Hammill, & Moats, 1999)	6:0–18:11 years
	Spelling Performance Evaluation for Language and Literacy—2nd Edition (SPELL-2; Masterson, Apel, & Wasowicz, 2002)	Grade 2–adult

School-Age Students: Phonological Awareness Interventions. When practitioners work with school-age students, they target PA skills with more intensity and make activities less gamelike. It should be clear to older students why they are working on PA. To increase self-awareness, practitioners teach metacognitive strategies to use when sounding out words. In the following example, the practitioner works with a student on decoding a word with an initial consonant blend:

> In this word, first you see three consonants grouped together: *spl*—that's a blend—and we pronounce it like /spl/. The next sound is *a*; that is a short vowel, /æ/. The next sound, *sh*, is a digraph; remember a digraph represents two letters together that make one sound. This sound is /ʃ/. Now let's blend the sounds together: /spl/—/æ/—/ʃ/. *Splash*, the word is splash! You try the next word; look for that *spl* blend.

Professionals sometimes use Elkonian boxes (see Figure 10.4) to teach students to move tokens and then letter tiles into boxes to represent sounds during phoneme identification, blending, and segmenting tasks. The words are made progressively more difficult to encourage students to listen to subtle sound changes. For example:

> Show me the word /sɪt/. Good. Now, show me the word /sæt/. What sound changed? Right! The middle vowel changed! Now, show me the word /fæt/. What changed? That's right. The first sound changed, didn't it?

SCHOOL-AGE STUDENTS: NARRATIVES

Children's narratives are an important link between oral and written language development. The **oral narrative** is a monologue describing a real or fictional event, organized into linked utterances with specific linguistic features. During a narrative, the speaker

Figure 10.4 **Elkonian Boxes**

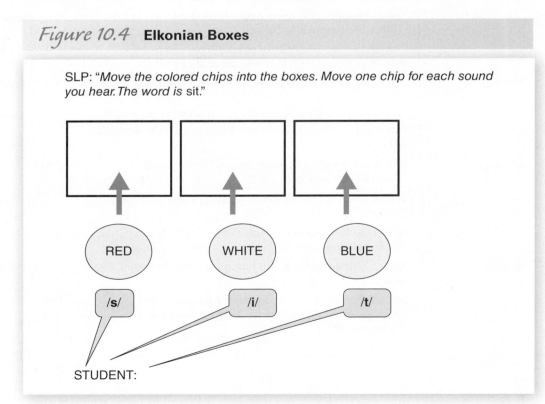

describes a thematic event—in other words, an event centered around one or more connected actions. Children who successfully produce oral narratives have a foundational skill that contributes to reading and writing. However, students with language impairments often struggle to produce oral narratives, and this impairment negatively impacts literacy development (Scott & Windsor, 2000).

Consider this example of an oral narrative from a 6-year-old girl. In this example, the student tells a story in response to a picture showing a spaceship landing in a park with children hiding behind a bush:

> A boy and the girl came out of the bushes. And they were in the bushes. And then they saw (an) a spaceship come down. And aliens come out. And then the girl wanted to go out and see them. And, the boy said, "Don't do it." And she kept looking. And (um) they came to stay. And the spaceship went up.

This child demonstrates beginning knowledge of aspects of narrative production, exhibiting both narrative microstructure and macrostructure.

Narrative microstructure features are internal linguistic features occurring within oral narratives. Microfeatures include students' use of increasingly complex syntax along with literate language features (i.e., decontextualized language, cohesive devices, descriptive vocabulary). As children move from kindergarten to upper elementary school, they increasingly include the required microstructure features needed to produce an effective narrative (Justice et al., 2006).

Narrative macrostructure refers to overall story organization. A story is not just a random collection of ideas. A story engages the listener with (a) a description of a particular event, (b) the actions that occurred in response to the initial event, and (c) the consequence of the subsequent actions. This linked series of events is called the **story episode**. A story episode contains three important components. The first component is the **initiating event** (IE) or problem that sets the story in motion. The second component is the **attempt** (A), an action that is undertaken by the story's character to solve the problem. The third component is the **consequence** (C); it is a description of the character's attempt to solve the problem. Children produce a narrative with episodic structure, sometimes called a *true narrative,* around the age of 4½ to 5 years. Figure 10.5 illustrates a child producing a true narrative. Prior to this point, preschool children often produce a narrative called a two-event narrative. A two-event narrative contains several sentences describing an event (e.g., "I walked the dog. He pulled me down."). Alternatively, young children may produce a disorganized or leapfrog narrative, jumping from one event to another and leaving out major events. Table 10.5 demonstrates the typical pattern of narrative development.

A true narrative, with story episodic structure, contains a cause-and-effect relationship between the initiating event, the attempt, and the story consequence. Subordinating conjunctions such as *because, since, then,* and *so* are used to indicate cause and effect. For example, consider the following narrative:

> The mother went to the store, but she forgot to bring her purse (IE). After waiting in line for some time, arriving at the cashier's station, she realized that she had no money. In confusion, she dropped her items on the floor and ran out of the store (A). Since she had made such a spectacle of herself, she felt she could never return to her favorite store (C).

In this example, the word *since* highlights the relationship between the attempt (e.g., dropping the items) and the consequence (e.g., her embarrassment at returning to the store). Children with language impairment have difficulty with subordinating conjunctions; this deficit further impairs narrative quality.

Figure 10.5 Three Components of a Narrative Episode

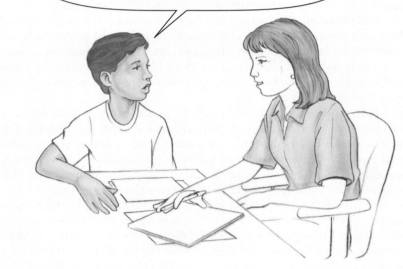

Last weekend my dad and I went fishing at the lake... **(initiating event)** And, suddenly, I felt something tugging really hard on the fishing line... **(attempt)** Finally, after a LONG time, we landed the fish! **(consequence)**

Table 10.5 Narrative Development

Age	Terms*	Characteristics
2–3	*Additive chains*, prenarratives, heap stories, descriptive or action sequences, two-event narratives, leapfrog narratives	• Additive chains: Child describes things he sees or hears in a sequence but does not describe causal relationships. ("I fall down, Mommy came outside.") • Heap story: Contains no central theme.

Age	Terms*	Characteristics
		• Leapfrog narrative: Disorganized narrative without temporal order; produced by children who are typically developing at young ages and older children with language impairments.
3–5	*Temporal stories*, sequence stories, primitive narratives, causal chains	• There is some linking of events in a temporal story, but there is typically no resolution and no character motivation.
6–7	*True narratives*, simple-causal narratives	• Episodic structure emerges (e.g., initiating event, attempt, consequence); the character's motivations are described.
>8	*Multi-causal*, complex narratives	• The story contains multiple embedded episodes. Narratives typically contain descriptive language.

*Italic term is most common; other terms also are used to describe narratives.
Source: Based on information from Roth, F. P. (2009). Children's early narratives. In P. Rhyner (Ed.), *Emergent literacy and language development* (pp. 153–191). New York: Guilford.

School-Age Students: Narrative Assessments. Assessors consider the use of both micro- and macrolevel features during school-age children's narrative analyses. Refer to Figure 10.6, a narrative decision tree, for a protocol to follow during macrostructure analysis. I also have provided examples of school-age narratives at the end of this chapter. Practicing narrative analysis is a very helpful activity for beginning SLP students because they must consider a child's overall ability to organize the narrative using story grammar and also evaluate microstructure features such as syntax and vocabulary use. Remember that children with LI typically have problems telling a sequenced story, and their stories often lack detail and cohesiveness (Curenton & Lucas, 2007; McCabe & Bliss, 2003).

Professionals sometimes elicit student narratives and complete an analysis much like the language sample analysis discussed in Chapter 3. Sometimes assessors use norm-referenced tests to complete a narrative assessment. An example of a norm-referenced narrative assessment is the Test of Narrative Language (Gillam & Pearson, 2004). To elicit the narrative examples at the end of this chapter, five children were asked to tell a story in response to a series of sequenced pictures. Prior to eliciting the narrative, the adult provided an example of an oral narrative.

Asking children to respond to a series of pictures is one way to elicit a student narrative. However, there are other approaches to eliciting a narrative, and different approaches

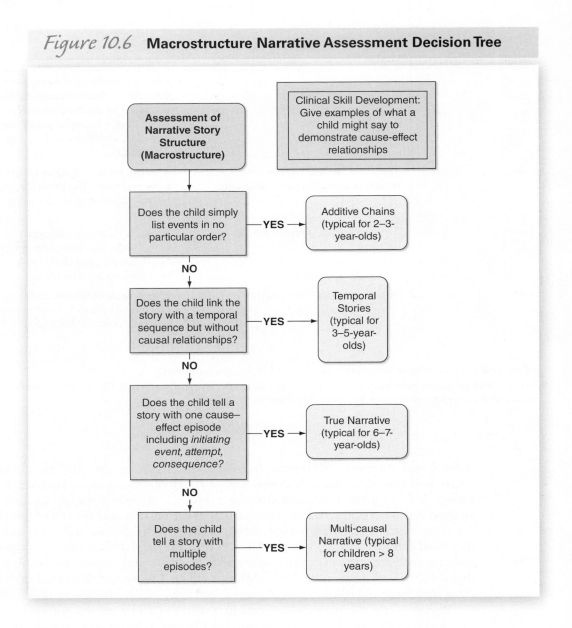

Figure 10.6 **Macrostructure Narrative Assessment Decision Tree**

place different demands on the child's narrative ability. For example, in a story-retelling narrative task, the assessor reads or tells a story (with or without illustrations) and asks the student to retell the story. This task is good for younger children or students with limited exposure to narrative language.

A more difficult narrative task is story generation. In this case, the assessor asks the student to make up a story with or without an accompanying illustration. Sometimes the assessor provides examples of narrative storytelling prior to soliciting a student's story, as the adult did when eliciting the narratives at the end of this chapter. A skilled assessor carefully considers a student's age, language abilities, and storytelling experience when choosing the approach to use for narrative elicitation.

School-Age Students: Narrative Interventions. Narrative intervention focuses on improving students' micro- and macronarrative features. At the beginning stages of narrative intervention, a practitioner selectively targets a single aspect of narrative production. If a student is mastering new microfeatures (e.g., descriptive vocabulary), the adult asks the student to produce the linguistic feature in a familiar narrative task. On the other hand, if the macro-level ability of story structure is targeted, the practitioner reduces the vocabulary or syntax demands during the story retelling. This dynamic relationship between different aspects of language should remind you of a statement introduced in Chapter 5: *Teach new forms within familiar functions.* Discuss with your classmates how you might apply this idea to develop narrative interventions for school-age students (see Focus 10.7).

Macrostructure is improved when children learn the underlying organization of a story episode. Awareness of macrostructure results in improved reading comprehension and written story organization (Westby, 2005). To facilitate macrostructure, a professional often uses symbols or written words (if the child is a reader) to remind the student

---

FOCUS 10.7   *Clinical Skill Building*

Balancing Macro- and Microstructure Demands during Narrative Interventions

As children learn a new linguistic task, they may not be able to process additional higher-order tasks at the same time. This idea is exemplified in the "bucket" theory, which suggests that there are trade-offs across language domains (Crystal, 1987). For example, there could be trade-offs in syntax production as children produce language containing story structure (e.g., characters, an initiating event). Application of this theory to narrative production suggests that a child attempting to produce increasingly complex narrative macrostructure may demonstrate reduced complexity at a microstructural level and vice versa. As the demands fill the linguistic bucket, the bucket overflows, and performance in one or more domains decreases. However, with practice, the child learns to produce combinations of linguistic skills.

How might the bucket theory affect language intervention for students working on other aspects of language production (other than narratives)? How can a language facilitator modify interventions to account for the bucket theory?

As a secondary (but related) issue, it has been suggested that during language assessment procedures, an SLP might want to stress the student's language system by intentionally but systematically tapping into multiple language domains and then observing how varying processing demands (i.e., requiring speeded performance or more complex language) affect the student's output (Lahey, 1990). Discuss how these two issues—(a) systematically reducing and then gradually increasing linguistic demands during intervention and (b) intentionally increasing processing demands during language assessment protocols—are "two sides of the same coin."

to include story setting, a main character, the initiating event, attempt, and consequence. Older children also learn metaskills to self-monitor story organization. Techniques such as using a checklist, story map, or rubric assist metadevelopment. An example of visual cues used to organize story structure is shown in Figure 10.7.

SCHOOL-AGE STUDENTS: SPELLING

Because spelling is a linguistic skill, children with language impairments have more difficulty with spelling tasks than do children with typical language (Larkin & Snowling, 2008). Accurate spelling involves skill development in several linguistic and cognitive domains. As demonstrated in Table 10.6, early spelling ability is closely linked to phonological awareness abilities. In later school years, spelling also requires morphological awareness. Both areas are potential areas of weakness for children who are language impaired.

Figure 10.7 Visual Cues to Enhance Narrative Production

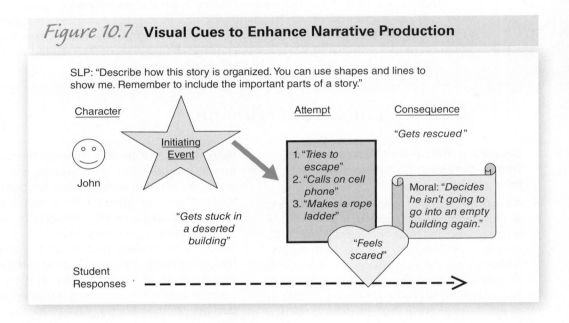

Table 10.6 Spelling Development

Age	Spelling	Spelling error examples
Preschool	Emergent/Preliterate Writing bears no letter–sound correspondence; children scribble, make letterlike shapes and some letters.	

Age	Spelling	Spelling error examples
Late preschool to mid-kindergarten	<u>Semiphonetic</u> Represents salient sounds; represents initial and final sounds in words; typically does not represent vowels.	S (seat) bk (back) Tf (teeth)
Mid-kindergarten to mid–first grade	↓ Developmental Path Varies Greatly ↓ <u>Phonetic Spelling</u> Represents all or most sounds in words; begins to represent vowels; does not demonstrate all spelling conventions.	fale (fail) plat (plate) jriv (drive)
Late first grade to second grade	<u>Within-Word Pattern</u> Represents most short vowels correctly, using but confusing long vowel patterns.	back (back) dinisore (dinosaur) chips (chips) driav (drive)
Mid–elementary school	<u>Syllable Juncture Stage</u> Children begin to pay attention to patterns such as doubling letters, stressed and unstressed syllable patterns.	funnier (i.e., double the final consonant of a syllable containing a short vowel before adding suffix)
Later elementary school	<u>Derivational Constancy Stage</u> Children understand word roots and use knowledge to spell.	exemption (i.e., derivation from word *exempt)*

Sources: Based on information from *Words Their Way: Word Study for Phonics, Vocabulary, and Spelling Instruction* (4th ed.), by D. R. Bear, M. Invernizzi, S. Templeton, and F. Johnston, 2007, Upper Saddle River, NJ: Pearson; "Meeting the Needs of Low Spellers in a Second-Grade Classroom," by J. Brown and D. Morris, 2005, *Reading and Writing Quarterly, 21,* pp. 165–185; *Learning About Print in Preschool: Working with Letters, Words, and Beginning Links with Phonemic Awareness,* by D. S. Strickland and J. Schickedanz, 2009, Newark, DE: International Reading Association.

Here, I briefly discuss foundational skills needed to become a proficient speller:

- *Phonological awareness* is a requirement for spelling as PA knowledge allows a student to segment words into individual phonemes. Phonological awareness proficiency is the best predictor of children's spelling development (Treiman & Bourassa, 2000). When a child spells *night* as *fite,* he or she demonstrates difficulty making a connection between the sounds and the letters representing the sounds.
- A student requires an ability to visually store images of words. *Visual storage* allows a student to form and maintain visual images for words, morphemes, and syllables. When a child spells the same word differently at different times (e.g., *lite, liet, light*), she demonstrates a weakness in visual storage ability (Masterson & Apel, 2000).
- A student needs *orthographic knowledge* to be a competent speller. Through development of orthographic knowledge, children learn to recognize that some letter

combinations are allowed and other letter combinations are never used. For example, the nonsense word *nuck* is a possible English letter combination, while the nonsense word *ckun* is not a possible letter combination in English because *ck* is never used in the initial position in words.

- *Morphological knowledge* involves the child's ability to identify base words and their inflected forms (e.g., *confess, confessor, confessional*). Inflectional morphemes are added to words, providing additional information about time (e.g., *ed, ing*) or quantity (e.g., plural *s*). Derivational morphemes, either *prefixes* (e.g., *un, re*) or *suffixes* (e.g., *tion, er*), change the word meaning or the word class (e.g., from *learn*, a verb, to *learn<u>er</u>*, a noun; Masterson & Apel, 2000).

School-Age Students: Spelling Assessments. Assessors typically begin a spelling assessment by collecting a sample of a child's spellings (Masterson & Apel, 2000). For example, a simple spelling assessment for young children consists of asking students to write the words *cat, nut, pit, mop,* and *bet.* The practitioner says a word slowly, stretching out the sounds, and then says the word normally. The student writes down the words; the practitioner gives the student a point for each letter spelled conventionally (i.e., the correct spelling) and a half point for a phonetically acceptable letter (i.e., KAT instead of CAT). There also are a number of norm-referenced spelling assessments. Examples are listed in Table 10.4.

School-Age Students: Spelling Interventions. A practitioner provides spelling intervention by focusing on a student's deficit areas: PA skills, orthographic knowledge, visual storage, or morphological skills. Deficit in phonological awareness is the most frequent cause of poor spelling; consequently, this is a frequently targeted skill for poor spellers. If, on the other hand, a student has weak orthographic knowledge, the practitioner focuses on teaching students to recognize viable and nonviable word combinations (e.g., *qu* is possible at the beginning of a word [*quick, queen, quiet*], but the letter *q* does not appear with any other vowels or in isolation in a word's initial position).

To improve visual storage skills, students practice identification of correctly spelled words from a list of foils (i.e., words that are similar to the target word but are spelled incorrectly). Finally, for students with morphological deficits, a practitioner focuses on teaching students to recognize and use frequent morphological patterns. Figure 10.8 demonstrates the clinical decision-making process used to identify the appropriate focus for a spelling intervention program.

The use of word sorts is an effective instructional strategy (Bear et al., 2007). During a word sort activity, a practitioner provides a child with a selection of written word cards demonstrating contrasting spelling patterns. For example, if the practitioner determines that the child does not demonstrate the short-vowel/long-vowel pattern, cards contain short- and long-vowel words such as *man, main; pan, pain; fin, fine; Tim, time; Sam, same.* Each card contains one word; in this example, the word sort consists of 10 cards.

To complete the word sort activity, the practitioner asks the child to sort the cards into short vowels and long vowels. A card pair can be placed out on the table to provide an example. In this example, the practitioner places two cards out and says, "This card is *man*—it has a short vowel; this card is *main*—it contains a long vowel. Now you sort out the rest of these cards into long- and short-vowel piles. I'll help you if you get stuck."

Figure 10.8   **Spelling Intervention Decision Tree**

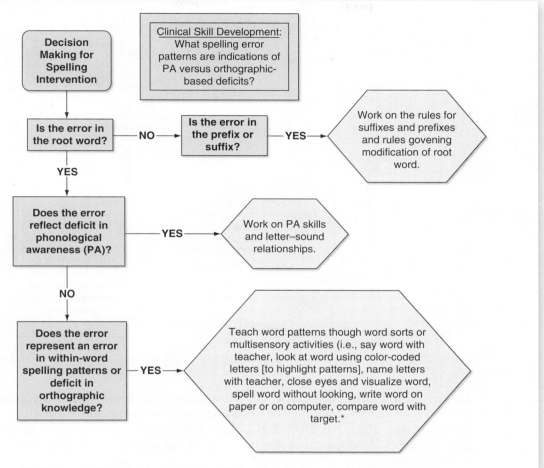

*Multisensory techniques (Beringer et al., 1998) are used to improve visual storage and othographic knowledge.
Source: Based on information from "Learning to Spell: Implications for Assessment and Intervention," by J. J. Masterson and L. A. Crede, 1999, *Language, Speech, and Hearing Services in Schools, 30,* pp. 243–254.

The practitioner supports the child's problem solving, guiding his meta-awareness of the long-vowel vs. short-vowel pattern. Figure 10.9 provides an example of an advanced word sort.

SCHOOL-AGE STUDENTS: READING COMPREHENSION

Comprehension is a complex combination of higher-level mental processes that includes thinking, reasoning, imagining, and interpreting (Kahmi, 2009). Reading comprehension becomes increasingly important as a reader moves from the early grades into high school.

Figure 10.9 Advanced Spelling Word Sort

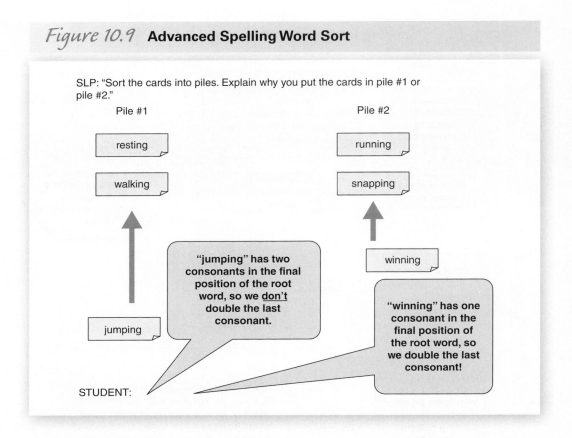

The foundation skills most closely aligned with reading comprehension are vocabulary development, narrative ability, and students' use of metastrategies during the reading process (Catts, 2009; NICHD, 2000). I have already discussed narrative performance and vocabulary development in this book; in the subsections below, I focus on reading comprehension.

School-Age Students: Reading Comprehension Assessments. To assess reading comprehension, practitioners typically have a student read text and then ask the student to answer questions about the text. McKenna and Stahl (2003) suggest asking questions at three levels of thinking: literal questions, inferential questions, and critical questions.

Literal questions require a student to recall a specific fact that is explicitly stated in the reading passage. **Inferential questions** are similar to literal questions in that they are fact based; however, the answer to an inferential question must be logically concluded from the text. For example, a practitioner may ask a student, "What do you think will happen next?" The student must use facts presented in the passage to make a prediction even though the outcome is not explicitly stated.

Critical questions draw on an individual's value system. To answer a critical question, a student must interpret factual information in keeping with his or her own morals or beliefs. The adult typically uses the word *should* when framing a critical question (e.g., "Should Mr. Scrooge have given the poor man more money?").

An SLP and a classroom teacher work together to determine whether a student meets the state's reading comprehension academic standards. As an example of reading standards from one state, consider the reading educational standards for Ohio's fourth and sixth graders. I have underlined the changes in the standards from the fourth- to sixth-grade levels:

- *Ohio Grade 4: Reading Literature.* The student can:
  - Standard Statements
    1. Refer to details and examples in a text when explaining what the text says explicitly and when drawing inferences from the text.
    2. Determine a theme of a story, drama, or poem from details in the text; summarize the text.
    3. Describe in depth a character, setting, or event in a story or drama, drawing on specific details in the text (e.g., a character's thoughts, words, or actions).
- *Ohio Grade 6 Reading Literature.* The student can:
  1. Cite <u>textual evidence to support analysis</u> of what the text says explicitly as well as inferences drawn from the text.
  2. Determine a theme or central idea of a text and how it is conveyed through particular details; <u>provide a summary of the text distinct from personal opinions or judgments</u>.
  3. Describe how a particular story's or drama's plot unfolds in a series of episodes <u>as well as how the characters respond or change as the plot moves toward a resolution</u>.

Professionals should be familiar with the student educational standards for reading comprehension along with other standards for reading and writing skills. Find out more about your state's educational standards for reading comprehension (see Focus 10.8) You will also want to understand how states are moving toward what is known as the "Common Core." Learn more about the Common Core in Focus 10.9.

FOCUS 10.8   *School-Based Issues*

Language Arts State Standards

Every SLP and educator should know how to locate the Language Arts State Standards for his or her own state. Language arts include reading, writing, and oral language at different grade levels.

Here's how I found the state standards for Wisconsin. First I typed "Language arts state standards Wisconsin" into Google. My search took me to the Wisconsin's Model Academic Standards for English Language Arts at http://dpi.wi.gov/stn_elaintro#content.

I scrolled down to the bottom on this page and saw performance standards for grades 4, 8, and 12. I chose the English Language Arts - Standard A - Performance

(continued)

Standards Grade 4 and found the following content standards:

By the end of Grade 4, students will:

A.4.1 Use effective reading strategies to achieve their purposes in reading.

- Use a variety of strategies and word recognition skills, including rereading, finding context clues, applying their knowledge of letter–sound relationships, and analyzing word structures.
- Infer the meaning of unfamiliar words in the context of a passage by examining known words, phrases and structures.
- Demonstrate phonemic awareness by using letter/sound relationships as aids to pronouncing and understanding unfamiliar words and text.

Find the content standards for your state. In class, discuss the professional's role in helping students achieve language arts standards. Consider the standards related to reading, writing, and oral language. How can an SLP write goals that will help students who are at risk target these standards? Practice writing intervention goals related to each of the relevant standards.

FOCUS 10.9   *Learning More*

The Common Core

The Common Core State Standards Initiative is a U.S. education initiative that seeks to bring diverse state curricula into alignment with each other by following the principles of standards-based education reform. This reform originated out of the "accountability movement" that began in the United States as states started to use mandatory tests of student achievement; the rationale was that students should demonstrate a common core of knowledge that all citizens should have to be successful in the workplace and that these standards should be consistent from state to state.

Standards were released for mathematics and English language arts in 2010, and a majority of states adopted the standards. States were given an incentive to adopt the Common Core Standards through competitive federal "Race to the Top" grants. With the implementation of new standards, states are also required to adopt new assessment benchmarks to measure student achievement.

The adoption of the Common Core Standards has been controversial. It has been argued that the program takes away innovation and decision making by teachers and enforces a "one-size-fits-all" curriculum that ignores cultural differences among classrooms and students. In addition, education experts have argued that the creation of Common Core Standards lacked adequate public input and was driven by corporate interests and policymakers. Critics have also said that the standards emphasize rote learning and uniformity over creativity and fail to recognize differences in learning styles, and they have said that the assessments are excessive and are not the right method for making decisions about student grade promotion, teacher job evaluation, and school closing. You can learn more about the Common Core Standards at www.corestandards.org.

School-Age Students: Reading Comprehension Metaskills Interventions. Practitioners help students improve reading comprehension strategies by explicitly teaching metaskills (Boardman et al., 2008). When working with students on comprehension metaskills, practitioners help students track comprehension by asking—and answering—literal and inferential questions. Students are taught to (a) make predictions and form questions prior to reading and (b) answer the questions as they read. This question-and-answer technique keeps students actively engaged with the reading task. When students feel confused, they learn to look up difficult words, summarize paragraph by paragraph, and modify predictions as needed.

Practitioners teach students to flexibly combine comprehension strategies. Students learn to activate prior knowledge by briefly listing what they know along with information they predict might be contained within the text. Students begin to use headers and pictures to predict the text's content. Students also look for topic sentences to determine key concepts.

Students learn to use graphic organizers and visual diagrams to organize important concepts. They use graphic organizers before reading to activate prior knowledge and refer to visual organizers to answer questions. After reading short passages, students learn to summarize the main ideas and reread, if necessary, to confirm their summarization. The goal is for students to apply strategies independently and automatically whenever they read (Boardman et al., 2008).

SCHOOL-AGE STUDENTS: WRITING

Writing involves three basic processes: (1) planning what to say and how to say it, (2) translating ideas into written form, and (3) reviewing writing to edit and improve what one has written. The first step, planning, requires the writer to set goals, generate ideas, and organize ideas into a logical pattern (Graham, 2005). Many students with language impairments or learning disabilities do not have the metaskills or executive functions to complete the needed steps for good writing. **Executive functioning** refers to the goal-oriented, purposeful behaviors that allow an individual to take a strategic approach to problem solving. Positive executive functioning includes behaviors such as inhibiting actions, attending selectively to the important information, setting goals, and planning and organizing behaviors.

A writing assessment can be criterion based or norm referenced. Norm-referenced writing assessments are listed in Table 10.4. There are several recommended approaches to criterion-referenced assessment (Espin, Weissenburger, & Benson, 2004). The first method is called *primary trait scoring*. In primary trait scoring, the adult evaluates the student's writing sample for specific traits (e.g., organization, use of topic sentences, grammar, use of cohesive devices) and compares the student's work against a grade-level standard. Typically, the assessor uses a rubric to rate each trait on a 4- or 5-point scale (e.g., 1 = unsatisfactory, 2 = minimal, 3 = satisfactory, 4 = elaborated, 5 = exceptional).

A second writing assessment approach mirrors the oral language sample analysis described in Chapter 3. This analytic approach considers quantitative features of the student's writing such as mean length of utterance, number of different words, and number of complex sentences. Analytic scoring techniques are more sensitive than primary trait scoring, but the disadvantage is that they are more time-consuming.

A final recommended approach is consistent with curriculum-based language assessment. In this approach, the assessor obtains a 3- to 5-minute writing sample in response to a curriculum topic. To analyze the writing sample, the assessor considers how well the student reflects curriculum goals in terms of vocabulary, content, sentence structure, spelling, and number of sentences written.

Writing intervention either focuses on specific foundation skills (e.g., spelling, punctuation, syntax) or targets the metaskills and executive function required for the writing process. The goal is to train students to use effective strategies as they complete writing assignments. Practitioners use a number of intervention techniques to enhance students' metaskills and executive functioning abilities:

- Students use story organizers to preplan writing tasks or summarize text. A student learns to organize story ideas or text with circles, boxes, and connecting lines. The use of story organizers facilitates brainstorming, hypothesizing, and prediction; activates prior knowledge; and heightens awareness of a story's underlying structure (Buis, 2004).
- Students learn to improve their self-editing and proofreading skills and learn to use an evaluative rubric. The use of an evaluative rubric or check sheet improves self-evaluation skills and independence.

I will be discussing more about a specific writing intervention, the writing lab approach (Nelson, Bahr, & Van Meter, 2004; Nelson & Van Meter, 2006a), in the final section of this chapter.

WORKING WITH TEACHERS

Literacy intervention for older school-age students focuses on a number of language-based academic skills. The reading and writing targets for older students center primarily on academic areas directly linked to classroom success. As you learned in Chapter 6, curriculum-based language assessment is a key component in this process. Once a student's curriculum-based language assessment is complete, the practitioner develops classroom-based interventions focusing on (a) increasing the student's underlying skills, (b) facilitating the student's meta-awareness of the processes required for successful completion of academic tasks, and (c) modifying academic tasks, instructions, or processes to increase student success.

In the best-case scenario, practitioners provide support facilitating classroom implementation of instructional strategies. I like to think of a school-based practitioner as an academic "coach" for students as well as teachers. When working with teachers, a practitioner balances coaching experiences to (a) develop teachers' content knowledge relating to language–literacy connections, (b) provide opportunities to model instructional strategies within the classroom, and (c) observe teachers implementing target strategies and provide feedback (Walpole & McKenna, 2004). The coaching should be interactive, with plenty of time for collaboration and discussion; both the practitioner and classroom teacher continuously reflect on the process. The best collaborative models are developed at a schoolwide level; the coaching is shared among all members of the educational team. The educational team includes the general education teacher, special educator, school psychologist, reading teacher, resource room specialist, SLP, and even school administrators. Expertise is shared, and responsibilities are negotiated on a case-by-case basis.

CULTURAL CONSIDERATIONS IN READING AND WRITING DEVELOPMENT FOR SCHOOL-AGE CHILDREN

As students move into later elementary, middle school, and high school grades, educators consider how a student's reading and writing is influenced by his or her culture (Ball, 2006). Experts describe a three-step process—accommodation, incorporation, and adaptation—to provide culturally sensitive education to students from nonmajority cultures (Klingner & Edwards, 2006):

- Accommodation requires practitioners to consider their students' communicative styles and home literacy practices. Practitioners should remember that home literacy, even when there is extreme poverty, is often a rich source of language and print experience.
- Incorporation requires reading/writing professionals to study community practices undervalued by schools and incorporate culturally rich literacy learning into the curriculum. It is important to build on communities' "funds of knowledge"—for example, incorporating family oral storytelling into language arts programs.
- Adaptation requires practitioners to help students and families gain access to the language and literacy culture associated with academic success. Culturally and linguistically diverse parents, parents living in poverty, and immigrant parents want to help their children succeed in school but are sometimes unsure how to work with school practitioners.

Educators sometimes overlook subtle skills affecting literacy learning for school-age children; we may assume that children know information we take for granted. For example, even a text's font conveys information. For example, certain font styles may be used in the United States in reference to Halloween or a horror movie. Italics are often used to add an air of formality, as in wedding invitations. In contrast, Times Roman font conveys an academic flavor to text (Hartley & Harris, 2001). How do you interpret the font styles in Figure 10.10? Skilled readers use cultural knowledge to assist their reading comprehension; if a student lacks cultural knowledge, he may be viewed as less intelligent or capable than he actually is.

Figure 10.10 Different Fonts Communicate Underlying Meaning

A font style might be used to look like something a teacher writes on a chalkboard; used to infer that the reader is a student in a classroom.

Italics may be used to convey a formal tone.

This Roman font is associated with academic text.

Reading and Writing Interventions for Students with Significant Levels of Impairment

Most of this chapter focuses on emergent literacy and reading and writing interventions for students who have mild-to-moderate communication impairments; the assumption is that individuals with mild-to-moderate impairments can become conventional readers but may require targeted interventions to become proficient.

Professionals also work with individuals with more significant levels of disability. While data suggest that individuals with significant levels of impairment (i.e., individuals with moderate-to-severe intellectual disability, individuals with moderate-to-severe levels of autism) may not become skilled conventional readers, experts suggest that all students should have opportunities to participate in reading and writing activities (Kaderavek & Rabidoux, 2004). When a practitioner is working with an individual with significant learning challenges, literacy goals may look different. For example, an adult with significant intellectual disability may have a literacy goal that includes supported interactive book sharing or functional writing opportunities. However, even if the activities are different, every individual should be able to participate in our society's "literacy culture." Below I describe a model of literacy intervention called the interactive-to-independent (I-to-I) model (Kaderavek & Rabidoux, 2004). The I-to-I model describes an approach to goal writing and intervention for individuals with significant learning challenges.

THE I-TO-I MODEL: OVERVIEW

The I-to-I model is based on Vygotsky's social interactionist theory, along with social participation theories (Rogoff, 2001). Social participation theory suggests that literacy is a socially constructed practice that should be accessible to all individuals, regardless of ability level. An individual's participation in literacy at any level should be valued and supported. By participating in meaningful interactive literacy experiences, many individuals gradually move toward more independent and conventional reading and writing competency.

A foundational principle of the I-to-I model is the recognition that reading and writing help the individual interact with his or her world. In order to interact with written text, individuals with significant disability are likely to need meaningful, concrete literacy experiences. With the I-to-I model, literacy is viewed as more than teaching individuals with disability to name letters, identify safety signs (e.g., STOP, EXIT, POISON), or repeatedly copy words. As an alternative to completing these rote tasks, the I-to-I model proposes that literacy activities, to be meaningful to individuals with significant disability, must center on shared interactions. The I-to-I model consists of five levels of communication partnership facilitating literacy development; each level represents a different level of social and environmental support.

I-TO-I MODEL: LEVEL I

The first level in the I-to-I model focuses on the individual's ability to maintain a joint focus of attention around a shared storybook or other literacy artifact. A literacy artifact can include family pictures, simple line drawings, or other meaningful written or graphic items (e.g., comic books, illustrations, postcard collections). An interaction with a book or other literacy artifact provides opportunities for meaningful interaction regardless of an individual's conventional reading ability. As Table 10.7 demonstrates, at Level I, the literacy goal focuses on keeping an individual with a significant level of disability increasingly engaged with the literacy artifact and encouraging back-and-forth turn-taking behavior by pointing at pictures or turning pages.

I-TO-I MODEL: LEVEL II

In Level II of the I-to-I model, a professional works toward balanced exchange during literacy interactions. Guided by social interactionist theory, the literacy partner builds on the individual's actions, vocalizations, and/or verbalizations and extends the communication elicited during the shared literacy interaction. Possible intervention goals for Level II are described in Table 10.7. A variety of literacy interactions (i.e., shared writing, looking at different types of written materials) should be included to maintain the individual's interest and engagement.

I-TO-I MODEL: LEVEL III

An individual operating within the I-to-I Model at Level I or II typically does not understand the symbolic nature of written language. Specifically, the individual may not recognize that written words represent meaning. For example, the individual does not recognize that the letters *C-A-T* represent the fuzzy animal that makes a purring sound. A Level III literacy partner begins to recognize some forms of conventional literacy; however, symbolic recognition may vary from that seen in a conventional reader.

For example, students with Down syndrome have achieved reading competency equivalent to that of fifth graders. Reading testing has confirmed, however, that many students with Down syndrome use visual recognition strategies (sight word recognition) as contrasted to a balanced strategic use of PA and visual recognition. Although sight word reading (by itself) is not a route to highly skilled conventional reading, in this case it resulted in functional reading ability. To achieve this level of reading proficiency, educators exposed children to sight words even before the children recognized all the alphabet letters (Layton, 2000).

A professional knows that a Level III student may recognize increasingly symbolic forms, such as icons, pictures, or sight words. Table 10.7 provides goals to build symbol use at this intermediate level. Typically at this stage, students require extended practice sessions and daily opportunities to use symbolic forms in real-life interactions.

I-TO-I MODEL: LEVEL IV

At Level IV, children perform conventionally literate tasks when supported by others, but their reading and writing abilities vary according to their strengths and weaknesses. For example, some children with autism demonstrate hyperlexia. As you recall, hyperlexia is the precocious ability to recognize written words significantly above an individual's language or cognitive skill level, often with minimal comprehension of the written text. In Chapter 9, I mentioned a young preschooler with hyperlexia; the preschooler had minimal ability to communicate with others day to day but could read aloud from the phonebook for extended periods (Kaderavek & Rabidoux, 2004). A professional worked with the preschooler by facilitating interactive and meaningful communication, focusing on illustrations in the phonebook's advertising section.

Students with strengths in sight word reading can be taught to recognize sight words by labeling everyday objects and attaching the written word to specific pictures or icons (Broun & Oelwein, 2007). Through repeated associations between pictures and written words, the sight words repertoire increases. Eventually, the professional encourages the Level IV reader to read beginning-level primer texts or read adult-made books containing familiar sight words. As reading new sight words becomes meaningful and motivating, adults work "backward" to teach concepts of individual letters and sounds from the known words (Broun & Oelwein, 2007). The range of literacy goals potentially targeted at the Level IV level is shown in Table 10.7.

I-TO-I MODEL: LEVEL V

A Level V reader can read conventionally but requires ongoing and varying levels of support to maintain reading and writing practices. For example, some individuals with intellectual disability may demonstrate more reading comprehension when they read aloud to others than when they read silently alone. Writing skills must be continually supported during everyday tasks. Remember that an individual with significant disabilities may vary in his or her literacy ability, depending on task familiarity and environmental support. For example, an individual may be able to read a daily schedule once it is familiar but may need additional support when new items are added to the schedule. Potential goals for a Level V reader and writer are shown in Table 10.7.

Table 10.7 **Interactive-to-Independent (I-to-I) Model of Literacy**

Level of the model	Associated literacy goals
Level I: Attention and responsiveness during literacy interactions	a. Student maintains attention to a literacy artifact and the literacy partner for _____ minutes.
	b. Student decreases off-task behaviors to no more than one per minute during a _____-minute storybook interaction.
	c. Student directs gaze at pictures, turns pages, and interactively manipulates flaps in a lift-the-flap book for _____ minutes.
	d. Student takes turns (using physical actions such as turning pages or pointing) during a shared storybook interaction _____ times during a _____-minute storybook interaction.
	e. Student uses emergent writing to tell a story or share an experience.
Level II: Balance and turn taking in literacy interactions	a. Student interacts with verbal, gestural, or signed communication within a shared literacy interaction.
	b. Student initiates communication during a literacy interaction.
	c. Student demonstrates a range of pragmatic communication skills (describing, requesting, responding, topic initiation and maintenance, etc.) during a literacy interaction.

Level of the model	Associated literacy goals
Level III: Symbolic understanding of written forms	a. Student uses sight words within the school or home setting in functional ways (recognizes own name, follows signs, picks out his own videos, etc.)
	b. Student matches representational symbols (line drawings) to real objects within a communication exchange. Student uses symbols to communicate needs in functional ways (e.g., pick a lunch menu).
	c. Student engages in communicative exchange in literacy interactions containing meaningful pictures and written words.
	d. Student identifies written words with pictures within a communicative literacy exchange (i.e., *not* rote picture-to-word drill).
Level IV: Conventional literacy supported by social interactions	a. Student uses familiar sight words to create novel sentences within a supported communication exchange.
	b. Student explains what was read to a naïve listener with support from the communication partner.
	c. Student dictates words to a communication partner to make a list of daily activities.
	d. Student writes notes to herself or himself as reminders about daily chores or activities with support.
	e. Student and communication partner create a scrapbook of favorite written materials (e.g., comic strips, TV guide, sports page) and add to it on a regular basis.
	f. Student and communication partner interactively read _____ new texts per week.
	g. Student and communication partner maintain a collaborative written diary illustrated with pictures of the student's activities.
Level V: Conventional literacy at independent level	Conventional literacy activities are introduced, with continued emphasis on social and interactive literacy use and function.

Source: Adapted from *Interactive to Independent Literacy: A Model for Designing Literacy Goals for Children with Atypical Communication* by J. N. Kaderavek and P. Rabidoux, 2004, Reading and Writing Quarterly, 20, pp. 237–260. Copyright © 2004 by Taylor & Francis Group LLC.

Intervention for Students with Reading and Writing Disability: Evidence-Based Practices

There are many different reading and writing programs for students with literacy learning deficits. I present two different programs below. I chose these programs because they were developed by SLPs and have documented efficacy. My goal is to show how a strong intervention has both a clear theoretical foundation and research documenting effectiveness.

EXPLICIT PHONOLOGICAL AWARENESS INTERVENTION

The explicit phonological awareness intervention (EPAI; Gillon, 2000) is based on several theoretical approaches that should be familiar to you. First, the approach is teacher directed and skill based rather than activity based. Thus, it reflects aspects of behaviorist theory; it is an approach that breaks down the complex behavior of reading by focusing on an individual component of the reading process.

EPAI, however, also draws from social interactionist theory in that the approach engages children in a complex task with the support of a more sophisticated partner. Shared participation in PA activities helps children discover the alphabetic principle.

The EPAI approach targets PA at the phoneme level rather than the word or syllable level. Gillon (2004) states that awareness at the word and syllable levels frequently develops from classroom-based activities. Classroom-based PA activities include rhyming games and clapping syllables. Although children should participate in activities at this level, for many children, implicit learning activities will not be sufficient. Children who are at risk for reading problems usually require more intensive and explicit instruction at the phoneme level to develop needed PA ability.

Gillon (2000) demonstrated the effectiveness of EPAI in a group of 23 children between the ages of 5 and 7 years. All the children had expressive phonological impairments (i.e., difficulty producing speech sounds). EPAI was implemented individually 2 hours per week; each child received 20 hours of intervention. Activities included letter–sound knowledge at the phoneme level, including phoneme identification, phoneme blending, phoneme segmentation, and tracking of sound changes in words.

Two examples of phoneme-level teaching techniques similar to those in the EPAI intervention are demonstrated in Table 10.8. Examples of intervention goals compatible with EPAI are provided in Figure 10.11.

Evidence Supporting the EPAI Approach. Gillon (2000) compared the pre- and post-intervention abilities of the 23 children receiving EPAI intervention with two comparison groups. A second cohort of 23 children also received 20 hours of intervention, but their treatment focused on oral speech production and expressive language abilities. A third group of 15 children did not receive treatment due to their inability to access treatment. This last group served as a no-treatment control group.

At the end of the 20-week intervention, the children in the EPAI group demonstrated significantly better ability to decode nonsense words than did the children in the other two groups. Importantly, the children in the EPAI group also showed better word recognition, reading accuracy, and reading comprehension. A follow-up assessment 11 months after the intervention indicated that PA, speech production, reading, and spelling development continued for the children in the EPAI group. The children in the other two groups made little or no reading progress (Gillon, 2002). These data demonstrate the effectiveness of

Table 10.8 **Example of Phonological Awareness Training Sequences**

Phonological awareness task	Activity	High- and low-support cues*
Recognition of initial sound in words	Show students a "mystery bag." Say, "We are going to guess whose picture is in the bag. I will give you some clues. The first clue is that the word starts with the /f/ sound. The next clue is that we just read about this animal. Sometimes this animal gets into the chicken coop. Can anyone guess what picture is in the bag?" 1st Child: "*Chicken!*" Adult: "*Good thinking, but let's listen to the first sound in that word: /tʃ/, /tʃ/, /tʃ/. We don't hear the /f/ sound in that one, do we?*" 2nd Child: "/f/ /f/ /f/" Adult: "*Good, you are thinking about that /f/ sound. The word starts with /f/.*"	• High support: "Let's listen to this word: *cow*. Do you hear the /f/ sound? No, you are right, there is not an /f/ sound in *cow*. It isn't a picture of a cow, is it? Listen to this word: *fox*. Do you hear the /f/ sound? You are right, there is an /f/ sound, and look—here is a picture of a fox in my bag!" • Low support: "Let me tell you the word slowly and see if you can guess: F-O-X. Does anyone know the word? Good, let's listen for the /f/ sound."
Onset-rime	Show children a picture and say, "Let's play 'I spy.' I will say a word in a funny way and you guess what I am looking at in the picture. I spy: *s-un*."	• High support: "Do you think I am looking at the sun or the moon? Listen: *s-un*." • Low support: "The first part of the word is /s/. Does anyone see a picture on this page that starts with /s/?"

*High support is provided when a child is learning the PA task; low support is provided as a child becomes more proficient in the PA task.

Figure 10.11 **Examples of Goals for Phonological Awareness Intervention**

Goal 1   Kirby will blend onset-rime words with picture cues. Kirby will correctly choose a target word from three pictures when given mild support four out of five times on 3 consecutive days. Mild support includes (a) up to three repetitions of a target word and/or (b) saying each of the pictured words with a prolonged initial sound.

Goal 2   Janice will identify the word that does *not* start with the target sound ("odd man out") four out of five times on 3 consecutive days given four words. The words will be no longer than three phonemes each, and the "odd man out" word will be dissimilar in manner and place of articulation (e.g., *man, mouse, car, mom*).

Source: Based on information from "Phonological Awareness Intervention: A Preventative Framework for Preschool Children with Specific Speech and Language Impairments," by G. T. Gillon, 2006. In R. J. McCauley and M. E. Fey (Eds.), *Treatment of Language Disorders in Children* (pp. 279–308). Baltimore, MD: Brookes.

PA intervention and underscore the connection between PA and reading ability. The use of a control group, but without randomization, places the level of evidence for EPAI at Level II.

WRITING LAB APPROACH

The writing lab (WL) approach focuses on improving students' writing processes and their oral language communication skills with computer support (Nelson et al., 2004; Nelson & Van Meter, 2006b). The term *writing process* describes the sequence of writing activities used by effective writers: topic selection, planning, organizing, drafting, revising, editing, publishing, and presenting. In the WL approach, SLPs work with general education teachers to facilitate students' meta-ability during the writing process and oral presentations. Students use computer software in many different ways during the writing and presentation sequence. Examples of software programs are shown in Table 10.9. Because WL targets a student's oral and written language skills, it is considered a cross-modality or multi-modality intervention approach.

Students' writing projects during the writing lab intervention are designed to be authentic; the goal is to have students work on a personally meaningful project that ultimately will be shared with an audience. Throughout the writing sequence, students use small-group interaction, peer and teacher conferencing, rubrics, check sheets or organizers, and computer software to plan, revise, and edit their papers. Each writing cycle is complete when the student orally presents his or her project to the group.

The WL approach is a top-down model. Students attempt to produce a high-quality project that communicates their ideas. Thus, students focus on a meaningful activity. As students revise and edit their papers, they focus on language subcomponents such as spelling, syntax, morphology, vocabulary, and story organization. Students are encouraged to use a recursive writing process; they write, share their writing, obtain feedback, and continue to revise and edit until they have a high-quality writing sample. Students practice oral communication skills in their small-group and one-on-one feedback sessions and during their final oral presentation. Students self-evaluate and receive teacher and SLP feedback on their oral and written communication. The goal is to have students cycle between the "top" (i.e., the written product and oral presentation) and the "bottom" (i.e., language subskills needed for an effective product).

The WL approach draws from social interactionist theory as an underlying principle; social interactionist principles are emphasized by the use of small groups and collaborative partnerships to facilitate students' oral and written communication. In addition, the WL approach reflects a second theoretical approach: information processing/connectionism theory. Information processing and connectionism theories suggest that language processing is interconnected and requires activation of areas of the brain responsible for specific language components (i.e., phonological, semantic, syntax). The assessment protocols associated with WL are naturalistic assessments, specifically curriculum-based language assessment (see Chapter 6 to review naturalistic/curriculum-based assessments and Focus 10.2 in this chapter).

The optimal schedule for the WL approach is a 1-hour session scheduled to occur in the general education classroom two or three times per week. Writing projects connect to ongoing classroom instruction, potentially including topics related to language arts, social studies, or science. An SLP and a teacher present mini-lessons that last no more than 10 or 15 minutes. A mini lesson introduces an aspect of the writing process such as (a) using brainstorming to find a topic; (b) using the computer thesaurus, spell check, or grammar

Table 10.9   **Software Examples Used in the Writing Lab Approach**

Writing skills	Processes supported	Software programs

Planning and organizing	• Organizing
	• Outlining
	  • Brainstorming
	• Illustrating
	
	• Drafting
	• Collaborating
		• Creative Writer 2 (Microsoft)
		• Microsoft Office (Microsoft);
		  AppleWorks for K–8 (Apple)
		• KidWorks Deluxe (Knowledge
		  Adventure)
		• ACDSee (ACD Systems)
		• Kidspiration 3 (Inspiration
		  Software)
		  • Google Docs and
		    Spreadsheets (Google)
		  • Pixie 3 (Tech4Learning)

Revising and editing	• Grammar, spelling, thesaurus,
	  editing
	• Rhyming
		• Microsoft Office (Microsoft);
		  AppleWorks for K–8 (Apple)
		• Storybook Weaver Deluxe
		  (The Learning Company)
		• The Amazing Writing
		  Machine (Riverdeep)
		• Stationery Studio (Fablevision)
		  • Ryme Genie (Freeware:
		    http://rhyme-genie
		    .en.softonic.com)

Desktop publishing	• Merge text and graphics
	• Add drawing and painting
	  tools
	• Modify text, margins, borders,
	  etc.
	• Create tables
		• KidWorks Deluxe
		  (Knowledge Adventure)
		  • Tux Paint (freeware; www
		    .educational-freeware.com)
		• HyperStudio (Software
		  MacKiev)
		• Kids Media Magic (Sunburst)
		• The Print Shop (Broderbund)

Sources: Based on information from *The Writing Lab Approach to Language Instruction and Intervention,* by N. W. Nelson, C. M. Bahr, and A. M. Van Meter, 2004, Baltimore, MD: Brookes; and 2013 Educational Software Review Rewards, retrieved from http://computedgazette.com/page3.html.

check; or (c) methods of story organization. Students spend the next part of the session writing on their own, conferencing with peers and teachers, and revising and editing work in progress.

Students develop author notebooks to organize materials and to maintain organizers to develop metaskills. Some students benefit from keeping word lists of confusing or difficult vocabulary (e.g., coordinating conjunctions, frequently misspelled words). To increase independence, students are encouraged to refer to their notebooks frequently. Completed projects are presented when the student takes the "author chair." Listeners provide feedback and ask questions. A teaching sequence is demonstrated in Figure 10.12. Intervention goals compatible with the WL approach are presented in Figure 10.13.

Figure 10.12 **Example of a Writing Lab Intervention Sequence**

Steps to Teach Student to Self-Evaluate Spelling and Punctuation

Spelling goal: Identification and consistent spelling of prefix words

- The student and adult are conferencing with regard to the student's writing project.

  Adult: *"What spelling rules have you been working on? Can you go through your paper and circle any of the words that we might need to take a look at?"*
  Student: *"I have been working on recognizing prefixes."*
  Adult: *"Can you give me some examples of prefixes?"*
  Student: *"Well, I have a list in my notebook. Like auto, and de, and com."*
  Adult: *"Exactly. Why don't you go through your paper and circle any prefix words and make sure you have spelled them all correctly. I'll come back in a few minutes and see how you are getting along."*

Punctuation goal: Correct use of quotation marks to indicate dialogue

- Two middle-school students (Josh and Sandra) are working together on a script for a short play to be presented to elementary school students. One of Josh's writing goals is to correctly use quotation marks to indicate dialogue.

  Adult: *"What do we call it when two people are talking to each other in a play?"*
  Josh: *"Dialogue."*
  Sandra: *"Like here, where they are talking."*
  Adult: *"Josh, can you explain to Sandra how we use punctuation in dialogue?"*
  Josh: *"We use quotes."*
  Adult: *"Sandy, do you understand how to show dialogue yet?"*
  Sandra: *"No."*
  Adult: (Supports Josh in his explanation of the use of quotation marks for dialogue. Students work together to use correct punctuation in their play with adult support.)

Figure 10.13 **Examples of Goals for Writing Lab Intervention**

Goal 1: Oral communication	During author group Sabrina will (a) maintain appropriate eye contact with her group members, (b) provide the peer author with one suggestion to improve his or her work, and (c) provide one positive comment to the author.
Goal 2: Text comprehension	Prior to reading an assignment, Caleb will (a) identify the headings and subheadings in the text and (b) summarize to his group members his ideas of what the article is about. While reading, Caleb will write down key words or sentences to use for his article summary.

Source: Based on information from *The Writing Lab Approach to Language Instruction and Intervention,* by N. W. Nelson, C. M. Bahr, and A. M. Van Meter, 2004, Baltimore, MD: Brookes.

Evidence Supporting the Writing Lab Approach. Nelson and her colleagues (2006) use a number of different measures to document students' improvement in written language. Some of the measures include (a) a word production fluency measure recording the number of words a student writes independently in a 1-hour written probe, (b) analysis of micro- and macrostructure features of oral and written narratives, (c) documentation of the number and type of conjunctions, (d) a count of the number of syntactically correct and incorrect sentences, and (e) computation of the percentage of words spelled correctly.

In one study, Nelson and colleagues (2004) implemented the WL approach with 53 third-grade students from three different classrooms. The students participated in WL 3 days a week—2 days in their classroom and 1 day in the school's computer lab. Students were from an inner-city school and included children at risk due to economic disadvantage, special educational status, or nonmajority cultural or racial status.

Assessors completed data probes at three points during the year. Figure 10.14 visually demonstrates the development in narrative story structure (i.e., macrostructure) for four groups of children. All students, regardless of special education status, demonstrated significant growth. Effect size for narrative development and the measure of word production fluency was large (Nelson & Van Meter, 2007). There was growth but not at the same high level in the other literacy measures. Because this study did not include a control group, the data reflect Level II evidence.

Figure 10.14　**Data Demonstrating Change in Narrative Ability during a Year of Writing Lab Intervention**

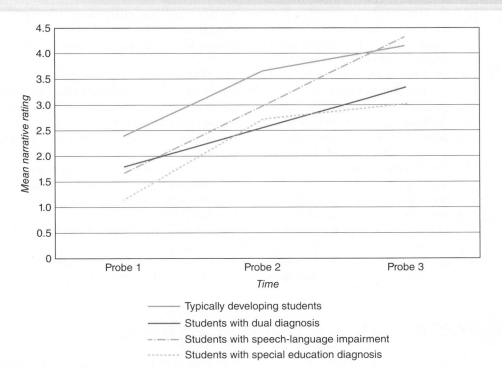

Source: From *The Writing Lab Approach to Language Instruction and Intervention* (p. 467), by N. W. Nelson, C. M. Bahr, and A. M. Van Meter, 2004, Baltimore, MD: Paul H. Brookes Publishing Co., Inc. Reprinted with permission.

Summary

- The American Speech-Language-Hearing Association (ASHA) strongly advocates that speech-language pathologists (SLPs) and special educators indirectly and directly incorporate reading and writing interventions into treatment programs. A preventive model of intervention is used with young children in keeping with the response to intervention approach.
- The most important emergent literacy targets include phonological awareness, print and alphabetic concepts, oral language skills, and early writing skills. Phonological awareness progresses from word- and syllable-level awareness to awareness of individual phonemes. With awareness at the phoneme level, a child learns to blend and segment words. Print referencing is an explicit teaching technique that facilitates children's development of print and alphabetic concepts. Early writing skills support children's literacy growth.
- The embedded-explicit model of early literacy intervention encourages SLPs to assist teachers in embedding literacy targets in child-directed and engaging classroom activities. SLPs and teachers provide regular explicit, adult-directed literacy activities in individual or small-group sessions to children who need increased learning opportunities.
- Foundational reading skills for school-age students include phonological awareness, reading comprehension, and reading fluency; these domains reflect a skill-based approach to reading development. Research indicates that professionals can improve students' reading comprehension through vocabulary building and by helping students learn comprehension metaskills. Spelling assessment and intervention include analyses of children's phonological awareness, visual storage, orthographic knowledge, and morphological knowledge. Word sorts are an effective intervention approach to improve spelling ability.
- Oral narrative development is an important language skill related to reading and writing development. Children develop both macro- and microstructure narrative features. Macrostructure includes story grammar; a mature narrative demonstrates thematic episode structure and contains an initiating event, an attempt, and a consequence. Microstructure includes literate language features that provide decontextualization, cohesion, and descriptive storytelling.
- The interactive-to-independent model of literacy intervention targets the individual with significant learning challenges. The model moves from highly interactive, shared literacy experiences (Levels I and II) to increasingly independent reading and writing with varying levels of adult support (Levels III–V).
- Two intervention programs are Gillon's phonological awareness intervention and Nelson's writing lab approach. The PA intervention provides explicit instruction in gamelike activities to enhance PA skills in young children. The writing lab approach uses the writing process to enhance the oral and written communication skills of older school-age children.

Discussion and In-Class Activities

1. In small groups, you will be assigned an emergent literacy domain (e.g., phonological awareness, print concepts, alphabetic concepts, oral language, writing) and a classroom theme (e.g., community helpers, seasons, farm and zoo animals, insects, rivers/lakes/streams, plants/flowers, healthy food, our bodies, machines). Develop three

different learning opportunities exemplifying your domain. At least one should be an explicit instructional activity, and one should be an embedded instructional activity. Each activity should use vocabulary, pictures, and activities that further the classroom theme. Consider how each activity could be modified for a child who struggles to perform this particular skill, and describe how the activity could be made more challenging for a child who has advanced skills.

2. Role-play an adult–student interaction using Elkonian boxes. Start with four boxes and colored blocks or chips. Give instructions for the following:

   - A CVC stimulus word (as in *bed*)
   - A stimulus word in which the client must change the initial or final consonant (e.g., *Ted* or *bet*)
   - A stimulus word in which the vowel is changed (e.g., *Tod*, *beat*).
   - A stimulus word in which a consonant is added to make a consonant blend (e.g., *bleat*).

   Make sure the adult gives appropriate feedback and reinforces the student's demonstration of sound modifications. Try it with different words; have the student leave the chips in place and add or delete chips to demonstrate how the sounds in the words change.

   Discuss in class the student skills required to complete this task. How could letters be used in this task instead of chips or blocks? When should letters be introduced? At what age would this type of activity be most useful? How could this activity be used to develop spelling ability?

3. Develop a word sort activity to teach a spelling rule. You can research spelling rules on the Internet. A good website is www.grammaruntied.com/spelling1.html.

4. Record or transcribe a story. Say to a friend or young child, "Tell me a made-up story; tell me the best story you can." What narrative features were demonstrated in the oral narrative? What features were omitted? Do you think the story was a good one? Why or why not?

5. Examine elementary textbooks (e.g., science, geography, language arts) for different grade levels. Develop strategies that might be used to increase a student's reading comprehension. Role-play with a student, with one of you taking the role of the professional and the other taking the role of the elementary-age child.

6. Use Figure 10.6 to help complete a macrostructure analysis of the narratives below. You should also consider microstructure features, including the children's use of cohesion devices, dialogic speech, and syntax. A helpful microstructure protocol is described in the article "A Scalable Tool for Assessing Children's Language Abilities within the Narrative Context: The NAP (Narrative Assessment Protocol)" (Justice et al., 2010). Download this article from your campus library, and use the NAP short form to score the following five narratives:

Kindergartener: Late for school	Second-grader: Aliens in the park
C: He got out of bed.	C: One day there was a boy and a girl playing tag in the park.
C: He spilled the milk on the table.	C: The boy was it.
C: And he got his shoes on.	C: And the girl was running from him.
C: And he ran to the bus.	C: Just then an alien spaceship landed on the Earth.
C: And then he went in school.	C: An alien family came out and talked a language they did not know.

C: After about a week, the aliens decided to go back home.
C: The girl wanted to touch them.
C: But the boy wouldn't let her.
C: When they left, they forgot their pets.
C: So the next day, they came back and took their pet with them.
C: Then they flew off into space again.
C: And lived happily ever after on their own planet.

Second-grader: Going to McDonald's	**Third-grader: Late for school**
C: As soon as Raymond and the little girl got home from school their mother said, "We're going to eat out tonight." C: "Where do you want to eat?" C: And the both of the children yelled out "McDonalds." C: So they hopped in the car. C: And their mother drove them to McDonalds. C: The girl couldn't make up her mind. C: Mother and Raymond knew what they wanted. C: The mother said, "I will have a salad with a drink." C: Raymond said, "I am going to have a hamburger with fries and a vanilla milkshake." C: The girl finally made up her mind. C: She said, "I want a hamburger with ketchup and a chocolate ice cream cone." C: Then the clerk said, "Will that be all?" C: They said, "Yes." C: And he said, "It will be twelve fifty." C: When the mother reached for her purse it wasn't there. A: Anything else? C: Um, no.	C: One day Mike was sleeping in bed. C: At seven thirty he woke up and looked at his clock. C: "Uh oh" he thought. C: He was late. C: He went downstairs and poured his milk for his cereal and made a big mess because he was looking at the clock. C: After he ate he went to his room and got dressed. C: Then he went downstairs and started tying his shoes C: But one of the laces broke. C: "Mmm," he thought. C: Finally he got his shoes tied and got his packed bookbag, and went and ran to the bus stop. C: But the bus was already leaving. C: "Oh no," he thought. C: So instead of riding the bus, he started running to school so he wouldn't be late. C: When he got there his teacher was standing outside the door and said that he was late.

Fifth-grader: Aliens in the park

C: A boy and a girl named Michael and Julie were walking on a path. C: They were trying to find a picnic table to eat their lunch. C: But they saw some smoke. C: And they didn't know what it was. C: So they went over to it. C: And it was a spaceship. C: And aliens started getting off.	C: And Julie thought it was kind of cool. C: So she grabbed Michael's hand. C: And she was going to go see them. C: But then they heard a lot of screeching noise. C: And they didn't know what it was. C: So they ran home and told their parents what they had found. C: And they tried to get back but something was in the way.

C: They were kind of scared.

C: But Michael almost ran.

C: But Julie grabbed his hand.

C: Michael wanted to go.

C: But Julie wanted to stay and see the aliens.

C: And so they couldn't go.

C: And their parents didn't believe them.

C: So they never saw the aliens again

Note: The transcripts were slightly modified in that word repetitions and fillers (e.g., *um*) were removed for purposes of this narrative assessment activity. C = Child, A = Adult.

7. Write three additional intervention goals consistent with Gillon's phonological awareness treatment. Then write goals for social communication skill, proofreading, brainstorming, and organizational strategy development for a student using the writing lab approach.

8. View a videotape of preschool children during adult–child book reading. Complete the early literacy observational checklist (Figure 10.1) together in class. What additional activities would you like to see in order to assess additional literacy skills? Develop a list of activities to elicit additional emergent literacy skills. As an outside assignment, you can audiotape or videotape interactions with a preschooler and document the child's ability using the observational form.

Chapter 10 Case Study

Ziquon is a third-grader whose oral reading is labored; he often guesses at the word from the first letter. He struggles when he reaches an unfamiliar word. His written work and spelling are poor. Spelling errors noted include PELN (for *plane*), BUP (for *bump*), and SESRT (for *sister*). However, Ziquon knows some sight words and pronounces these immediately and correctly (McKenna & Stahl, 2003).

Questions for Discussion

1. What assessments would you recommend for Ziquon?
2. What reading subskills do you think may be most impaired? Why?
3. Consider Ziquon's spelling errors. What evidence do they provide?
4. Describe an intervention program for Ziquon. What are primary targets for instruction?

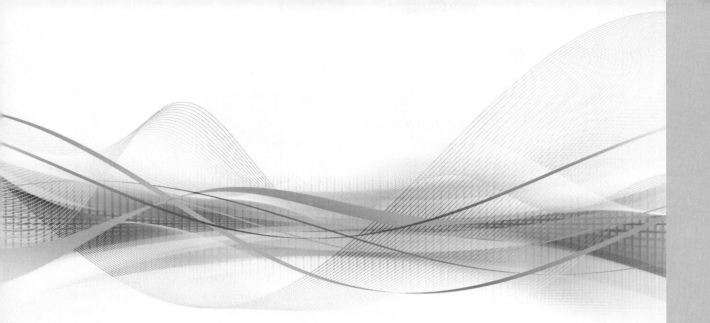

11

Augmentative and Alternative Communication (AAC) and Children with Language Disorders

—Julia M. King

Chapter Overview Questions

1. What is an augmentative/alternative communication (AAC) intervention approach?
2. What are the components of an AAC system?
3. What is *not* considered AAC?
4. What should be included in an assessment of language and communication for a potential AAC user?
5. What are some examples of using AAC as a part of language treatment?
6. What are the multicultural implications when working with families from nonmajority cultures and making a decision about including AAC in a language intervention program?

FOCUS 11.1 *Learning More*

Children with Physical Impairments

Children with physical impairments some-times have CCNs. You will learn more about how to support communication with

individuals with physical impairments in other coursework or textbooks on AAC. Cerebral palsy is a common cause of phys-ical impairments in children.

Individuals with language disorders, either receptive or expressive, may have **complex communication needs (CCNs)**. Many developmental disabilities such as Down syndrome, autism, and cerebral palsy are associated with communication impairments. People who have a communication impairment affecting daily communication are said to have CCNs. For children, CCNs can occur when there is difficulty with processing, comprehending, or producing language, resulting in unmet communication needs. For example, a young child understands his parent when asked what game he wants to play but has difficulty formu-lating his response because he does not know the name of the game or how to describe it. When semantic, syntactic, morphologic, phonologic, or pragmatic impairments impact the success of a child's communication, unmet communication needs prevent successful exchanges. An intervention approach used to address language development and commu-nication needs is an **augmentative/alternative communication (AAC) approach**. An AAC intervention approach compensates and facilitates, either temporarily or permanently, for the impairment and disability patterns of individuals with expressive and/or language comprehension impairments. AAC strategies and techniques may support language learn-ing for children with impairments in gestural, spoken, and/or written language modalities.

An AAC intervention approach can benefit children with language impairments as well as those with speech impairments, intellectual disability, or physical impairments (see Focus 11.1). In this chapter, I focus on aspects of AAC that support and enhance language development in children with CCNs. At the end of this chapter, I include a *Connections* section in which I discuss the multicultural issues that should be considered when work-ing with an individual from a nonmajority culture.

Background and Description

AAC refers to an area of clinical and educational practice, as well as an area of research (ASHA, 2005b). An AAC approach to assessment and treatment addresses temporary or permanent impairments, activity limitations, and participation restrictions of individuals with CCNs. CCNs may stem from language comprehension and production impairments in spoken and written language (ASHA, 2004d). Language impairments may affect the quality and frequency of an individual's communication participation in the activities of daily living. See Focus 11.2 for the WHO-ICF model, which describes activity limitations and participation restrictions.

AAC SYSTEM

Recall the aspects of language form, content, and use presented in Chapter 1. The domains of form, content, and use also are relevant for an AAC system. An AAC system includes rules for combining symbols to create a maximally intelligible and comprehensible

FOCUS 11.2   *Activity and Participation Issues*

World Health Organization

The World Health Organization (WHO) developed a framework to provide a standard language to describe health-related states (WHO, 2002). This framework is called the International Classification of Functioning, Disability, and Health (ICF). Although language impairments may not be considered health-related conditions, such impairment could affect a child's ability to use language in various communication activities and participate in life activities. The ICF framework defines *activity* as the execution of a task or action by an individual, and it defines his or her participation as involvement in life situations. The WHO framework focuses on documenting real-life changes in an individual's ability to communicate.

(i.e., understandable) message for the broadest audience of communication partners (i.e., form). It also relies on conventions relative to the selection and organization of vocabulary and communication messages (i.e., content). Finally, AAC systems are designed to maximize language use so that the individual communicates effectively and efficiently with as many people, and in as many activities, as possible (i.e., use). An AAC system is part of an AAC intervention approach. See the AAC System Components section later in this chapter for more information related to systems.

MULTI-MODAL COMMUNICATION

An AAC system is part of a multi-modal view of communication. **Multi-modal** refers to the use of multiple modalities when a person communicates (e.g., gestures, speech, facial expressions, writing, drawing, AAC system). How often do you use gestures or facial expressions to convey a message? Have you used a code when text messaging to represent words (e.g., *lol* for "laugh out loud")?

Children often use multiple modes of communication as they develop, even before they produce speech (e.g., crying, cooing, gazing, pointing). The use of pointing with voicing for a young child is very effective. For example, imagine that a child drops a cracker from her high chair, points to the cracker on the floor, and then vocalizes. It is likely that the communication partner will understand this action and vocalization as (a) a request to pick up the cracker or (b) a comment that the cracker is on the floor. We all use multiple modes of communication on a regular basis, sometimes simultaneously and sometimes one mode at a time. AAC systems offer modes of communication for children who require support for their language development and communication needs.

AAC System Components

AAC systems are comprised of four critical components: symbols, aids, strategies, and techniques (ASHA, 2004d, 2005b).

AAC SYMBOLS

Symbols can be graphic, auditory, gestural, textured, or tactile representations used to represent language concepts in AAC systems. Figure 11.1 shows examples of different symbols representing the same concept. An individual can use many different symbols

Figure 11.1 **Different Types of Symbols Representing the Same Language Concept/Communicative Message: "Hello"**

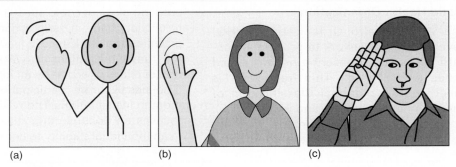

(a) (b) (c)

Sources: (a) Line drawing, Picture Communication Symbols (© 1981–2009 DynaVox Mayer-Johnson) used with permission. All rights reserved worldwide. (b) Line drawing, Picture Communication Symbols (© 1981–2009 DynaVox Mayer-Johnson) used with permission. All rights reserved worldwide. (c) From Signing Illustrated by Mickey Flodin, copyright © 1994 by Mickey Flodin. Used by permission of Perigee Books, an imprint of Penguin Group(USA) LLC.

to communicate. For example, a young child may use the manual sign for *hello* when he greets a friend on the bus. In other situations, he may point to a drawing representing *hello* to greet someone. The manual sign and the drawing are both examples of symbols. The first is an example of an **unaided symbol** because the child does not need any prosthetic (or external) support to convey his message. The second example demonstrates the use of an **aided symbol** because the child uses a support (i.e., drawing) to convey his message. For a more extensive summary of symbol types, see *Augmentative and Alternative Communication* by Beukelman and Mirenda (2013).

AAC AIDS

The second component of an AAC system is an aid. An **AAC aid** is a device that can be used to send or receive messages. The aid can be nonelectronic, such as a series of photographs, a collection of objects, or a series of black or color line drawings. Examples of nonelectronic aids are shown in Figure 11.2. Nonelectronic aids are also referred to as low, or light, technology.

Alternatively, an aid can be electronic and refer to simple devices such as talking photo albums or complex devices such as speech-generating devices (SGDs), as shown in Figure 11.3.

Electronic aids are referred to as high technology. Many AAC systems have both low- and high-technology components. An illustration of a child interacting with his language facilitator with an AAC system is shown in Figure 11.4.

People are also using everyday technology as AAC aids. For example, digital cameras, smartphones, and tablet computers are common types of technology that many people use on a daily basis. Using this technology for language learning and for communicative purposes is occurring with increased frequency in homes, classrooms, and

Figure 11.2 **Examples of Nonelectronic AAC Aids**

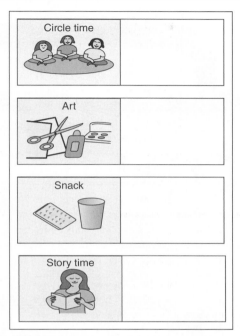

(a) Schedule board with line drawings.

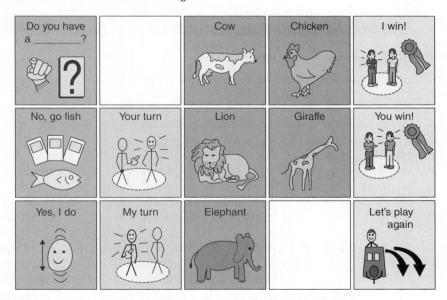

(b) Static paper communication display board with line drawings.

Sources: (a) Courtesy of Picture Communication Symbols from Mayer-Johnson Boardmaker; and (b) The Picture Communication Symbols © 1981–2009 by Dynavox Mayer-Johnson LLC. All rights reserved Worldwide. Used with permission.

Figure 11.3 **An Example of an Electronic AAC Aid**

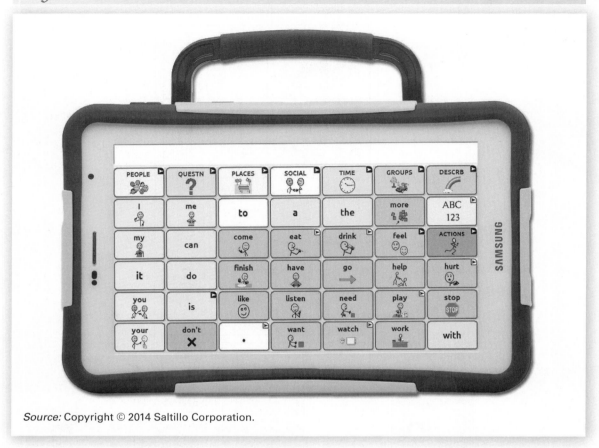

Source: Copyright © 2014 Saltillo Corporation.

therapy sessions. Vocabulary and communicative messages are represented with digital images captured with a camera (whether the camera is used independently or as part of a smartphone or tablet computer). These images can be imported into AAC aids for use as symbols or visual scene displays (VSDs). (See the Intervention section for more information on VSDs.) A group of researchers from Penn State is studying how just-in-time (JIT) programming can use digital images to represent new vocabulary and experiences (Light, 2012). For more information about JIT programming, read Focus 11.3.

Apps are also being used as AAC aids. Some apps are designed to support language and literacy development, supplement difficult-to-understand speech, and/or enhance communication skills. Unfortunately, because of the significantly lower cost of apps and everyday technology compared to dedicated SGDs, some parents and caregivers have been purchasing the former type of technology prior to participating in an assessment to determine which technology best matches the needs of their child. With any intervention strategy, technique, or tool, including apps, it takes training and experience to select the appropriate one. Learn more about some of the problems associated with caregiver-selected apps for individuals with CCN in Focus 11.4.

Figure 11.4   **Child Using His SGD (AAC Aid) When Interacting with His Language Facilitator**

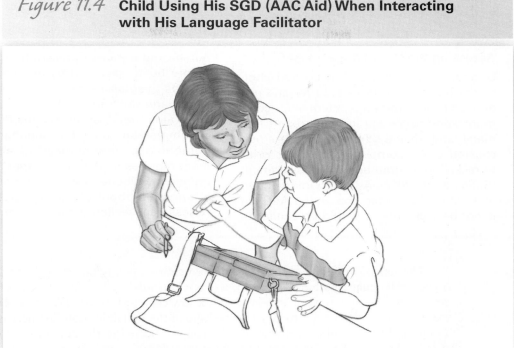

FOCUS 11.3   *Research*

Just-in-Time Programming

A new type of programming, called *just-in-time* (*JIT*) programming, is being investigated in AAC technologies (Light, 2012). JIT programming reduces the amount of time needed to program messages into an AAC aid and dynamically captures experiences and vocabulary items in real time during authentic communication interactions. This technology supports easy and quick importing of photos for VSDs by taking photos using a cell phone with a Bluetooth connection. JIT also has a simplified menu system that allows the communication partner to make photographs responsive via a touch screen (i.e., voice output names the picture when the student touches the screen). Light and colleagues (2012) compared interactions of young children when JIT programming was used with those using a traditional AAC system. They found that children took significantly more turns and had access to significantly more vocabulary concepts during interactions when JIT programming was utilized than they did with traditional systems. This exciting new technology has the potential to increase the opportunities for language learning for children with complex communication needs. Go to the Penn State Early Intervention site for young children with autism, cerebral palsy, Down syndrome, and other disabilities, at http://aackids.psu .edu/index.php/page/show/id/1, to learn about guidelines for early intervention. Review Steps 1 through 5 on the website and discuss how you might implement this program with a child who has a disability.

FOCUS 11.4 *Learning More*

Assessing the Use of Apps for AAC

Dunham (2011) stated that trained clinicians should assess the need for and use of apps to maximize the potential for communication success. Clinicians report that many families and school districts are purchasing tablet computers and apps prior to receiving a communication assessment (Shane et al., 2012). Adapting intervention to an already-selected app and/or AAC aid is not best practice. It would be similar to purchasing a pair of prescription glasses before being assessed by an eye doctor. Just as eyeglasses need to be individualized and customized for each person, AAC aids need similar consideration. Recommending apps for language development and communication enhancement requires an AAC assessment from a trained practitioner. You will find out more information about assessing apps in the Assessment section of this chapter.

The use of mobile devices and communication apps is rapidly evolving. If you, as a speech-language pathologist (SLP), work with individuals with CCNs, you will need to continually update your expertise and knowledge in this area. A good place to start exploring the AAC field is to go to the website of the Rehabilitation Engineering Research Center (RERC), a collaborative research group dedicated to the development of effective AAC technology. You can access this site at http://aac-rerc.psu.edu.

AAC STRATEGIES

The third component of an AAC system is strategy. An **AAC strategy** refers to methods used to communicate effectively and efficiently. AAC strategies support message timing, grammatical formulation, spelling, and communication rate (Beukelman & Mirenda, 2013). Some examples of strategies to enhance communication include prediction and encoding. The prediction strategy is "a dynamic retrieval process in which options offered to an individual with CCN change according to the portion of a word or message that has already been formulated" (Beukelman & Mirenda, 2013, p. 68). An example of prediction is when your computer shows you your most recently used files before showing you older or unused files. Young children with language impairments may benefit from letter and word prediction. Letter prediction can support spelling if the child knows the first letter of the word (see Focus 11.5). Prediction software also supports syntactical development as the program predicts the next word, based on the syntactic rules of English.

Encoding (i.e., using a code) is another effective AAC strategy. Encoding can help an individual quickly express a lengthy message. Young children may use color coding and symbol coding as they are developing language. Color coding can be used to designate a part of speech (e.g., yellow for nouns) or to highlight a type of communicative act, such as commenting. Symbol coding is used for quick communication. For example, if a child wants to tell his friend what he did last weekend without having to type each word or does not know how to spell the message, an entire communication message can be programmed into an SGD and represented with a symbol. A photo of the child's grandparents' home can be added to the display with the communicative message "I went to visit my grandpa and grandma this weekend. I had so much fun!" The entire communicative message is encoded by touching the photograph. Some encoding systems available in AAC devices,

FOCUS 11.5   *Learning More*

Word Prediction

You may be familiar with word prediction if you program names in your cell phone. The software predicts the name of the person, based on the letter you have typed.

For example, I start entering the letters *B-a-r,* and the predicted name *Barbara* is available for selection. This predicted name saves me four keystrokes because I do not have to enter the *b-a-r-a.*

such as alphanumeric coding, place high cognitive demands on the learner to remember the code and the corresponding message. Encoding improves communication efficiency when it is matched with each individual's capabilities (Beukelman & Mirenda, 2013). A child's cognitive ability must be considered when deciding on a coding system (Light et al., 2004).

AAC TECHNIQUES

The fourth component of an AAC system is technique. An **AAC technique** refers to how a message is conveyed. Some individuals who have an AAC system use their finger to point to symbols or look directly at their intended object (i.e., eye pointing). This technique is referred to as *direct selection* because the person directly selects a symbol. Pressing the numbers on a telephone is an example of direct selection. This strategy is often the most efficient. However, some individuals who cannot directly select a symbol because of a physical impairment must use scanning, another selection technique.

Scanning is most often used by individuals with physical limitations. Scanning involves a communication partner or an electronic aid that displays symbols in a predetermined pattern (Beukelman & Mirenda, 2013). Partner-dependent scanning involves a facilitator who scans through symbol choices until the child indicates his or her choice; the child communicates his or her choice by blinking, pressing a switch, vocalizing, or producing a predetermined physical movement. Electronic aids can also be used to scan choices with lighted displays. Again, the child waits while the aid scans through the symbols until the target symbol is illuminated. The child then produces a movement to select the target symbol.

AAC SELECTION SET

Many AAC components must be combined to develop an effective communication system. A practitioner creates an AAC system by combining symbols, aids, strategies, techniques, and selection set. An **AAC selection set** includes the messages, symbols, and codes that are available to a child at one time (Beukelman & Mirenda, 2013). Many AAC selection sets include a visual display; however, for individuals with visual impairments, auditory and tactile displays can be provided. A selection set can have fixed displays, dynamic displays, or visual scene displays (Beukelman & Mirenda, 2013).

Fixed displays have symbols and messages that do not change after the person selects the location. Think about ordering at a restaurant. The waiter cannot hear you because of the noise level, so you indicate your choice by pointing to the picture or words on the menu; nothing changes on the page. You have used a static (fixed) display to communicate your food choice.

In contrast, **dynamic displays** change after a location is selected. You have likely used dynamic displays on your cell phone or an ATM machine. A dynamic display AAC is

FOCUS 11.6   *Learning More*

Go to Dr. Dowden's website (http://depts.washington.edu/enables/) and find a myth and fact about AAC that you had not considered before. How can you help dispel myths about AAC?

often a portable tablet-style touch-screen computer that runs specially designed software. The software provides numerous communication displays that can be set up for the user. When an individual touches the computer screen, the software automatically changes the selection set to a new set of programmed symbols (Beukelman & Mirenda, 2013).

The final display type, **visual scene display (VSD)**, is a picture, photograph, or virtual environmental that depicts and represents a situation, place, or experience. I will discuss the use of VSDs in the Intervention section of this chapter.

WHAT IS *NOT* CONSIDERED AAC?

Now that you understand what an AAC intervention approach is and know about the components of AAC, I want you to know what is *not* considered AAC. Hopefully, as part of this discussion, you also have considered overarching issues about alternative modes of communication. Many professionals (i.e., therapists, teachers, administrators) have misconceptions about AAC. Dr. Pat Dowden at the University of Washington has a website that dispels some common myths about AAC and promotes the facts. She addresses misconceptions about topics such as the compatibility of AAC and intervention strategies and how AAC is more than assistive technology (see Focus 11.6).

AAC is not an intervention approach used to replace speech; instead, it is an approach that *augments* an individual's available skills and provides *alternative* communication strategies as needed. AAC is more than the use of "fancy, talking computers." AAC enhances input (i.e., understanding) as well as the output of language (i.e., expression). An AAC intervention approach can be used in combination with other language intervention approaches.

AAC does not hinder language or speech development. Blackstone (2006) reported, "AAC interventions can have significant benefits on the development of communicative competence and language skills" (p. 3). Blackstone's report as well as other published research studies reduce anxiety often expressed by parents about the implications of AAC interventions (see Focus 11.7). Concerns about AAC replacing traditional modes of

FOCUS 11.7   *Research*

In 2006, Millar, Light, and Schlosser completed a meta-analysis to determine the effect of AAC on the speech production of individuals with developmental disabilities. The research team found 23 studies examining the relationship between speech production and the effects of AAC intervention. The researchers concluded that speech increased in a majority of individuals (89%) with AAC intervention and that no individuals "showed a decrease in speech production as a result of AAC intervention" (Millar et al., 2006, p. 254).

communication are unwarranted. "AAC interventions are typically implemented to build communication and language skills through a range of modalities (including signs and aided AAC systems as well as natural speech), rather than to increase speech production alone" (Millar, Light, & Schlosser, 2006, p. 257; see also Romski et al., 2010).

Assessment

Assessment is a team effort. Considering AAC options during an assessment requires each team member to contribute information about a child's capabilities and needs. Family members are a very important part of the team. A child's use of AAC occurs at home, at school, and in the community. Accordingly, the family plays a key role in the intervention process (Granlund et al., 2008). In addition to members of the child's family, potential AAC assessment team members could include an SLP, the child's teacher and educational assistant, an occupational therapist, a physical therapist, a rehabilitation engineer, the child's nurse or physician, and (as the child becomes old enough) the individual himself or herself.

A comprehensive AAC assessment includes additional components over and above those in a standard language assessment (covered in Chapter 3). Language capabilities as well as capabilities in the areas of literacy, hearing, vision, oral-sensorimotor system, speech, cognition, and physical skills must be documented. Adaptations are made if the individual has a physical impairment that limits his or her participation in the language assessment (see Focus 11.8). The additional required components are identification of communication needs, identification of participation patterns, assessment of symbols, feature matching, and AAC system trials.

IDENTIFICATION OF COMMUNICATION NEEDS AND PARTICIPATION PATTERNS

To implement a high-quality AAC assessment, an assessor follows the participation model of assessment (Beukelman & Mirenda, 2013). A decision tree demonstrating the participation model is presented in Figure 11.5. The American Speech-Language-Hearing Association endorsed this model in 2004.

The participation model "provides a systematic process for conducting AAC assessments and designing interventions based on the functional participation requirements of peers without disabilities of the same chronological age as the person with CCN" (Beukelman & Mirenda, 2013, p. 108). Practitioners use this model to determine both intrinsic and extrinsic factors contributing to an individual's CCNs.

Why is functional participation important to AAC assessment? In Focus 11.2 I described the ICF framework from the World Health Organization (WHO, 2002). As you recall, the WHO-ICF framework considers an individual's everyday functioning in his or

FOCUS 11.8   *Clinical Skill Building*

Language tests often require a child to point to pictures. How could you adapt a language test for a child who has a physical challenge and cannot point with his or her finger? How might adapting a language test for a child with physical challenges impact the results, or your interpretation of the results, from a standardized test?

Figure 11.5 **AAC Participation Model**

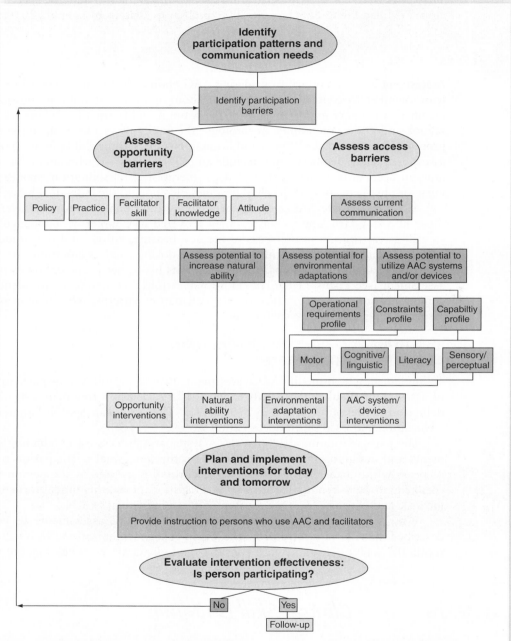

Source: Reprinted by permission from Beukelman, D. R., & Mirenda, P. *Augmentative and Alternative Communication: Supporting Children and Adults with Complex Communication Needs* (4th ed.). Baltimore: Paul H. Brookes Publishing Co., Inc.

her community, school, or job. The WHO-ICF framework underscores the importance of an individual's overall communication.

An assessor may not capture an individual's everyday communication patterns within the confines of a traditional language assessment (using norm-referenced assessments and one-on-one interactions). Everyday communication patterns are documented when the assessor observes the individual at school, during social activities, and in a variety of interpersonal interactions. Observing everyday communication routines also helps the assessor identify barriers that potentially limit the individual's communication.

The WHO-ICF framework also guides questioning during an AAC assessment to determine an individual's communication needs. For example, the assessor questions the individual, family, teachers, and/or caregivers to determine:

1. Communication or academic expectations (e.g., silent reading during quiet time in a second-grade classroom)
2. Important communication environments (e.g., Cub Scouts, Special Olympics, school, home)
3. Typical communication partners (e.g., parents, grandparents, siblings, friends, educational assistants, teacher, coach)
4. Activities and routines of daily living (i.e., Does the child participate in kindergarten morning circle time?)
5. Regularly required communicative messages (e.g., messages to support sharing at circle time or checking out books from the school library)

Two goals underlie the information-gathering protocol listed above; the first goal is to identify the child's participation patterns, and the second is to compare the child's communication patterns with communication patterns of same-age peers.

To complete the second goal, team members fill out a participation inventory (Beukelman & Mirenda, 2013). The participation inventory documents the child's communication patterns in everyday interactions; team members also describe same-age peers' communication patterns within each interaction. Team members then compare the optimal level of participation (i.e., peers) to that of the child to identify participation barriers as possible intervention targets.

The results from the communication assessment may lead to one or more of the following conclusions:

- The individual may benefit from an AAC approach to intervention (Beukelman & Mirenda, 2013).
- The individual's natural communication abilities should be targeted for intervention.
- The individual may benefit from environmental changes to facilitate communication.

The conclusions listed here are not mutually exclusive. An individual with language impairment may benefit from an AAC approach in combination with an intervention focusing on improving language skills and communication abilities.

SYMBOL ASSESSMENT

A comprehensive AAC assessment also includes a symbol assessment. Recall from the beginning of the chapter that there are many types of symbols. The goal of a symbol assessment is to "select the types of symbols that will meet the individual's current communication needs and match his or her current abilities, as well as to identify symbol options that might be used in the future" (Beukelman & Mirenda, 2013, p. 158).

AAC symbol assessment considers both unaided and aided symbols. The assessor documents the individual's use of unaided symbols (i.e., gestures, vocalizations, and/or manual signs) along with the individual's understanding and use of aided symbols (i.e., photographs, line drawings, orthography). For example, a common sign recognized by many is a stop sign. Four symbol options for *stop* are shown in Figure 11.6. Does the shape of the sign, the color of the sign, and/or the word *stop* represent the concept to an individual? A symbol assessment determines which type of symbol is meaningful to each child. As a next step in symbol assessment, you determine the student's ability to use symbols within natural interactions (Beukelman & Mirenda, 2013). With modeling and prompting, you demonstrate how selecting the symbol results in a desired activity (i.e., "I want to stop this game."). It is also crucial that you train others to offer opportunities as well. Interactive opportunities extend the assessment process into the student's daily life. This "trial intervention" provides valuable information, allowing you to make recommendations regarding the type of symbols appropriate for the child's AAC system.

AAC assessments can be natural extensions of more traditional communication assessments. Extending symbolic use to represent language for input as well as output eliminates barriers and provides opportunities for children with language impairments to participate in everyday communication activities.

Figure 11.6   **Different Symbols Representing the Concept *Stop***

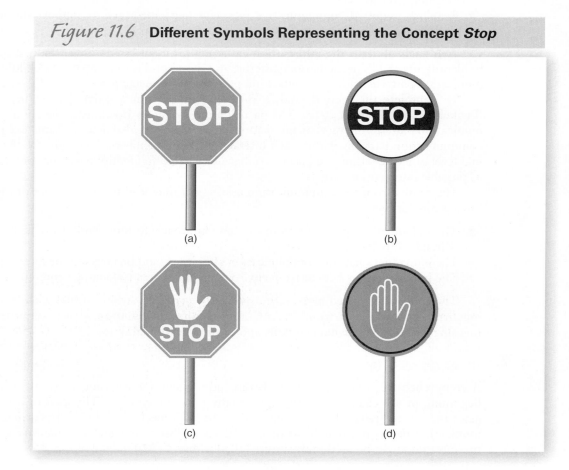

FEATURE MATCHING

Another component of a comprehensive AAC assessment includes a match of AAC system features with the capabilities and communication needs of the child. AAC system features refer to the components previously discussed: symbols, aids, strategies, and techniques. Specifically, an individual should have opportunities during an assessment to try different types of displays (e.g., static, dynamic, visual scene) and selection sets. The assessor provides opportunities for the child to try varied features of AAC systems in meaningful, age-appropriate contexts.

Results from an AAC assessment include recommendations for an AAC system and training. The AAC system is part of a multi-modal approach to language intervention. The system is a tool that can enhance effective communication when the features match the child's needs and capabilities. Intervention must include appropriate teaching to ensure that the child and others understand how the system augments and/or provides an additional mode of communication. See Focus 11.9 for more about assessment protocols used during an AAC assessment.

FEATURE MATCHING, MOBILE TECHNOLOGY, AND COMMUNICATION APPS

An AAC assessment that includes feature matching should occur prior to purchases of mobile technology and communication apps. However, as you read earlier, this practice is not happening because sometimes families and caregivers are purchasing technology and then asking an SLP to make the system work for their child (AAC-RERC, 2011; Shane et al., 2012). Consider the case study presented in Focus 11.10 and discuss the clinical questions posed at the end of the case study.

A number of clinical features should be considered when selecting an app for use with mobile technology. Important features include identifying the purpose of the app, speech output capability, speech settings, display and feedback features, rate enhancement, access, required motor competencies, levels of support needed to use the app, and cost. I provide a definition of each clinical feature and an example of clinical questions that might be considered for each feature in Table 11.1. These features should match the

---

FOCUS 11.9   *Learning More*

Social Networks: A Communication Inventory for Individuals with Complex Communication Needs and Their Communication Partners (Blackstone & Hunt Berg, 2003) is a commercially available assessment and intervention planning tool that can help you investigate a child's communication needs. The Social Networks tool facilitates and guides a clinician and an AAC team to identify (a) the skills and abilities of the child and communication partners; (b) the child's modes of expression; (c) appropriate augmentative and alternative symbols, aids, strategies, and techniques; (d) potential topics of conversation; and (e) levels of support needed to communicate. This information is used to plan ongoing intervention, maximizing the child's communicative effectiveness and independence.

FOCUS 11.10 *Clinical Skill Building*

Jayden is a 10-year-old boy who has been diagnosed with cerebral palsy. He uses a wheelchair for mobility and has difficulty producing clear, intelligible speech because of the motor challenges in his face, mouth, neck, and torso. Jayden speaks in one- to two-word utterances because he does not have enough breath support to say longer sentences. Jayden's family members understand about 75% of what he says. People Jayden doesn't know well or has never met have a very difficult time understanding Jayden when he talks. Because of this challenge when communicating, Jayden finds it frustrating to talk to people at school and in the community. Jayden has used an SGD at school for 5 years but has not used the device in the community. Because it is difficult to transport Jayden's SGD for everyday activities and weekend outings, Jayden's father often left the device at home, limiting Jayden's ability to communicate effectively with other people.

Jayden's father wondered if there was an AAC system that was more portable and easier to take out into the community. He bought a tablet computer and a communication app for his son. The app Jayden's father purchased speaks key phrases aloud with the tap of a picture. The pictures were very different from the pictures/symbols used in Jayden's SGD. Without consulting Jayden's SLP, Jayden's father programmed a few phrases for his son to use in a number of situations where the SGD was challenging for the family. Jayden's father was happy that he had thought of another solution for his son. However, when Jayden tried to use the app and mobile technology, his fingers pressed more than one key at a time. The speech output was also difficult to hear in noisy environments. Jayden was frustrated by these challenges and did not want to continue using the mobile technology.

After reading this case study, discuss the following clinical questions: What problems might occur with Jayden's father selecting and programming key phrases in the app? Did this AAC system make Jayden more independent? What do you think might have happened if Jayden had participated in an AAC assessment before his father had bought the mobile technology and app?

features identified as necessary for a child to participate in intervention sessions targeting language and communication activities.

The number of apps available is increasing daily, so a list of communication apps would be quickly outdated. However, you can look to resources on the Internet that provide current names, descriptions, and prices for apps designed to enhance language and communication. Some of these resources also allow you to compare features of apps to one another (King, 2013). AAC TechConnect (www.aactechconnect.com) provides a list of communication apps that are categorized by features (e.g., speech output, word prediction). Try searching for communication apps in app stores such as the iTunes App Store or Google Play and see how many apps you can find that support drawing, speaking, or writing.

Table 11.1 **Clinical Features to Consider When Selecting a Communication App**

Clinical feature	Definition	Clinical questions to consider
Purpose of use	Description of the app's purpose	Was the app created for the purpose of expressive, receptive, and/or organization of communication? How does this app fit the student's communication needs?
Output	The type of output provided by the device (e.g., speech, text, or both)	How can this student most easily and quickly communicate? What communication parameters are expressed by the family?
Speech settings	The prosodic features of the speech output (e.g., pitch, volume, rate) as well as the ability of the device to speak an entire phrase or sentence	Are the student and the family comfortable with the speech output? Can the characteristics of the speech output be modified as the individual matures to represent age and gender?
Display	The layout of the app, including the size, font, and color of symbols	How can the display be customized (e.g., font size, borders, colors) to enhance the individual's ability to use the app? Is it possible to import and modify icons as needed?
Feedback features	The ability of the icon to zoom, enlarge, or vibrate when the communicator touches the screen	How can the feedback features be modified (e.g., highlight/zoom/enlargement of an icon, auditory review) when an icon is selected (e.g., tactile /vibration feedback) to enhance communication? Do the customization options include the ability to turn them on or off?
Rate enhancement	The ability of the app to be modified to increase the rate of communication	What rate enhancement features are available to increase the rate of communication output (e.g., word prediction, abbreviation expansion, recently used lists, grammar prediction)? Do the customization options include the ability to turn them on or off?
Access	How the user interacts with the device in terms of item selection (e.g., direct selection, scanning)	Is the individual required to touch the screen to select an item? What customization features are available, and can they be turned on and off? Can the selection features be modified as the user's skills develop?
Required motor skills	The motor abilities of the user required to access the device	Can the timing for accessing the communication target be modified to adapt to a slower or less accurate motor response?
Competencies support	Support provided by the app publisher for resolving technical issues	Will the individual or family be able to access support independently of the SLP? How quickly and in what manner are technical issues resolved?
Cost/ miscellaneous	Cost and additional options that are available with the app	Is there a good cost–benefit ratio for this particular app?

Source: This information is summarized from Gosnell, Costello, and Shane (2011).

Intervention

AAC intervention approaches vary from structured behavioral teaching models to child-centered interactive and social pragmatic models (Beukelman & Mirenda, 2013; Light & Drager 2006). A practitioner matches the best intervention strategies for each child, based on results from the assessment. Family members and other communication partners are involved in the AAC intervention program. Parents and caregivers are trained to facilitate the child's language and communication development during everyday interactions (Light & Drager, 2006). Light and Drager (2006) described the initial results of a study in which very young children (ages 8–40 months) were introduced to appealing, easy-to-use AAC technologies in meaningful social contexts. The children's parents were simultaneously taught to model the use of the AAC device during interactive play, social routines, games, and reading activities. Results were impressive: Noted improvements in communication skills occurred with respect to (a) turn-taking behaviors, (b) semantic development, (c) vocabulary acquisition rate, and (d) ability to combine concepts to express complex messages. In addition, the researchers reported that the children used their AAC systems to communicate, play, and learn new concepts in addition to developing phonological awareness and literacy skills.

Below I present three AAC intervention approaches: the System for Augmenting Language (SAL), visual scene displays (VSDs), and Picture Exchange Communication System (PECS). For more information on different AAC interventions, you can check out the book *Pragmatically Speaking: Language, Literacy, and Academic Development for Students with AAC Needs*, edited by Soto and Zangari (2009).

THE SYSTEM FOR AUGMENTING LANGUAGE (SAL)

The **System for Augmenting Language (SAL)** is a total-immersion approach to teaching language comprehension and use (Romski & Sevcik, 1996). With the SAL approach, practitioners introduce symbols gradually and avoid teaching language in a structured fashion (Drager, 2009). Instead, students are encouraged to use their AAC system in realistic spoken communication situations to produce both referential and **regulatory communication acts**. Regulatory communication acts are completed when an individual indicates his or her own needs in routines of daily living. The five components of SAL are listed in Figure 11.7.

Several studies provide evidence that supports the use of SAL with individuals with a range of disabilities; these studies represent evidence of intervention effectiveness at Level III. Cafiero (2001) presented a case study of a middle-school student with autism. The practitioner engaged the student in conversation and modeled and expanded any of the student's communication attempts with his communication board. After implementing the intervention, the student showed improved receptive and expressive vocabulary as well as more positive interactions.

In another study, SAL-trained communicators (with 5 years of AAC experience) were compared with two groups of non-SAL-trained communicators, including both "speakers" and "nonspeakers" (Romski et al., 2005). All three groups consisted of participants with moderate-to-severe intellectual impairment. The results of the study supported the use of the SAL approach. Compared to the nonspeakers, the SAL communicators had higher-quality interactions and a higher level of conversational appropriateness in an interaction with an unfamiliar communication partner. In comparison with the "speakers," the

Figure 11.7 **SAL Components and Instructional Strategies**

1. The student is provided with a speech-generating device (SGD) to use within the natural communication environment.
2. Symbols are displayed on the SGD, with the English word printed above; the symbols are selected to improve social communication and to meet individual communication needs.
3. The communication partner encourages the child to use symbols by teaching symbol use in loosely structured, naturalistic communicative activities (e.g., "Tell me what you want, *water* or *juice*?")
4. Communication partners are trained to use symbols in their communication with the student (i.e., both partners use symbols during interactions).
5. The professional provides ongoing support to the student and his or her communication partners as a resource for using the approach.

Source: Based on information from *Breaking the Speech Barrier: Language Development through Augmented Means,* by M. A. Romski and R. A. Sevcik, 1996, Baltimore, MD: Brookes.

SAL users were described as being "less fluid." However, the SAL communicators demonstrated an advantage over the speakers in that they used more specific references during their interactions.

The SAL approach has also been implemented with young preschool children. Drager and colleagues (2006) investigated a modeling intervention with two preschoolers with ASD using a single-subject, multiple-baseline design. The intervention consisted of engaging the children in interactive play activities and providing symbols on their language boards. For example, the practitioner pointed with an index finger to a ball in the classroom and then sequentially pointed (within 2 seconds) to a graphic symbol *ball* while simultaneously vocalizing the word *ball*. Four symbols were introduced during each play activity, and each was modeled four times per session. The results indicated that intervention was effective, with increasing symbol comprehension and increasing symbol production (i.e., object labeling) in both children.

Romski and colleagues (2010) also reported positive outcomes from augmented language interventions for toddlers. Parents were taught how to interact and use communication strategies with their children and randomly assigned to augmented communication input, augmented communication output, or spoken communication groups. Vocabulary size was larger after the augmented language interventions, both input and output. These results support the benefit of augmented communication strategies and provide more evidence to dispel the myth that AAC hinders speech development.

VISUAL SCENE DISPLAYS (VSDs)

Visual scene displays (VSDs) can be used in an intervention program to support language by organizing vocabulary and communicative messages schematically rather than semantically (Beukelman & Mirenda, 2013). I described VSDs earlier in the chapter, when I discussed AAC selection set.

Beukelman and Mirenda (2013) describe a visual scene display as "a picture, photograph, or virtual environment that depicts and represents situation, a place, or an experience" (p. 77). Children use VSDs to explore, learn, and communicate with parents and other communication partners (Light & Drager, 2006). The arrangement of language concepts and communicative messages in a VSD is very different from that in the traditional AAC communication board. A traditional AAC display represents language concepts and communicative messages with symbols, photos, and words organized into rows and columns. In contrast, a VSD provides contextual support in comparison to a traditional grid display.

VSDs use photographs or pictures instead of individual line drawings to symbolize language concepts and communicative messages. VSDs can be used with low- or high-technology AAC devices. When a high-tech VSD is used, typically "hot spots" are created within each visual scene to represent messages that support the student's learning or communication. For example, in Figure 11.8, if the picture were used with a high-tech VSD device and the hot spot were located on the blue pail, the device could be programmed with the name of the object (i.e., to enhance semantic knowledge) or programmed with a communication message such as "I poured the pail of water on my cousin's head" to support a student's syntax and pragmatic skills.

A VSD also can be used in a low-technology display. In this case, the visual scene of the children playing in the water would be transferred into an SGD or used in a communication book. In either case, a skilled practitioner would use the contextually rich display to represent meaningful and authentic interactions, enhancing the student's language learning (Light & Drager, 2007).

What other hot spots could be programmed with concepts or communication messages using a high-tech VSD and the visual scene shown in Figure 11.8? Examples might include water, children, playing, fun, and summer. Identifying communication messages requires a practitioner to learn background information about the photos and generate communication messages that are meaningful to the child. Does the child want to

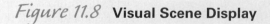

Figure 11.8 **Visual Scene Display**

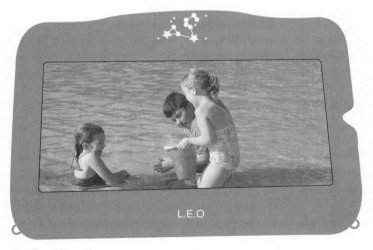

Source: Photo by Don King.

comment on what happened during her vacation? Does the child want to tell a story about her vacation? Does the child want to ask students in her classroom if they can guess what the children were building or what game they were playing? Just like typically developing children, children with complex communication needs and language challenges should be able to participate using a full range of pragmatic functions.

To determine what communicative messages might be relevant for a student, begin by asking the family questions such as "Where was the photo taken?" "Who is in the picture?" "When did this experience take place?" and "Why is this image meaningful to the child?" Another example of a communicative message that might be associated with a hot spot on the face of the boy would be "My cousin said 'Hey, what are you doing with that?' right before I dumped it on his head." On a traditional display, symbols of the three children would likely be represented in three different locations, along with symbols representing the water, the pail or toys, and perhaps a game. The traditional display would be less intuitive and more abstract to use than a VSD. Examples of other VSDs are available at the AAC website at the University of Nebraska–Lincoln, at http://aac.unl.edu/intervention.html.

The advantages of VSDs are that the realistic nature of the scenes maximizes meaningfulness and organizes language concepts within categories. Also, VSDs facilitate children's use of speech-generating devices. Young children often find SGDs difficult to use (Light & Drager, 2007). It is suggested that using a VSD can act as a springboard for young children, who then may eventually use other types of AAC devices. Additional ideas to be considered when recommending AAC devices for young children are provided in Focus 11.11.

PICTURE EXCHANGE COMMUNICATION SYSTEM (PECS)

The **Picture Exchange Communication System (PECS)** is a popular treatment approach used frequently with children who are on the autism spectrum. In recent years, PECS also has been used with children and adults with other diagnoses. "The primary goal of PECS is to teach functional communication" (Bondy & Frost, 2009, p. 298). PECS is based on principles of applied behavior analysis. The protocol has six phases; see Table 11.2 for a summary of each phase of PECS.

Despite the popularity of PECS, there is limited research to support the use of this language intervention approach. Schlosser and Wendt (2007) conducted a systematic review to determine the effectiveness of PECS instruction on prelinguistic behaviors,

---

FOCUS 11.11   *Clinical Skill Building*

- When recommending AAC technology as part of an intervention plan, remember to consider a child's developmental level and what you would expect other children that age to do. What would a typically developing 3-year-old child be doing? Think of the participation model to keep your expectations and goals realistic and natural.
- AAC intervention should be multi-modal. What does this mean? What are different modes of communication? What would be appropriate modes of communication for a 2-year-old? How about for a 5-year-old?

Table 11.2 **Phases of the PECS Protocol**

Phase	Description
I. Teaching the communicative exchange	The child learns how to request by selecting a picture of an item he or she desires and giving it to or exchanging it with a communication partner for the chosen item. The picture is a graphic symbol that represents the object.
II. Teaching persistence	The child learns how to exchange pictures with increasing distances to communication partners and/or to the communication pictures.
III. Discrimination training	The child learns how to discriminate between two choices.
IV. Teaching "I want" sentences	The child learns how to use a picture that represents *I want* before selecting the desired object.
V. Teaching a response to "What do you want?"	The child learns to respond to the question "What do you want?"
VI. Teaching use of additional sentence starters	The child learns new sentence starters such as "I see" to develop commenting.

Source: Based on information from "The Picture Exchange Communication System," by A. Bondy and L. Frost, 2009. In P. Mirenda and T. Iacono (Eds.), *Autism Spectrum Disorders and AAC* (pp. 279–302). Baltimore, MD: Brookes.

speech production, expressive social regulation, and communicative functions of children with ASD. They reviewed 12 studies with a total of 105 participants; their results indicated that PECS only improved the communicative function of requesting in a small number of the studies. As you recall from Chapters 1 and 2, requesting is a pragmatic function used to regulate or control the actions of others.

Wendt (2008) conducted another systematic review of research investigating AAC intervention using graphic symbols for children with autism spectrum disorder (ASD). His review of 15 studies found strong evidence that graphic symbols improved children's ability to request; however, no evidence indicated that certain graphic symbols worked better than others. Wendt also concluded that the available evidence did not support a specific intervention approach for teaching children to use graphic symbols. Wendt summarized his results by stating that when an interventionist develops graphic symbol intervention for a child with ASD, the interventionist should consider the iconicity of symbols, along with the child's information-processing abilities, learning style, and cognitive abilities.

*Connections**

As you recall, throughout this book, the sections called *Connections* are used to highlight issues with broad applications across the range of communication disorders. In this *Connections* section, I highlight issues related to multicultural mismatch. Children with SLI, children with intellectual disability, children on the autism spectrum, and children

*Portions of the *Connections* section of this chapter were written by Stephanie M. Curenton.

with CCNs come from a variety of ethnic or cultural groups. Your cultural expectations and experiences may be very different from a child's family experiences and expectations. Reflect on how the information presented below might affect your decision making with respect to all the language impairments discussed in this book.

Sometimes an SLP is presented with a multicultural challenge because there is practitioner–client ethnic mismatch. As you learned earlier in this book, ethnic mismatch occurs when there are conflicting expectations for a student's communication or behavior. Below I discuss some of the major multicultural challenges faced by SLPs who work with individuals from various cultural groups.

MULTICULTURAL CHALLENGES

The first multicultural challenge is that more than half of children in the United States who receive services for speech and language are from ethnic minority groups (U.S. Department of Education, 2002). The high occurrence of nonmajority children receiving speech-pathology services may result in ethnic mismatch; more than 90% of SLPs are women of European descent (ASHA, 2006b). The match between practitioner and client is important because although some nonmajority families do not believe an SLP's ethnicity matters (Roseti, Tellis, & Gabel, 2001), other families may mistrust practitioners who are European American. So as practitioners, our presence might have a positive or neutral effect on some clients but a negative effect on others. Consequently, it is important for you to consider issues related to ethnic mismatch.

The second challenge is that all practitioners, regardless of their ethnicity, are unintentionally operating from the European cultural framework because they have been trained to use language philosophies, assessment instruments, procedures, and intervention practices stemming from a European tradition (see Hwa-Froelich & Vigil, 2004). Practitioners must realize that they are operating from European traditions and understand the implications of socioeconomic and regional differences. There is a need for the qualified practitioner to have increased self-awareness that considers the traditions, values, and experiences of multiple cultural groups.

Cultural self-awareness begins when a practitioner examines the values, beliefs, and patterns of behavior that are part of his or her own cultural identity. Self-awareness recognizes that one's own beliefs and behaviors are not inherently right but rather represent only one perspective. So, for example, if an individual from a different cultural group said, "Children should only talk when they are first addressed by an adult," you would not want to immediately say, "Oh no! A child should be able to talk whenever he wants to!" Your reply of "oh no!" would demonstrate ethnocentrism. **Ethnocentrism** occurs when a member of one culture judges an individual from another culture solely by the values and standards of his or her own culture. In this case, different cultures have varying pragmatic expectations about politeness. Children from collectivist cultures, as most ethnic minority children are, are socialized to be quiet when communicating with adults and may not be expected to talk unless directly addressed by an adult (Hwa-Froelich & Vigil, 2004). **Collectivist cultures** focus on interdependence among group members and the well-being of the extended family; a child raised in a collectivist culture is likely to communicate more frequently to peers than to adults. In most collectivist cultures, elders are the leaders of the family (Cheng, 2002). There are aspects of individualism and collectivism in all cultures, but each culture has a primary orientation; African, Asian, Latino, and Native American cultures value collectivism.

In contrast, in an **individualist culture,** the focus is on the individual and his or her immediate (nuclear) family. European tradition is a more individualistic culture. In an individualistic culture, it is often expected that in an adult–child interaction, the adult or more competent communicator should modify or limit his own level of language output and encourage the less competent speaker (the child) to communicate.

As mentioned above, collectivist cultures tend to place less importance on an individual's independence. In this case, you may find that when working with a nonmajority family member, some of your suggestions are not implemented. So, for example if you emphasize how an AAC system may increase the student's independence when communicating, your suggestion may be ignored. On the other hand, if you emphasize how the AAC system will help the student interact with his extended family, your suggestion may be welcomed. Also, in some cultural groups, drawing attention to a child's disability in public places may not be considered appropriate (Soto, 2012). Therefore, understanding the dynamics of the home communication system is a critical element when recommending and designing AAC systems for clients (Parette, Brotherson, & Huer, 2000).

Finally, to be culturally responsive, a practitioner should ask for family input about the home language and communication needs, the nature of disability, and the level of participation they expect to contribute to the intervention. Cultural differences influence not only the roles that the parents are willing and able to take in teaching their child, but also those they are expecting the professional to fulfill (Hwa-Froelich & Vigil, 2004; Soto, 2012). Here are some questions to ask to assess a family's view on communication (Soto, 2012):

- When do you want the child to communicate when he is with the family?
- Who does the child usually play or interact with?
- What are the family routines when your child talks to adults?
- Who is "in charge" of family decisions?

When you make recommendations about an AAC system, make sure to assess how the family feels about the recommendations and whether the recommended strategies fit within the family's dynamics. It has been reported that some nonmajority families do not desire to use an AAC system at home. Researchers have reported that family members sometimes feel that they are already able to communicate at home without using AAC strategies and techniques (McCord & Soto, 2004). It is important to work within the family's expectations while also advocating for a child's communication participation.

In summary, suggestions for developing culturally responsive intervention should include (a) acknowledging and collaboratively developing goals for the intervention; (b) arranging meetings at times and locations convenient to family members; (c) seeking family member's input on whom to invite to meetings (e.g., extended family, siblings, trusted professionals); (d) balancing the ratio of family and professional participants at trainings; (e) allowing time for family members to understand the different components of the AAC system; (f) considering the level of formality that may be expected in the family–practitioner interactions and asking how each family member prefers to be addressed; (g) developing or purchasing manuals and training materials in the home language and targeting home routines that are identified by the individual and family; (h) providing an interpreter at all meetings; and (i) offering ongoing support to family and the individual with CCN as the student matures and develops, resulting in changes to the AAC system to meet new situations or changes in communication needs (Soto, 2012).

Summary

- In this chapter, I introduced AAC as an approach for improving children's language and communication. The evidence is clear that children with language concerns and complex communication needs often benefit from an AAC approach. AAC interventions (a) enhance participation in meaningful activities, (b) help meet an individual's communication needs, (c) facilitate language and literacy development, and (d) improve an individual's language skills.
- The benefits of an AAC approach are numerous. Examples include language learning in supported natural activities, increased use of multiple modes of communication, increased participation in communicative interactions, and increased interactions with peers in a variety of different environments.
- When an individual has communication needs that are not being met, these needs are called complex communication needs (CCNs). CCNs may stem from language comprehension and production impairments in spoken and written language. Language impairments may affect communication opportunities and social participation.
- AAC systems are composed of four critical components: symbols, aids, strategies, and techniques. Symbols can be graphic, auditory, gestural, and textured or tactile and are used to represent language concepts. An AAC aid is a device that can be used to send or receive messages. An AAC strategy refers to methods used to communicate effectively and efficiently. AAC strategies support message timing, grammatical formulation, spelling, and communication rate. Technique refers to how a message is conveyed. Some individuals who have an AAC system use their finger to point to symbols or look directly at the intended object; scanning is another AAC technique. An AAC system is part of a multi-modal view of communication. Multi-modal refers to the use of multiple modalities when a person communicates.
- AAC is not an intervention approach used to replace speech but rather to augment the skills a child has and to provide alternative strategies and techniques when needed to enhance language development and overall communication skills. It is a common misconception that the use of AAC will hinder speech and language development; recent research demonstrates that this is not true.
- Additional assessment components for a potential AAC user include (a) the identification of participation patterns, (b) the identification of the individual's communication needs, (c) a capabilities assessment, (d) a symbol assessment, and (e) feature matching.
- The System for Augmenting Language (SAL) is a total-immersion approach to teaching language comprehension and use. The SAL approach uses graphic symbols to help students communicate for social purposes. Students who use SAL learn to use referential and social-regulatory symbols in a variety of communication environments. Visual scene displays (VSDs) can be used in an intervention program to support language by organizing vocabulary and communicative messages in a scene display rather than in a grid format. The advantages are that VSDs use scenes representing familiar events and activities; this maximizes meaningfulness and preserves the authenticity of everyday life. There is evidence that the Picture Exchange Communication System (PECS) helps children learn to request by exchanging a picture system for a desired object. There is limited evidence supporting PECS as a language development intervention program.
- An ethnic group is a group of individuals who share a common language, heritage, religion, or geography/nationality. More than half of SLPs' clients are non-European

American ethnic minorities; however, the majority of SLPs are of European American descent. This variation in practitioner–student cultural experience can result in ethnic mismatch.

Discussion and In-Class Activities

1. In the past, AAC was thought of as an approach of last resort. Results from numerous studies provide evidence that using an AAC approach supports language development and provides another mode of communication. Interview an SLP. Ask if he or she has used an AAC approach to support language. If so, how did he or she measure progress? Did he or she have support from the family? Did he or she use any of the AAC interventions introduced in this chapter? What were the outcomes?

2. Go to the website developed by Drs. Janice Light and David McNaughton at http://aacliteracy.psu.edu to learn about the evidence and resources supporting literacy development for children with CCNs.

3. Role-play a discussion you might have with a classroom teacher. The teacher is concerned that using an AAC system with a child in her classroom might limit the child's efforts at verbal speech.

4. Role-play a scenario in which a grandparent, an aunt, and an uncle accompany the parents to the child's AAC assessment. It is clear that the parents defer to the grandparents and the uncle. After the role-play interaction, discuss the session. Brainstorm other possible ways the session could have been handled. Invite an individual from a collectivist culture to class and have him or her view the role-play. Ask for feedback regarding techniques that may have facilitated the interaction.

5. Go to the website of the AAC-RERC and view the webcasts "AAC interventions to maximize language development for young children," at http://aac-rerc.psu.edu/index.php/webcasts/show/id/7, and "Maximizing the literacy skills of individuals who require AAC," at http://aac-rerc.psu.edu/index.php/webcasts/show/id/1. Take the quiz and submit it as a class assignment, or discuss one of the webcasts with your classmates.

Chapter 11 Case Study 1

Background. Ben is a 4-year-old boy who lives with his parents and 6-year-old brother. Ben's mother reports having had a normal pregnancy with no complications and an unremarkable birth at 39 weeks. Ben has a history of multiple ear infections and has been diagnosed with spastic cerebral palsy. Ben is ambulatory, with the assistance of a walker. He uses speech to communicate, but he has dysarthria, which results in imprecise articulation. Ben's parents report that they understand his speech about 50% of the time, but other communication partners understand only 25% of his speech. Ben's parents are concerned because Ben often gets frustrated when he has difficulty expressing himself and when he is not understood. Ben is starting prekindergarten soon, and the parents are concerned about how his communication challenges will impact his academic success and social interactions. Consider the questions presented in Focus 11.12.

Ben's Assessment.   Ben is referred to you, the school SLP. First, you plan your assessment. Refer to the Assessment section of this chapter for the components of a comprehensive AAC assessment. Let's walk through the steps of an AAC assessment together, using Ben as an example:

1. Gather case history information. I provided background information in the earlier description. These are questions I ask myself as I prepare for an assessment: When did Ben get the diagnosis of cerebral palsy? Has he received any services, medical or therapy, for symptoms related to his cerebral palsy? What modes of communication does Ben use (e.g., facial expressions, gestures, signs, speech)? Has he had his hearing tested? How many ear infections has he had? (What do you think when you hear that Ben has had multiple ear infections? How can ear infections affect language development?) Does Ben have a motor speech disorder (i.e., dysarthria)? Does Ben have feeding or swallowing difficulty? Who does Ben communicate with? Where does Ben communicate? What does Ben communicate about? Are those topics similar to those of other 4-year-old boys?

2. Identify participation patterns. How will you do this? Why is it important for you to know about typically developing 4-year-old children? How will you determine if there are any barriers affecting Ben's participation in life situations?

3. Complete a communication needs assessment. You will need to interview Ben's parents and observe and interact with Ben at his home. Let's say you discover that Ben communicates in the following environments, with the following partners, and about the following topics. What other information might be missing?

Current Partners	Environments	Topics
Parents	Home	Toys
Sibling	Relatives' homes	Food
Grandparents	Parks	Books
Friends	Church	TV
People from church	Stores	Family
People in the community	Restaurants	

FOCUS 11.12   *Clinical Skill Building*

Can you think of any other questions you would want to ask before you begin the assessment? Why is it important to gather this information before you begin your assessment with Ben?

4. Complete a capability assessment. For this example, assume that your capability assessment reveals the following:

   a. Ben passed his hearing screening.
   b. Ben's parents report that Ben had his vision checked recently, and there are no concerns.
   c. Ben's receptive language skills are at expected levels for his chronological age; his expressive language is delayed, and he has an MLU of 2.2. Examples of Ben's utterances include "Where doggie?" "Doggie running" and "Play car."
   d. Ben recognizes 75% of the letters in the alphabet.
   e. Ben's speech is characterized by imprecise articulation and low volume from a moderate spastic dysarthria.
   f. The occupational therapist (OT) and the physical therapist (PT) report that Ben is right-hand dominant but uses both hands for gross and fine motor tasks. Ben holds and uses large crayons and large pencils with built-up grips. He ambulates with the assistance of a walker. A basket could be mounted on the front of Ben's walker to hold an AAC system.

5. Complete a symbol assessment. You find that Ben successfully understands and uses symbols representing concepts in photographs, as well as both black-and-white and colored line drawings. He does not read words at this time.

6. Remember to include AAC system features trials in your assessment:

   a. **Symbols:** Interactive play activities are used to teach Ben the meaning of symbols and provide opportunities for him to use the symbols. Given the results of the symbols assessment, colored line drawings with the printed word are used in each activity.
   b. **Aids:** Different types of aids are used to augment Ben's input (i.e., teach Ben new vocabulary) and facilitate his participation in play activities. A nonelectronic communication board, an SGD with digitized speech (i.e., human-recorded speech), and an SGD with synthesized speech (i.e., computer-generated speech) are all tried with Ben during the assessment. Ben uses all types of aids successfully during the assessment. He independently communicates messages and answers questions using an electronic SGD with speech output.
   c. **Strategies:** Ben is taught and uses symbols to generate sentences using the sequencing of two or three symbols, is taught to use symbols to represent entire messages for quick communication (i.e., encoding), and is given opportunities to use VSDs to facilitate understanding of language concepts and expression of ideas from family photos from a recent vacation.
   d. **Techniques:** Ben is successful with directly selecting symbols and areas on both nonelectronic aids and electronic aids with his right index finger. His accuracy for selection is 100%.

e. **Selection set:** Ben is successful using static displays during interactive activities to request activities, answer questions, and express his feelings. He also is successful using a dynamic display as he navigates between pages with minimal prompting to talk about his interests, request an activity, and participate in a card game. Ben uses VSDs successfully during the assessment session. He demonstrates understanding of language concepts displayed on visual scenes, uses the display to request activities, and initiates a topic regarding a recent family trip (using a family photograph Ben's parents have brought to the assessment).

Writing an Intervention Plan.   You learned about Ben's current communication. Now it is time to formulate an intervention plan. You know Ben has complex communication needs (CCNs) secondary to his dysarthria and expressive language impairment. Why would Ben benefit from an AAC approach to treatment? An AAC approach would facilitate his expressive language development, meet his current communication needs, and address participation patterns for now and in the future.

Based on the assessment results, a multi-modal communication intervention approach including an AAC system is recommended. Answer these questions: Which modes of communication does Ben use? How might an AAC system augment his current modes of communication and add an alternative mode? What AAC features did Ben have success using during the assessment? What AAC features would enhance Ben's communication? How might an AAC system facilitate participation in life situations for Ben? (See Focus 11.13 for more issues that should be considered). We know Ben successfully uses the following AAC features: color line drawings with the printed word, direct selection, encoding, speech output, and all types of displays. There are several different SGDs with these features, as well as mobile technology with a communication app. Your job is to match the features Ben uses successfully with an available AAC system and provide a trial period of use for him during your intervention program. Remember that AAC assessments are dynamic and ongoing. The best intervention plan will include extensive opportunities for Ben to learn his AAC system and use it in naturalistic situations.

FOCUS 11.13   *Clinical Skill Building*

What do you think when you hear that Ben gets frustrated when he experiences difficulty communicating? How is language expression different from speech production? How could difficulty producing speech impact language development?

Chapter 11 Case Study 2: Focus on Multicultural Issues

Remember that cultural awareness applies to children with a range of communication impairments. This case study features Laurimar, a child with a hearing loss (see Chapter 7 for information on hearing loss); it is provided here to foster a discussion of the application of cultural awareness with children from a nonmajority culture. Consider the questions posed in this chapter: When do you want the child to communicate when he is with the family? Who does the child usually play or interact with? What are the family routines when your child talks to adults? How might these questions guide your interactions with Laurimar's family?

The early intervention team for Laurimar, a 3-year-old with a moderate hearing loss, was meeting to discuss her goals for the coming year. Each professional spoke briefly about Laurimar's accomplishments to date, her strengths, and the areas that required continued attention. Laurimar's speech therapist was excited: "I have to admit I was really reluctant at first to meet with Laurimar at her child care center. I thought it would be too distracting, but it's really working out well." Laurimar's father was thrilled and said, "So you're helping her to talk to the other kids?" The speech therapist looked confused for a moment. "Well, in the long run. But for our weekly sessions, I've arranged to meet in a room down the hall." Laurimar's father disagreed, saying, "That's not the point of having you come to the center. We want her to be able to talk to the other kids, to make friends. You're not helping her do that when you take her out of the room!" Laurimar's mother spoke up as well: "We don't care if she doesn't sound perfect. All that matters is that she's able to play with other kids, that they understand her. What are you going to do about that?"

Questions for Discussion

1. If you were Laurimar's parents, how would you feel during the discussion above?
2. If you were a member of Laurimar's early intervention team, how would you respond to her mother's question?

Source: This Before the ABCs: Promoting School Readiness in Infants & Toddlers, by R. Partkian, 2003, Washington, DC: Zero to Three Press. Case study was written by Stephanie M. Curenton.

Appendix A

A Tutorial: The Meaning of Standard Scores

1. To begin this example, imagine that I want to find the "worst" softball throwers so that I can provide extra coaching. First, I take the children out of their classroom (by age) and measure how far each child can throw the softball. I find out that 6-year-old girls can throw the softball an average distance of 40 feet (the mean). Some girls are very good throwers; a few girls are very poor throwers (Figure A.1).

2. Then I have 10-year-old girls throw softballs. They can throw the balls farther; the mean throw for the 10-year-old girls is 60 feet (Figure A.2).

   At this point, I am a bit confused because I want to identify the girls who need the most help across the age groups. I am going to need

Figure A.2

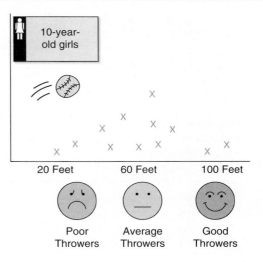

Figure A.1

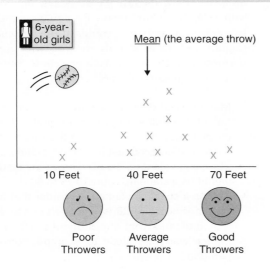

to organize the data so that I can easily determine whether each girl is a good thrower, an average thrower, or a poor thrower. I decide to give any girl who throws the ball to the mean distance (for girls her age) a score of 100 (see Figure A.3).

Remember: This *does not indicate* that the girl threw the ball 100 feet. Instead, I am assigning a score of 100 to any 10-year-old girl who throws the softball the mean distance (for 10-year-olds, a distance of 60 feet). I then assign scores to all the other 10-year-old girls to indicate how close (or far away) each girl threw in relation to the mean.

3. Now, there are several points to consider in Figure A.4. First of all, I have overlaid a

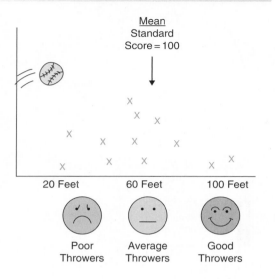

Figure A.3

bell-shaped curve over the data points. (In real life, the normative distribution would be statistically computed.) If I were to continue to document many throws by many 10-year-olds, I would end up with data that would

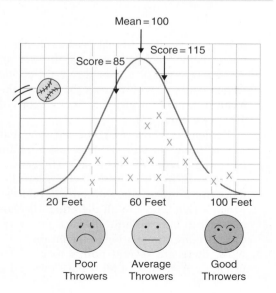

Figure A.4

resemble this curve. The height of the curve at the midpoint (the mean) indicates that more girls threw the ball this distance. As the distance gets longer (moving to the right on my graph), the curve is lower because fewer girls can throw a longer distance; the curve is lower on the left because only a few girls have significant difficulty throwing the ball. In nature, when individuals are sampled (for any behavior), this is the result. Most of us perform at an average level at most tasks. A few people are somewhat better than average, a few are somewhat worse than average; a very few are much higher than average (i.e., superior performers), and a few individuals will be much lower than average (i.e., individuals with a disability at the targeted task).

Next, in Figure A.4, I have begun to assign scores that represent each girl's throw *relative to the mean for the 10-year-old girls*. A score of 85 is less than average, and a score of 115 represents a score that is better than average. These converted scores are called *standard scores*. A standard score (SS) does not indicate the distance the ball is thrown; instead, standard scores are converted scores that allow me to document individual performance relative to same-age peers.

4. In Figure A.5, I have added standard deviations to demonstrate how the measurements are distributed. A standard deviation is the average distance a score falls from the mean score. In a normative sample, approximately 68% of the girls fall ±1 standard deviation (SD) from the mean. By going to the left approximately 1.5 standard deviations (Figure A.6), I can identify the girls who are performing at the lowest 10th percentile compared to their same-age peers.

Many school districts require a student to fall 1.5 SD below the mean to qualify for special education services. If the mean of a norm-referenced test is 100, the standard score equivalent for 1.5 SD below the mean would be a standard score of 79 to 80.

As a specific example, consider that a standard score of 98 is a converted score that indicates that the student's performance was very close to average, compared to her peers.

Figure A.5

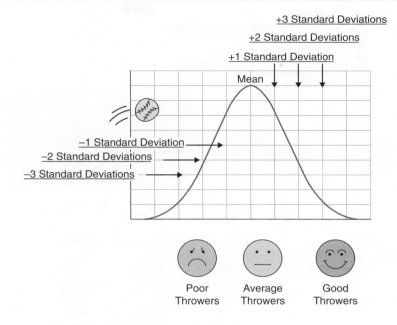

Figure A.6

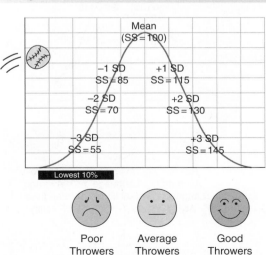

Standard scores also can be converted to percentile rank—an indication of an individual's relative standing in terms of percentage. The percentile rank indicates the percentage of people or scores that fall at or below a specific score on the bell-shaped curve. If an individual achieves a percentile rank of 60%, it means that 40% in the sample had higher scores.

5. I hope it is clear by this point that using standard scores allows me to use the same scoring system for children of different ages. Remember that a score represents where a child performs relative to her peers. So, a score of 100 for a 6-year-old girl indicates that she was able to throw the ball 40 feet (refer to Figure A.7), whereas a score of 100 for a 10-year-old girl indicates that she threw the ball 60 feet (Figure A.7).

In both age groups, if I select the girls who receive a standard score below 80, I will have identified the girls who are the most in need of some additional coaching to improve their skills.

6. In Figure A.8, I demonstrate how this example pertains to children with a language disorder. Using a norm-referenced test, I can identify where a child performs on a tested language skill compared with other children her age. If

Figure A.7

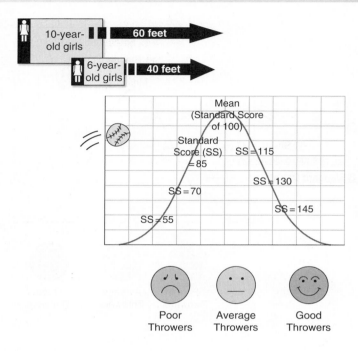

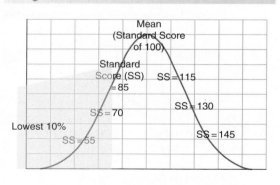

the standard score is between 85 and 115 (±1 standard deviation), I know that the child's language ability is average. If she falls higher than 115, her language ability is higher than average. If her standard score is between 80 and 85, her language ability is somewhat below average. A standard score below 80 indicates that the child is performing at the lowest 10th percentile compared to other children her age.

It is important to note that not all norm-referenced tests have a mean of 100; some tests, for example, have a mean of 50. Regardless of the conversion that is used, the standard score reflects how close (or far away) the child's performance is compared to that of her same-age peers.

Figure A.8

Mean
(Standard Score
of 100)

Standard
Score (SS)
= 85   SS = 115

SS = 130

SS = 70

Lowest 10%   SS = 145

SS = 55

Below-
Average
Language
Ability

Average
Language
Ability

Above-
Average
Language
Ability

Appendix B

T-Unit Analysis*

As you learned in Chapter 3, once a student begins to communicate in longer utterances, the assessor uses an alternative technique called T-unit analysis instead of computing mean length of utterance. In Chapter 3, I provided a brief discussion of T-unit analysis. In this appendix, I provide a more step-by-step description of the process.

1. Adolescents in the school setting typically can be engaged in a story retelling based on favorite movies, books, or television shows. It also is a good idea to obtain a spontaneous writing sample to include in an analysis; the writing sample can be analyzed in the same way as an oral sample, and the T-unit productions can be compared. Obtain a language sample of at least 50 utterances by audiotaping a one-to-one interaction with a student.

2. Transcribe and type the utterances on a computer for readability. Syntactical structures are analyzed in terminable units. A *terminable unit* (*T-unit*) is a main clause with all subordinate clauses embedded in it. To get started, you should first look for coordinating conjunctions—*and, but, or, so*—to divide your sentences into T-units. A T-unit should be able to stand on its own and make sense.

3. Count the number of T-units. Then count the number of words (not morphemes) in each T-unit. Complete your T-unit analysis by completing the following steps: (a) separate the sample into T-units whenever there is a coordinating conjunction, (b) count the number of words in each T-unit, (c) compute the mean T-unit score by dividing the total number of words by total number of T-units, and (d) consider how many T-units contain complexity (described later in this appendix). Incomplete sentences that answer questions are excluded when counting T-units.

Normal development of syntax includes simple, compound, and complex sentences. One type of complex sentence is sentences containing subordinating clauses (marked with [ ] in the examples below). In a T-unit analysis, when you divide up the T-units, *first* you look for compound sentences so that you can separate a compound sentence into multiple T-units, and *then* you look for T-units that contain complexity (e.g., subordinating clauses, gerunds). A complete list of syntax forms that are considered to represent complex syntax can be found in Chapter 3. The following are examples of how you divide up sentences into T-units:

- **Simple:** There's a traffic jam today. (1 T-unit)
- **Simple:** She could take the freeway or the turnpike. (1 T-unit)
- **Compound:** There's a traffic jam today // <u>so</u> I will be late for work // <u>and</u> my boss will be mad. (3 T-units)

*Courtesy of Maryjane Palmer

- **Compound:** There's a traffic jam today // <u>and</u> I saw a car crash on the way to work. (2 T-units).
- **Compound:** There is a traffic jam today // <u>but</u> it didn't make me late for work. (2 T-units).
- **Compound:** I can drive to work via the freeway // <u>or</u> I can drive to work via side streets. (2 T-units).
- **Complex:** [If there is traffic jam today], I'm going to find a different way to drive to work [since I don't want to be late]. (1 T-unit)
- **Complex:** Drivers get frustrated [whenever there is a traffic jam]. (1 T-unit)

After you have separated the sentences containing coordinating conjunctions, you look for complex sentences containing subordination, using words such as *after, although, as, as if, because, before, even if, if, since, unless, until, when, whenever, wherever, whereas,* and *while*. In the examples above, the last two sentences demonstrate the speaker's use of complex sentences. In a T-unit analysis, you do not separate a sentence containing a subordinating clause, because subordinating clauses cannot stand on their own. You are interested in looking for T-units that contain subordinating clauses because they provide evidence that the student can produce complex sentences. Students with language impairment have difficulty formulating subordinating clauses and complex sentences. A student with a higher mean T-unit will be producing more complex sentences than a student with a lower mean T-unit.

4. Compare the average number of words in the elicited language sample to the average number of words for spoken samples and written samples. Determine whether the student's mean T-unit is below what you would expect for his or her peer group using the data provided in Table B.1.
5. This is an example of a T-unit analysis:

SLP: Do you have any pets?
Student:

   a. *3 cats* / **not a T-unit**
   b. *One got run over by a car* [*when I was younger*] / **T-unit, 11 words** (Note use of passive verb phrase, subordinating clause[*])
   c. *One just ran away* / **T-unit, 4 words**
   d. *Um* <u>and</u> *the cat this year got eaten somehow* / **T-unit, 8 words** (Note use of the filler *um*)
   e. *We let him out of the house* / **T-unit, 7 words**
   f. <u>and</u> *we guess that a coyote found him* / **T-unit, 8 words** (Note use of *that* as an object)
   g. *They live like in a canyon out there* / **T-unit, 8 words** (Note use of the filler *like*, prepositional phrase)
   h. *I guess like back of the field* / **T-unit, 7 words** (Note use of the filler *like*, prepositional phrase)
   i. *I've never been there exactly* / **T-unit, 5 words**
   j. <u>but</u> *I hear coyotes at night* / **T-unit, 6 words** (Note use of prepositional phrase)

Average words per T-unit: 7.1 (64 words / 9 T-units = 7.1). The student is in eighth grade. Is his mean T-unit within normal limits?

---

[*]During the school-age years, students developing typically will begin to use a variety of more sophisticated syntax forms, including appositives, elaborated subjects, and other features such as nonfinite clauses, prepositional phrases, and relative clauses. It is beyond the scope of this undergraduate text to define all these grammatical forms; this will be an area of focus in your future training as a speech-language pathologist or educational practitioner.

Table B.1   **Mean Number of Words per T-Unit in Spoken and Written Samples**

Grade	Spoken samples	Written samples
7	9.72	8.98
8	10.71	10.30
9	10.96	10.05
10	10.68	11.79
11	11.17	10.67

Source: Information from *Language Development: Kindergarten through Grade Twelve*, Research Report No. 18, p. 35, by W. L. Loban, 1976, Urbana, IL: National Teachers of English.

6. To understand why the use of complex sentences will result in a higher mean T-unit score, complete the following exercise. First, watch the fun video *Beatbox Brilliance*, at www.youtube.com/watch?feature=player_embedded&v=GNZBSZD16cY#at=118.

After watching the video, work in a group to make different levels of language samples. Some groups should write 10 complex sentences such as "Tom Thum is able to use his voice and sound as if he is playing an instrument." Other groups should write 10 compound sentences such as "Tom Thum uses his voice in an interesting way, and I liked to hear the different sounds." Finally, some groups should write 10 simple sentences such as "Tom Thum makes a lot of interesting sounds." Switch language samples (so that each group is computing a T-unit analysis from one of the other groups). Compare the final results. Which group has the highest mean T-unit? How do the mean T-unit scores from the simple sentence group and the compound sentence groups compare?

7. Remember that the reason you use T-unit analysis with older school-age students is that students with language impairments often talk in long sentences, but the sentences do not contain complexity (e.g., subordinating conjunctions).

Report Writing

SPEECH AND LANGUAGE ASSESSMENT REPORT

	Comments on report
Client's Name: Thad Smith **Parent's Name:** Ms. Jane Jones **Address:** **Phone Number:** **E-mail:** **Chronological Age:** 5:6 **Date of Birth:** **Date of Evaluation:** **Name of Evaluator:**	• The required demographic information is typically specified by the school, hospital, or clinic. Fill in as required.

I. CASE HISTORY INFORMATION AND STATEMENT OF PROBLEM:

Thad is a male, 5 years and 6 months old, seen for a speech-language evaluation at XXXX clinic. His mother, Ms. Jones, stated that Thad has difficulty understanding others and communicating his ideas. She stated that Thad has problems "putting his words together in a coherent fashion."

Ms. Jones's pregnancy was unremarkable. At birth, however, Thad was suspected as having meningitis. He was tube-fed for 1 week. Final testing for meningitis was negative. At age 2 years, Thad had a high fever virus that caused two consecutive seizures; he was hospitalized for 3 days. No other medical concerns were noted.

Ms. Jones reported that Thad achieved all physical milestones as expected. She first noted Thad's speech delay when he was 2 years old. Thad began to use single words at age 2½ and two-word combinations at 3½. Presently, Thad uses one- or two-word combinations to communicate. No other members of the family have a history of speech or language delay.

Thad is in a preprimary full-day program for children with special educational needs at XXX school.

• Be as concise as possible, but include all relevant information.

EXAMINATION FINDINGS

II.   ASSOCIATED AREAS

Thad's hearing was screened and was within normal limits for both ears.

    The examiner completed an oral-facial examination to assess Thad's oral mechanism. Structure and function of articulators (lips, tongue, jaw) were normal. Thad was able to rapidly repeat syllables ("*pa-ta-ka*") in imitation of the examiner.

    Thad's voice quality was assessed informally and was within normal limits. Fluency and rate of speech were normal. Cognitive abilities were informally assessed in play and with drawing tasks; Thad performed at levels consistent with his chronological age.

    Gross and fine motor skills were informally assessed and were within normal limits; Thad was able to hop on one foot, walk a straight line, and hold a pencil in the proper position as he copied a letter *T*.

- Hearing, oral-motor, voice, fluency, cognitive, and fine/gross motor skills were assessed informally.

III.   SPEECH

The examiner administered the Goldman-Fristoe Test of Articulation–2 to assess Thad's production of consonants in the beginning, middle, and final positions in words. Thad substituted /w/ for /r/ in all positions in words and /d/ for /th/ at the beginning of words. Thad achieved a percentile rank of 54%, indicating that his ability to produce sounds in words is within normal limits. The noted sound errors are not produced correctly until ages 6 to 7 for many children developing typically.

- The purposes of the test are described briefly.
- The writer clarifies why the noted speech errors are not considered to be a deficit area.

IV.   LANGUAGE

Language use (pragmatics)

Thad's ability to communicate his needs was accomplished both verbally (single words and some word combinations) and nonverbally (pointing, gesturing, sounds). During play, Thad was able to greet the examiner, label items, request help, comment on actions (he said "oh-oh" when the blocks fell down), request information and objects, and deny (said "no" when asked if he wanted to play with the doll). He took turns during block play. He stayed in the

- The writer defines pragmatic use and gives examples to clarify terms as appropriate.
- The writer included a description of the earliest pragmatic skills (turn taking, eye contact) as well as pragmatic skills typically seen in toddlers and preschoolers (requesting, labeling, etc.)
- Because Thad is at the one-to two-word level, later-occurring discourse skills (e.g., clarifying topic) were not addressed.

interaction with the examiner, demonstrated appropriate eye contact, and had appropriate facial expressions and affect (i.e., smiling, laughter). Thad demonstrates appropriate use of early-developing pragmatic skills.

Language content (semantics) and following directions

Thad's understanding of word meaning was assessed both formally and informally.

The examiner administered the subtests of the Clinical Evaluation of Language Function–Preschool 2 (CELF-P-2) to evaluate Thad's use and understanding of words and his ability to understand and follow concepts and directions. Subtest scores are as follows:

CELF-P-2 semantic subtests	Standard score (SS) & percentile	Normal range percentile
Concepts & Following Directions (receptive)	4 (SS) 2%	Above 10th percentile
Word Classes Total (receptive & expressive)	4 (SS) 2%	Above 10th percentile
Expressive Vocabulary	3 (SS) 1%	Above 10th percentile

Informal assessment during the play session confirmed the results of the CELF-P-2. Thad was able to follow one-step but not two-step commands. Thad was able to name seven body parts and count to 10 by rote but had difficulty understanding descriptive words (e.g., "Show me the biggest truck," "Show me the old shoe") or following directions containing prepositions ("Put the ball under the table," "Show me the book that is on the box.")

Thad's use of words to communicate and express meaning was noted during the play session. Thad's mean length of utterance (MLU; average number of words used to communicate) was 1.9. This MLU places Thad at Brown's Stage I, a level typically achieved by children between 18 and 24 months. Children

- Thad's standard score and percentile are provided. The normal range is given to aid interpretation. On the CELF-P-2, the subtest mean is 10 and one standard deviation is ± 3 (i.e., scores between 7 and 13 are within 1 standard deviation).
- The results of the informal assessment elaborate and clarify the results of the norm-referenced testing. The writer gives examples so that the reader can understand the implication of Thad's difficulties with understanding word meanings.
- Because Thad is at Brown's Stage I, (MLU 1–2), his use of word combinations is discussed in this section of language content (i.e., semantics). For an older child who is beginning to use morphology, MLU and the language sample analysis information would be included under language form (i.e., syntax).
- Thad's MLU is used to gauge where he is on Brown's stages. Comparison information is provided to aid the reader's interpretation.
- Number of different words (NDW) is provided.
- This description of MLU and NDW describes Thad's quantitative data for his language sample analysis.

who are age 5 with typical language development are generally at Brown's Stage V+ and have an MLU of 4+ words.

Thad's vocabulary consisted primarily of concrete nouns (e.g., *truck, block, ball, shoe, tummy, cracker*), with limited verb use. Only the verbs *want, go, give,* and *night-night* ("me night-night") were noted. Modifiers consisted of *my* and *no* (e.g., "no dolly," "my shoe"). In total, Thad used 45 different words in a 100-utterance language sample. By age 6, children developing typically generally use 117 words in a 100-utterance sample.

Language form (syntax) and morphology

Syntax refers to word order, and morphology refers to grammatical forms (plural *s*, past tense *ed*). Thad's spontaneous speech did not contain age-appropriate syntax or morphological complexity. The earliest forms of grammatical complexity produced by children developing typically include plural *s*, possessive *s* (e.g., "mommy's shoe"), the *ing* verb (*walking*), and irregular past tense verbs (*ate, went*). Thad did not use these morphological forms generally produced by children between 2 and 3 years old. Thad used unmarked verbs and nouns (i.e., root word with no morphological endings).

Thad used an early-developing pattern for question forms. For example, he used voice inflection ("*Me go?*") rather than the more advanced syntax ("*Can I go?*"). Thad did not use auxiliary verbs (i.e. helping verbs, as in "Dog is going.").

The following expressive subtests on the CELF-P-2 corroborate the analysis obtained by Thad's spontaneous language sample.

CELF-P-2 syntax subtests	Standard score (SS) & percentile	Normal range percentile
Word Structure (expressive)	4 (SS) 2%	Above 10th percentile
Sentence Structure (expressive)	4 (SS) 2%	Above 10th percentile

- This description of Thad's difficulties with morphology and syntax reviews the qualitative data from his language sample analysis.
- The morphological structures documented within Brown's stages are listed for the reader so that the writer can describe Thad's complexity as compared to a child developing typically.

- Interrogative reversals are often very difficult for children with language impairments (LI), because they require a variation of the typical subject–verb–object word order and require the use of the auxiliary verb *can* (in this example). You will learn more about the syntax problems of children with LI in Chapter 5.
- The summed scores on the CELF-P-2 reinforce the information reported in the rest of the report. If there were discrepancies between subtest scores or if there were inconsistent results between the naturalistic assessments and the norm-referenced findings, the writer would clarify the results.
- The confidence ranges for the percentile score refer to the standard error of measure (SEM). Because a student's score is not "absolute," his performance can vary. The testing manual provides a numeric value that is subtracted from and added to the child's standard score to obtain a range of scores at a 90% confidence interval. This means that one can be 90% sure that the child's true score (i.e., the range of possible scores he could obtain if tested repeatedly) would fall between the reported percentile range.

Combined scores for the CELF-P-2. Overall, Thad's combined core language score was 71, interpreted as a percentile rank range of 1%–7% (90% confidence interval). His receptive score for the CELF-P-2 was a standard score of 69 and a percentile rank range (90% confidence interval) of 1%–5%. His expressive combined standard score was 67, interpreted as a percentile rank range (90% confidence interval) of 1%–4%.

In summary, Thad's observational assessments, language sample analysis, and results on the CELF-P-2 indicate a severe receptive-expressive language impairment in the areas of semantics (word meaning), syntax (word order), and morphology (grammar forms).

V. CONCLUSIONS AND RECOMMENDATIONS

Thad presents as a child who has cognitive skills that are within normal limits but with a history of language delay. Formal and informal assessments demonstrate an average level of speech production ability (i.e., ability to produce sounds) but severely impaired receptive and expressive language skills.

Thad is able to use verbal and nonverbal skills to communicate his needs. He does, however, demonstrate significant delays in vocabulary growth. His utterances are reduced in length and complexity.

Because Thad (a) was able to sustain attention to a task and (b) has positive family support, the prognosis for language improvement is good with regular (two to three times weekly) intervention and a home language stimulation program.

Recommendations include:

1. Increase production and comprehension of vocabulary, particularly focusing on action words (i.e., verbs), modifiers, and early-developing prepositions (*in, on*).
2. Increase word combinations through interactive play and book reading, using modeling, recasting, and elaboration of Thad's productions.

- There should be no surprises in the summary section or in the recommendations. That is to say, the writer cannot make a recommendation for a language domain that has not been justified in the preceeding report. So, for example, in the recommendations, it would be inappropriate to make a recommendation to provide speech intervention because, in the report, the writer indicates that Thad's speech is within normal limits.

- The rationale for any intervention must be substantiated by data results in the body of the report.
- The need for ongoing formative assessment (using language sample analysis) is highlighted. It is likely that once intervention begins, Thad's expressive skills may change rapidly. The professional will monitor his progress and alter the focus of intervention (potentially focusing

3. Introduce early-developing morphemes (*ing, ed,* plural *s*) when Thad begins to produce two- to three-word combinations spontaneously.
4. Continue to monitor Thad's ability to produce sounds in speech and reevaluate his use of modifiers, auxiliary forms, and pronouns, etc., with periodic language sample analysis.
5. Meet with Thad's preschool teacher to coordinate language programming in his preschool program.

more on syntax and morphology) as Thad's utterance length improves.

Language Sample Analysis Worksheet

Child's Name:	Chronological Age:	Language Sample Analysis (LSA) Step # 1 (Quantitative Analysis)								
Examiner:	Date of sample:	LSA Step #2 (Qualitative Analysis) Notes								
List Utterances Below:	(A) Pragmatic Functions (✓ Check one)							(B) Semantic Roles and Relations (Describe)	(C) Bound Morphemes and Brown's Stage Morpheme Typically Appears	# of morp.
	Requests	*Declarations*	*Answer questions*	*Agree/disagree*	*Social speech*	*Imitation*	*Other*	Examples Agent Action Object Modifier Negation Agent + Action Action + Object Agent + Action Modifier + X Negation + X X + Location	Examples of bound morphemes Present progressive (*ing*) Prepositions (*in, on*) Plural (*s*) Present tense aux. (*can, will*) Possessive ('*s*) Irregular past tense verb Articles (*a, the*) Copula and auxiliary "*BE*" Regular past tense verbs (*ed*) 3rd-person singular verb (*s*)	

Possible intervention goals include:

American Speech-Language-Hearing Association. (2003). American English dialects [Technical Report]. Available from www.asha.org/policy.

Appendix E

Tutorial on African American English and Identifying a Language Disorder vs. a Language Difference

Before you begin this tutorial, go to the University of North Carolina website (www.learnnc.org/lp/pages/4816) and *read the information and watch the video* on African American English (AAE). Note that AAE has phonological, lexical (i.e., vocabulary), pragmatic, and morphosyntax variations compared to General American English (GAE). However, in this tutorial I concentrate solely on the morphosyntax differences between AAE and GAE.

Review important terminology:

- **African American English (AAE):** The variety of English used by many (but not all) African Americans.
- **Code switching:** The practice of moving between variations of a language in different contexts. Many African Americans switch between GAE and AAE, depending on the social situation.
- **Contrastive morphosyntax features:** Morphosyntax features unique to AAE (e.g., zero copula, zero third-person present tense, zero past tense). The implication of contrastive features is that an individual who uses AAE may not use the copula verb, third-person regular verbs, past tense *ed* verb endings, etc., but regardless have typical language development.
- **Dialect or linguistic patterns:** The various language forms are arranged in regular and predictable ways.
- **Dialect:** A form of a language spoken by a group of people from the same regional or cultural background. Everyone speaks a dialect, but some dialects are more noticeable than others.

- **General American English (GAE):** A variety of English that is taught in school. In the United States, the Midwest typically is identified as where GAE is spoken.
- **Noncontrastive morphosyntax features:** Morphosyntax features are shared between GAE and AAE (e.g., pronouns, articles, demonstratives, complex sentences). The implication of noncontrastive features is that if an individual who uses AAE has problems using pronouns, articles, demonstratives, or complex sentences, he or she may have language impairment.
- **Optional use:** Refers to a speaker's use of a particular linguistic structure at some times and not others.

Consider the policy of the American Speech-Language-Hearing Association (ASHA, 2003b):

> It is the position of the American Speech-Language-Hearing Association (ASHA) that no dialectal variety of American English is a disorder or a pathological form of speech or language. Each dialect is adequate as a functional and effective variety of American English. Each serves a communicative function as well as a social-solidarity function. Each dialect maintains the communication network and the social construct of the community of speakers who use it. Furthermore, each is a symbolic representation of the geographic, historical, social, and cultural background of its speakers.

Consider the following concern, challenge, and clinical problem. There is *concern* regarding assessment of children who are African American, because although there are approximately 70,000 speech-language pathologists (SLPs) registered with ASHA, fewer than 3% of them identify themselves as African American (ASHA 2004e; 2006c). This number is significantly less than the 13% of the general population that identifies itself as African American (Charity, 2008). The *challenge* is that it can be difficult for a GAE-speaking SLP to differentiate a child with a language disorder from a child with a language difference (e.g., a child who uses AAE). Often children who speak AAE are misdiagnosed. For example, African Americans are overly identified as having special educational needs (Charity, 2008; Seymour, 2004).

Dr. Harry Seymour (2004) suggests that the *clinical problem* is that the linguistic features of AAE can be similar to patterns of a language disorder. AAE is characterized by optional use of certain linguistic structures, particularly morphological inflections. The term *optional* refers to a speaker's use of a particular linguistic structure at some times but not at others. For example, AAE speakers may or may not produce a present tense sentence without a copula verb (i.e., "zero copula," *He is nice → He nice*), zero third-person present tense agreement (*She cooks → She cook*), and zero past tense *ed* (*He played yesterday → He play yesterday*). Because a language-disordered child may delete the copula *is*, third person *s*, and past tense *ed*, it can be difficult for an SLP to differentiate disordered patterns from the typical patterns spoken in AAE.

Below are the primary listed morphosyntax features sometimes mistakenly regarded as errors according to the rules of GAE. Remember that the use of these AAE features is rule governed and systematic (Bland-Stewart, 2005):

- **Zero copula** (or the deletion of the verb *be* and its variants). For example, *He a good student* (AAE) vs. *He is a good student* (GAE).
- **Lack of the past tense marker (*ed*).** For example, *Yesterday he walk home* (AAE) vs. *Yesterday he walked home* (GAE).
- **Absence of possessive *s*.** For example, *Here is Mama purse* (AAE) vs. *Here is Mama's purse* (GAE).
- **Irregular verb form.** Sometimes a past tense verb is used in place of a past participle and

vice versa—for example, *She seen him* (AAE) vs. *She saw him* (GAE) or *She knowed he was there* (AAE) vs. *She knew he was there* (GAE).
- **Absence of plural *s* marker** (with nouns of measure, such as numbers); for example, *James got 5 toy* (AAE) vs. *James got 5 toys* (GAE).
- **Use of negation in AAE.** (A) The use of ain't is permissible—for example, *She ain't coming home today* (AAE) vs. *She isn't coming home today* (GAE); (B) multiple negation—for example, *She ain't got no time for nobody*.
- **Inflection of *be*.** Using *be* to indicate a habitual action or something that occurs all the time—for example, *We be working* (AAE) translates to *We work all the time* (GAE).

Consider the possible answers to these concerns. One can follow a number of alternative approaches to distinguish a disorder from a difference in an AAE speaker (Bland-Stewart, 2005):

1. Perform a contrastive analysis on the child's language sample.

   - The SLP elicits a naturalistic language sample from the child and then analyzes the child's use of morphosyntax. In using the contrastive analysis method, the clinician separates expressive speech-language patterns that are consistent with a client's AAE dialect (e.g., use of zero copula) from patterns that represent true errors (e.g., improper use of pronouns, lack of articles, absence of complex sentences). If the language patterns are consistent with the client's dialect, then a difference, not a disorder, is indicated. If, however, the language patterns are inconsistent with the client's dialect, then they constitute "true errors," and a disorder may be suspected.

2. Evaluate the complexity of the child's utterances.

   - Consider the frequency of complexity in a child's communication unit. A child with increasing levels of sentence complexity as he or she matures is likely to be developing language in a typical fashion. (Read more about this procedure in Chapter 3.)

3. Carefully use standardized tests.

   - Use standardized tests with modifications for dialectal features, such as the *Diagnostic Evaluation of Language Variation* (DELV; Seymour, Roeper, deVilliers, 2005). The DELV is designed for children between the ages of 4 and 9 and is nondiscriminatory to non-GAE users.

4. Use alternative approaches.

   - Support test results with dynamic assessment (see Chapter 3), and use the response to intervention (RTI) approach (see Chapter 4) to determine how children progress once they are provided high-quality instruction. Allow extra time for a child's response; increase the number of practice/trial items; remove potentially culturally biased items; ask a child to explain incorrect responses; and conduct observations in the child's classroom, home, and other environments where interactions can be observed.

AAC aid A device used to send or receive messages. The aid can be nonelectronic (such as a series of photographs, a collection of objects, or a series of black-and-white or colored line drawings) or electronic.

AAC selection set How visual symbols are presented; a selection set can include fixed displays, dynamic displays, hybrid displays, or visual scene displays.

AAC strategy Methods used to communicate effectively and efficiently; used to support message timing, grammatical formulation, spelling, and communication rate (Beukelman & Mirenda, 2005). Some examples of strategies to enhance communication include prediction and encoding.

AAC technique How a message is conveyed. Some individuals point or look at their symbol; other individuals use techniques such as scanning.

Accent Speech and language patterns that reflect regional differences in phonology and semantics.

Accommodation The Piagetian concept of cognition that is demonstrated when prior schemata are adjusted to incorporate new information.

Achieving Communication Independence A comprehensive assessment for individuals with moderate to severe intellectual disability.

Adaptive behavior Conceptual, social, and life skills.

Adult-directed intervention An intervention in which the adult leads the interaction by (a) choosing the stimulus items; (b) regulating how the child will respond; (c) prompting particular responses through pointing, modeling, or the use of questions; and (d) providing direct feedback on the child's performance.

Aided symbol A symbol that requires a support (i.e., drawing) to convey the message.

Alphabetic awareness An individual's understanding of letter names and the connections between letters and sounds.

Antecedent event A stimulus that precedes a behavior; a term linked to behaviorist theory.

Applied behavior analysis (ABA; or discrete trial or Lovaas therapy) A set of principles that guide behavior-based intervention for individuals on the autism spectrum.

Assertiveness–responsiveness scheme A scheme that profiles an individual according to levels of social participation; an assertive communicator initiates conversational turns, and a responsive communicator responds to others' communication attempts.

Assimilation A Piagetian concept of cognition that is demonstrated when a child takes in new information and incorporates it into his or her existing schemata.

At risk The potential to develop a disorder, based on specific biological, environmental, or behavioral factors.

Attempt A component of a narrative story episode; it is the action that is undertaken by the story's character to solve a problem.

Attention The ability to orient and react to a specific stimulus.

Attention-deficit/hyperactivity disorder (ADHD) A disorder in which a student exhibits behaviors of impulsivity, high activity, and distractibility.

Auditory neuropathy/dys-synchrony (AN/AD) A disorder of the auditory nerve fibers at the connection point with the cochlea (synapse) or higher that causes variable hearing thresholds and reduced word recognition.

Auditory processing disorder (APD) Impaired ability to make use of spoken language and other auditory signals, despite normal hearing thresholds.

Augmentative/alternative communication (AAC) approach Systems that compensate and facilitate, temporarily or permanently, for the impairment and disability patterns of individuals with severe expressive and/or language comprehension deficits. AAC may be required for individuals demonstrating impairments in gestural, spoken, and/or written modalities.

Autism spectrum disorder (ASD) The preferred term used to describe the range of disorders in social and communication functioning.

Autistic savant An individual on the autism spectrum who has a unique talent. The unique ability is likely to be in mathematics (e.g., "lightning calculation"), memory, geography facts, or artistic/musical ability.

Backward design   An approach to decision making that advocates considering the desired results for a particular student before setting an intervention goal; after describing the ultimate goal, an SLP identifies interventions needed to equip students to achieve the ultimate goal.

Baseline   The data obtained prior to intervention; documentation of the occurrence of the target behavior before intervention.

Behavioral chaining   Reinforcement of a number of linked substeps with the goal of training a complex behavioral sequence.

Behavioral phenotype   The connection between a person's genetic endowment and observable outcome.

Behaviorism   A theory that learning occurs when an environmental stimulus triggers a response or behavior.

Bilingual-bicultural approach   An approach in which persons align themselves with the Deaf culture and communicate via sign language, learning written English as a second language.

Bilingualism   The ability to read, speak, understand, and write in two languages.

Blinding   A process whereby an individual who assesses subjects in a research study is not the same individual who directs the study or provides treatment.

Bottom-up learning (or data-based learning or data-based processing)   Learning guided by perceptual processes, interpreted as they are passed up to higher-order levels; specific subskills needed to accomplish an overall task.

Buildup/breakdown   A language modeling technique in which an adult deconstructs a sentence into its separate components (e.g., noun phrase, verb phrase, prepositional phrase, adverb, and adjective clauses) and then builds the sentence back to its original form.

Case grammar   A semantic theory, proposed by Fillmore, which states that children's semantic use of words precedes syntax and is guided by universal concepts.

Case history   A review of the written documentation of a child or student to obtain background information on developmental, medical, and educational history.

Central auditory processing disorder (CAPD)   Refers to the efficiency and effectiveness by which the central nervous system uses auditory information.

Chaining   A complex behavioral sequence is broken down into smaller units so the child can be trained to complete a multistep task.

Child-directed intervention   An intervention in which an adult follows a child's lead, responds contingently to the child's responses, and waits for the child to respond before initiating another conversational sequence.

Chronic otitis media   Repeated or ongoing inflammation of the middle ear caused by infection.

Chunking   Organizing items into familiar, manageable units.

Classroom-based model of service delivery   The practitioner works with a student in the classroom; the curriculum materials or ongoing classroom activities are the stimulus for communication.

Classroom discourse   Academic discourse is often characterized by the teacher's initiation of a question, the teacher's evaluation of the student's verbal contribution, and the teacher's control of the conversational topic; classroom discourse also is viewed as the mechanism that facilitates students' high-level thinking skill.

Cochlear implant   A device implanted in the cochlea of an individual with significant hearing loss that enables access to auditory signals.

Code switching   An individual's ability to alternate between formal and informal language; it also refers to an individual's ability to vary between dialectal language patterns and General American English.

Cognitive perceptual processing skills   Attention, discrimination, organization, transfer, and memory.

Cognitive theory   Based on the writings of Jean Piaget, a proposed sequence of progressively more sophisticated cognitive abilities from sensorimotor stage to advanced cognitive ability in the formal operations stage.

Cognitive verbs   Verbs used to describe the actions and thoughts of characters in text; includes words like *thought, knew, remembered, decided, imagined, forgot, asked, told, explained, called,* and *yelled.*

Cohesive language   Language features that require a speaker or writer to use words linking information from one sentence to another. Includes linkage between an introduced referent and a pronoun referring back to the referent and subordinating conjunctions, such as *because, so, then,* or *therefore.*

Collectivist culture   A culture that focuses on interdependence among group members and the well-being of the extended family.

Communication   Transfer of symbolic and nonsymbolic information (i.e., facial expressions, body language, gestures) between interaction partners.

Communication forms (or communication means) The way in which a child communicates, including gestures, nonlinguistic sounds, spoken or signed word or pictured symbols, and combinations of words or signs.

Communication functions (or communication intentions or communication acts) The goal of a communication attempt, such as requesting, commenting, refusing, protesting, sharing emotion, initiating a topic, or continuing a topic.

Communication intent Intent demonstrated when an individual exhibits (a) gestures, vocalization, and/or eye contact to direct the attention or actions of a communication partner; (b) joint visual attention; (c) waiting after a communication attempt (i.e., expecting the partner to respond); or (d) persisting in a communication attempt that is not understood.

Communication means see *Communication forms*

Communication modality The method one uses to exchange information or ideas. May include spoken language and/or sign language.

Communication probe An interaction designed to elicit a specific child response.

Communication subdomains An elaborated version of the form–content–use chart developed by the author; used to explain how the speech-language pathologist prioritizes the language domains when working with an individual who has a language disorder.

Communication temptations Orchestrated situations in which the situation is "sabotaged," heightening the child's need to communicate (e.g., favorite toys are placed out of reach, desired items are placed in containers requiring adult assistance).

Complex communication needs (CCNs) Needs of children who have difficulty with processing, comprehending, or producing language, resulting in unmet communication needs.

Composition skill An individual's ability to integrate pragmatic, syntax, and semantic language domains to formulate and express thought.

Conductive hearing loss A hearing loss that results from diseases or obstructions in the outer or middle ear.

Consequence A component of a story episode underlying narrative structure; the result of the character's attempt to solve the problem.

Construct validity The underlying theory on which an assessment instrument is based.

Content validity The degree to which test items represent a defined domain.

Contingency The semantic and pragmatic links between a language facilitator's communication and a child's output.

Continuous reinforcement A system in which every correct response is followed by an event, increasing the probability that the response will be repeated.

Continuum of naturalness A continuum of behaviors describing treatment intervention ranging from a strong adult (clinician)–directed approach (typically in a one-to-one adult–child interaction) to an approach that is child directed and takes place within the child's everyday interactions.

Conventional reading An individual's ability to decode unfamiliar words and draw meaning from written text.

Conversational assertiveness The ability to initiate conversational turns.

Conversational discourse Unstructured or unplanned spoken interactions that occur between two individuals.

Conversational recast treatment (CRT) An intervention in which the targeted grammatical feature is produced very frequently during the intervention session; the adult uses sentence recasts.

Conversational repair strategies Verbal behaviors exhibited by a speaker or listener during a communication breakdown.

Conversational responsiveness The ability to respond to others' communication attempts.

Coordinating attention Following an infant's focus of attention and matching a child's communication to his or her eye gaze.

Criterion-referenced assessment Assessment that is used to evaluate an individual's ability relative to a predetermined level of performance, often used to measure progress in intervention.

Criterion-related validity The degree to which results on one test align with those of another test measuring the same construct.

Critical question A question that demands that an individual draw on his or her value system for an answer.

Cultural self-awareness A trait that begins when a practitioner examines values, beliefs, and patterns of behavior that are part of his or her own cultural identity.

Cultural sensitivity Awareness and lack of judgment about the cultural practices of various groups.

Curriculum-based language assessment An assessment process that considers the academic content and social interaction demands of the curriculum, the skills the student brings to the curriculum, the knowledge and skill needed to succeed academically, and identification of instructional modifications to enhance a student's academic success.

Cyclic goal attack strategy   A strategy in which several goals are targeted, each for a specified time period independent of accuracy, with a repeating sequence.

Data-based processing   Processing that is based on incoming data; it is sometimes called bottom-up processing.

Data collection   Clinical procedures that (a) allow an SLP to track a student's progress from one session to another, (b) document the effectiveness of an intervention approach, and (c) maximize the effectiveness of the intervention.

Deaf culture   A system of customs and beliefs shared by individuals with prelingual hearing loss.

Decibel (dB)   A unit of measurement related to hearing threshold.

Decision tree   A graphic illustration of the alternatives in the decision-making process.

Decoding   The ability to translate a word from print to speech, usually by employing knowledge of sound–symbol correspondences. It is also the act of deciphering a new word by sounding it out.

Decontextualized language   Language features that allow the listener to understand what is spoken or written without background information or environmental cues.

Deep structure   Chomsky's principle describing the underlying meaning of the sentence the speaker wants to produce.

Degree of hearing loss   The severity of hearing loss (e.g., mild, moderate, severe, profound).

Delayed language development   A child's language abilities do not follow the typical developmental timetable.

Descriptive-developmental approach   An approach that describes an individual's language use by focusing on his or her level of language development and functioning within natural contexts.

Developmental synchrony   A cumulative practice of auditory and language brain centers to perfect a developing skill such as listening.

Diagnostic and Statistical Manual of Mental Disorders, Fifth Edition (DSM-5)   A handbook, published by the American Psychiatric Association, that is used most often in diagnosing mental disorders in the United States.

Dialect   A form of speaking that has distinct syntactic, semantic, and phonetic features. Dialects within a language are usually comprehensible by those who speak other dialects.

Dialogic speech   A linguistic form found in text; language quoted or spoken by a character in a story.

Differentiated instruction   An approach to teaching that includes planning and executing various educational approaches to meet individual learning needs of students.

Direct service classroom-based approach   An approach in which a practitioner (a) collaborates with a teacher, using a team-teaching method, or (b) takes turns with the teacher, providing specific lessons to the entire class.

Directive language   Adult-directed language that occurs when a parent asks a child to say or do something or asks many questions.

Disability   An umbrella term that covers impairments, activity limitations, and participation restrictions.

Discourse   Connected and contingent flow of language between two or more individuals.

Discrepancy criterion model   A model that requires that a child have a significant difference between IQ (i.e., overall cognitive ability) and school achievement.

Discrete trial   see *Applied behavior analysis*

Discrimination   The ability to attend to specific stimuli in a field of similar stimuli.

Disequilibrium   A Piagetian term that describes a cognitive process in which a child recognizes that two schemata are contradictory. Reorganization to higher levels of thinking is motivated by this disequilibrium.

Distributed practice   An intervention approach that provides children with opportunities to practice a skill frequently throughout the day; associated with classroom-based intervention approach.

Dominant culture (or mainstream culture)   The traditions, values, beliefs, and behaviors associated with European American culture.

Dosage   The frequency, intensity, and duration of services required to achieve optimal intervention outcomes.

Drill   An adult-directed intervention approach that elicits a high number of child responses; typically produced in response to adult questions and followed by adult reinforcing statements and feedback.

Drill play   An intervention activity that is somewhat more natural than drill but still highly structured;

in drill play, an element of a play routine is used to increase motivation.

Dual language program   An academic program in which the goal is for students to maintain the first language (L1) while learning English as a second language (L2).

Dyadic interaction   A two-person communication.

Dynamic assessment (DA)   A process-oriented measure that evaluates a child's ability to learn via a test–teach–retest approach.

Dynamic display   An augmentative communication device in which the symbol position changes after a location is selected (e.g., a prediction device allows the more frequently chosen symbols to occur at the top of the possible items to be selected).

Dysarthria   A motor speech disorder in which the muscles of the mouth, face, and respiratory system may become weak, move slowly, or not move at all after a stroke or other brain injury; the type and severity of dysarthria depend on the area of the nervous system affected.

Echolalia   Repetition or echoing of verbal utterances made by another person.

Ecological approach   A theory that acknowledges variation in individual, family, community, and cultural modes for dealing with challenges; it considers the impact of an individual's communication impairment in relation to functioning and relationships within the family and community.

Effect-size estimates   Metrics designed to characterize results in more functional and meaningful ways; effect-size data indicate the magnitude of an effect in addition to estimates of probability.

Effectiveness   In describing experimental research, the extent to which a specific intervention results in a positive outcome when it is used in routine practice.

Efficacy   In describing experimental research, the extent to which a specific intervention, procedure, or service produces a beneficial result under ideal conditions.

Efficiency   In describing experimental research, the extent of the resources that are required to produce a beneficial result within the domain of evidence-based practice.

Embedded intervention   A contextualized, child-centered activity that takes place during ongoing classroom routines.

Embedded learning opportunity   An intervention that takes place as part of children's self-initiated, naturalistic, and contextualized interactions as they occur in the classroom.

Emergent literacy   The skills, knowledge, and attitudes that are precursors to conventional reading and writing.

Empathizing (or theory of mind or mindblindness)   Perceiving another's motives or thoughts as well as the ability to understand how another person might feel in a particular situation. Empathizing deficits are characteristic of autism spectrum disorder.

Engagement   A child's duration and complexity of play and quality of interaction with others.

Enhanced milieu teaching (EMT)   A naturalistic approach that is appropriate for children who are able to imitate sounds and words, have a vocabulary of at least 10 words, and have an MLU between 1.0 and 3.5 words.

Epidemiology   The scientific study of factors affecting the health and illness of populations; epidemiologic studies are descriptive or analytic, with the goal of identifying causal factors.

Equilibrium   A balance between assimilating new information into old schemata and developing new schemata through accommodation.

Ethnic group   A group of individuals who share a common language, heritage, religion, or geography/nationality.

Ethnic mismatch   A situation in which a student's home culture and the service provider hold conflicting expectations for the student's communication or behavior.

Ethnocentrism   A member of one culture judging an individual from another culture solely by the values and standards of his or her own culture

Etiology   The cause of a disorder or disease.

Exclusionary criteria   Other possible causes of language impairment that must be eliminated as possible reasons for a child's language delay to meet criteria for specific language impairment.

Executive functioning   Goal-oriented, purposeful behaviors that allow an individual to take a strategic approach to problem solving.

Expansion   A modeling technique in which an adult repeats a child's preceding verbalization, along with adding one or more morphemes or words to make the sentence an acceptable adult sentence.

Explicit intervention   Structured, sequenced, adult-directed instruction in which an adult selects a particular language/literacy target and carefully sequences the child's exposure.

Expository narrative   An informational narrative genre in which an individual describes a sequential event within a domain of academic content (e.g., science experiment, historical incident).

Expressive language An individual's ability to express himself or herself and communicate meaning using language.

Expressive vocabulary The words a child produces.

Extended optional infinitive theory The theory that young children with language impairment persist in using unmarked verbs (e.g., *walk* vs. *walking*, *walks*, or *walked*) well beyond the point when children with normal language discontinue this pattern.

Extension A language modeling technique in which an adult repeats a child's preceding verbalization and adds additional information related to the ongoing event.

External evidence Evidence supporting the use of a specific intervention approach based on the results of well-designed experimental studies.

Extinction Lack of reinforcement, with the goal of eliminating an unwanted behavior.

Fading A technique in which an adult's prompting is reduced and the behavior is gradually shaped to occur naturally within a social context.

Far transfer Learning applied to different contexts.

Fast mapping A vocabulary-learning process in which young children learn a new word with only minimal exposure.

Fidelity The degree to which an intervention in a research study is carried out as described.

Figurative speech Words or expressions that are used nonliterally, such as metaphors, idioms, and proverbs.

Fixed displays Symbols and messages that do not change after a person selects a location on an AAC device.

Focused stimulation A modeling procedure in which a child is exposed to multiple examples of a linguistic target within a meaningful communication context.

Formative assessment An evaluation of performance in a real-life context; formative assessment allows the assessor to gather information and make adjustments to assist student learning.

Frequency The number of vibrations or the number of repetitions of a complete wave form in cycles per second; an acoustic measure that correlates to the perceptual quality we call *pitch*.

Functional assessment (or functional analysis) An assessment in which a professional gathers information about a student's behavior in order to identify the function or purpose of an aversive behavior and uses the information to develop behavioral-change interventions.

Functional communication Communication events that occur during daily activities; forms of behavior that express needs, wants, feelings, and preferences that others can understand.

Functional communication training (FCT) A behavioral intervention that replaces maladaptive behaviors with more socially acceptable communication options.

Gene duplication Any duplication of a region of DNA that contains a gene; Down syndrome is sometimes caused by gene duplication.

Generalization The ability of an individual to apply a learned skill in a novel situation.

Generalization probe A probe in which an interventionist evaluates the use of a target behavior as it occurs in a natural context or as it is independently produced by the student.

Genotype An individual's genetic endowment.

Giant words Two- or three-word combinations that a child hears frequently; a phrase treated as a polysyllabic single word. The words are not used separately or in novel combinations with other words.

Goal attack strategy The way in which multiple goals are approached or scheduled in an intervention session.

Goal attainment scaling (GAS) (or functional communication measure; performance rating system) An individualized, criterion-referenced approach that documents a student's baseline performance and numerically records behavioral changes from a –2 to a +2 level.

Goal An intervention objective that is made up of three components: a *do* statement, a *condition* statement, and a *criterion* statement.

Graph A visual representation of the occurrence of a behavior over time.

Hand leading Using another's body to communicate (e.g., moving the mother's hand toward an object), often instead of pointing.

Hearing age The number of years between the time a person was treated for hearing impairment (e.g., hearing aids fitted and intervention initiated) and his or her chronological age.

Hearing threshold The lowest level at which a sound signal is audible.

Horizontal goal attack strategy A strategy in which several goals are repeatedly targeted within every session.

Hybrid intervention An intervention approach in which a clinician focuses on a small subset of language behaviors and focuses a great deal of attention on identified targets in an intervention session; a midpoint intervention approach on the continuum of naturalness.

Hyperlexia The precocious ability to recognize written words significantly above an individual's language or cognitive skill level; often children with hyperlexia minimally comprehend what they read.

Idiopathic intellectual disability An intellectual disability whose cause is unknown.

Image rehearsal A learning strategy in which an individual aids recall by associating task components with pictures.

Imitation When one communication partner copies another's actions or sounds.

Impairment A problem in body function or structure.

Incidental teaching A strategy in which a language facilitator manipulates the environment to increase the likelihood that a child will communicate.

Inclusion Federal law that mandates that children with disabilities are educated in the same context as nondisabled peers to the degree possible.

Indirect service classroom-based approach An approach in which an SLP or a special educator serves as a consultant to a classroom teacher so that instructional methods can be adjusted to meet a child's special needs.

Individual growth and development indicators (IGDIs) Child performance measures designed to help guide intervention decisions and provide information about children's development.

Individualist culture A cultural characteristic in which the focus is on the individual and his or her immediate (nuclear) family.

Individualized Education Program (IEP) A plan that outlines special education and related services and is specifically designed to meet the unique educational needs of a student with a disability.

Individuals with Disabilities Education Act (IDEA) A U.S. law that guarantees all children with disabilities access to a free and appropriate public education.

Infant-directed talk (or motherese) Characteristics of child-directed communication that enhance an infant's ability to learn language.

Inferential question A question form that demands that an individual make a logical conclusion from the text in order to answer the question.

Information-processing theory (or connectionism) A model of cognition and language that compares the human brain to a computer and considers that cognitive ability is achieved by linked neuronal components.

Initiating event A component of a story episode that underlies narrative structure; it is the problem that sets the story in motion.

Intellectual ability Mental capability that involves an individual's ability to reason, plan, solve problems, think abstractly, comprehend complex ideas, learn quickly, and learn from experience; this capacity is often represented by an IQ score. Also defined as the ability to apply knowledge in order to perform better in an environment.

Intellectual disability (ID) A disorder originating before age 18 and characterized by significant limitations in intellectual functioning, along with limitations in adaptive behavior.

Intensity Sound level, measured in decibels or other scales; the psychological correlate is loudness.

Intermediate-level intervention goal A goal highlighting grammatical categories, operations, or processes.

Intermittent reinforcement (or partial reinforcement) A system in which only some correct responses are followed by the reinforcing event.

Internal evidence Evidence supporting the use of a specific intervention approach based on (a) an individual client's perspective and beliefs and/or (b) an SLP's clinical expertise.

Interrater reliability The reliability index that documents that when different assessors give the same test there will be similar results.

IT's Fun program A performance-based intervention for school-age students with intellectual disability.

Joint visual attention Following the direction of a communication partner's gaze or pointing or showing an object with the intention of drawing the communication partner's attention to the object or event.

Knowledge-based processing Processing that is based on an individual's previous experience or knowledge; it is sometimes called top-down processing.

Language A complex and dynamic system of conventional symbols used for thought and language expression that can be expressed orally, through writing, pictured symbols, or manually.

Language–age match A comparison of a chronologically younger individual who has an equivalent MLU as the student with language impairment.

Language content Semantics.

Language delay Language development that mirrors typical development but at a delayed rate of acquisition.

Language difference A variation of a symbol system used by a group of individuals that reflects and is determined by shared regional, social, or cultural/ethnic factors.

Language disorder Impaired comprehension and/or impaired use of spoken, written, and/or other symbol systems.

Language expansion The adult repeats the child's verbalization and adds morphemes or words to make the sentence an acceptable adult sentence.

Language extension The adult repeats the child's verbalizations and adds semantic information to the child utterance.

Language form Phonology, morphology, and syntax.

Language function or language use Pragmatics.

Language-learning disability Language-based learning disabilities are problems with age-appropriate reading, spelling, and/or writing; typically used to refer to school-age students with a primary language impairment and associated literacy deficits.

Language sample analysis (LSA) An evaluation of an individual's spontaneous or self-generated speech; this type of analysis has both quantitative and qualitative components.

Late language emergence A young child (2 to 3 years old) who exhibits a developmental lag in language.

Late talker A young child under age 4 who has a language delay.

Least restrictive environment (LRE) A learning plan that provides the most time possible in the regular classroom setting.

Level I evidence Evidence resulting from randomized experimental research; this is considered the best, or "gold standard," research design in the levels of evidence for scientific studies.

Level II evidence Evidence reflecting high-quality, but nonrandomized, experiments in the levels of evidence for scientific studies.

Level III evidence Evidence reflecting well-designed nonexperimental studies and case studies in the levels of evidence for scientific studies.

Level IV evidence Evidence representing experts' opinions in the levels of evidence for scientific studies.

Levels of evidence A tiered approach to evaluating external evidence when implementing evidence-based practice.

Ling Six Sound Test A method of determining hearing aid, cochlear implant, or other device function, based on a person's responses to six sounds (i.e., /oo/, /ah/, /ee/, /sh/, /s/, /m/) that span the human speech frequencies. Named after Daniel Ling, who described the approach.

Linguistic chauvinism One dialect being seen as superior and proper.

Listening and spoken language specialists (LSLS) Specialists who help children who are deaf or hard of hearing develop spoken language and literacy, primarily through listening.

Literacy orientation Aspects of children's temperament, motivation, and attention in response to book reading or other literacy interactions.

Literacy socialization A learning opportunity that includes activities such as shared book reading and shared writing activities.

Literal question A question form that requires a student to recall a specific fact explicitly stated in the reading passage.

Literate language Frequently occurring syntax and morphological features that occur in written text or formal spoken language.

Loudness The perceptual correlate of *volume*; relates to the decibel level of an acoustic signal.

Macrosystem Part of the ecological model that summarizes society's cultural views and practices regarding individuals with intellectual disability.

Mainstream culture see *Dominant culture*

Mainstreaming Having students with disabilities spend a portion of their school day in the general education program and a portion in a separate special education program. (This is not a preferred term. The term *inclusion* is now used instead.)

Maladaptive behaviors Socially inappropriate or self-injurious behaviors such as tantrums, hitting, or head banging.

Mand-model A strategy in which a language facilitator uses a verbal prompt in the form of a question ("What do you want?"), choice ("Do you want _____ or _____?"), or mand ("Tell me what you want.").

Massed practice Intervention provided in less frequent and longer sessions.

Massed trials An intervention approach in which the individual participates in intensive one-on-one training to increase accuracy and recall of a targeted behavior.

Mean A statistical average of all the scores in a sample.

Means–end A Piagetian principle in which a child demonstrates intentionality; it occurs when a child identifies a problem and makes a plan to solve the problem.

Mediated learning phase   The middle phase of dynamic assessment (i.e., test, teach, retest), during which an assessor teaches a child a skill; the child is monitored for attention span, planning, self-regulation, motivation, and response to the intervention.

Mediation   An adult's manipulation of a task to increase the learner's success and self-efficacy.

Memory (or working memory)   Current information retained to carry out everyday tasks.

Mesosystem   Part of the ecological model that includes school, neighborhood, community organizations, and workplace.

Meta-analysis   A specialized form of systematic review in which the results from several studies are summarized using a statistical technique that results in a single weighted estimate of the findings.

Meta-awareness   Self-reflection that demonstrates the learning process.

Metacognition   Conscious awareness of the thinking process.

Metalinguistics   An individual's ability to focus on and talk about language.

Macroanalysis   An analysis in which the assessor considers an individual's ability to interact during a conversation; a focus on discourse skills.

Microanalysis   A fine-grained analysis in which the assessor considers the student's verbal output at an utterance-by-utterance level.

Microcephaly   An abnormally small head.

Microsystem   Part of the ecological model that includes family and caregivers.

Mixed hearing loss   A hearing loss that refers to a combination of conductive and sensorineural loss and means that a problem occurs in both the outer or middle ear and the inner ear.

Modeling   A technique in which an adult talks and a child listens; it provides an opportunity for the child to induce linguistic structures because the communication partner provides multiple examples of the language target. The language facilitator notes the child's focus of attention and provides a language model that reflects the child's interest.

Morphology   The language domain that governs the structure of words and the construction of word forms.

Morphosyntax   The combined features of morphology and syntax.

Motivation (or mastery motivation)   Goal-directed behaviors undertaken to achieve positive feelings associated with task competency.

Motor apraxia   The inability of a person to perform voluntary and skillful movements of one or more body parts although there is no evidence of underlying muscular paralysis.

Multi-modal   Including multiple modalities in communication (e.g., gestures, speech, facial expressions, writing, drawing, AAC system).

Narrative macrostructure   The overall organization of a narrative; the story structure.

Narrative microstructure   Internal linguistic features that occur in narratives; the narrative microstructure includes the syntax, vocabulary, and literate language used within narratives.

Nativist theory   A theory connected to the writings of Noam Chomsky that proposes that children have an innate ability to learn language.

Naturalistic assessment   An assessment in which an observer provides multiple opportunities for an individual to perform skills across domains (i.e., social, cognitive, motor, communication).

Near transfer   Learning applied to closely related contexts.

Negative reinforcement   An unpleasant stimulus that is removed when the targeted behavior is performed.

Neural maturation   An accumulating body of science that explains the relationship between language and brain development in young children.

Neurological soft signs   Behaviors consistent with a neurological impairment; however, the brain scan of an individual with neurological soft signs does not show hard evidence of neurological damage.

Neuroplasticity   The brain's capacity (e.g., the neural auditory system) to be molded or reshaped.

Nonverbal IQ (or performance IQ)   A measure of one's ability to carry out motor tasks or analyze and solve problems using visual reasoning.

Nonword repetition task   Repetition of nonsense words; used as a nonlinguistic processing task to diagnose language impairment.

Norm-referenced assessment (or normative referenced assessment)   An assessment in which ability is compared to a larger standardization group, usually resulting in a standard score; often used to determine eligibility for services.

Normal distribution of scores   Statistical description of how behaviors cluster around the mean score on a norm-referenced assessment; results in a bell-shaped distribution of scores.

Number of different words (NDW)   A quantitative analysis of semantics (language content); the number of different words that occur in a 100-utterance language sample.

Object constancy   A Piagetian principle that describes how a child learns that he or she is viewing the same object, regardless of distance, light, or different viewing angle.

Object permanence   A Piagetian principle that describes a child's realization that an object exists even when he or she cannot see it.

Objective data   Data that are based on observable phenomena (e.g., ratings scales, behavioral/classroom observations, test scores).

Obligatory context   The conversational context that calls for the use of a specific grammatical form.

Onset-rime   The initial consonant sound of a syllable (the onset of *bag* is *b-*, of *swim* is *sw-)* and the part of a syllable containing the vowel and all that follows it (the rime of *bag* is *-ag*, of *swim* is *-im*).

Open combining   A sentence-combining approach in which a student combines simple sentences to make a longer, more complex sentence.

Oral narrative   A monologue that describes a real or fictional event, organized into linked utterances with specific linguistic features.

Organization   The ability to systematize incoming information to speed processing and facilitate retrieval.

Otitis media   Inflammation of the middle ear caused by infection.

Paradigm shift   A radical change in thinking that leads to new approaches.

Parallel talk   A modeling technique in which an adult uses language to describe what a child is thinking, feeling, and doing.

Parent–child communication routines   Play routines that involve action patterns and facilitate child participation.

Partial reinforcement   see *Intermittent reinforcement*

Peer confederate training   Training in which students with typical language are taught to use strategies to encourage communication from students with communication disorders.

Phenotype   The observable characteristics or physical manifestation of one's genotype.

Phonics instruction   Letter–sound relationships needed to read or spell words.

Phonological assessment   An evaluation of the rules that govern the sound combinations in speech production; it considers sound error patterns.

Phonological awareness (PA)   The ability to reflect on and manipulate phonemic segments of speech; PA is highly correlated with early reading skill.

Phonological awareness deficits   Problems detecting, segmenting, and blending sounds.

Phonology   The sound system of a language and the rules that govern the sound combinations.

Phrase structure grammar   A Chomskian description of the basic syntax structure of a sentence, regardless of the language being spoken.

Piagetian theory   Developmental theory based on the work of Jean Piaget (1896–1980), who developed principles of cognitive processes.

Picture Exchange Communication System (PECS)   A six-phase intervention program designed to teach functional communication.

Pitch   The perceptual correlate of acoustic frequency (e.g., the individual perceives a tone as high pitch vs. low pitch).

Play-based assessment   A form of naturalistic assessment that considers a child's ability to use objects in functional ways, play symbolically, and communicate in a familiar context.

Positive reinforcement   A stimulus that increases the frequency of a particular behavior, using pleasant rewards.

Practice   The repetition of a task to gain proficiency.

Pragmatics   Context-related features of language; principles governing language use.

Predictive validity   How well a test score will predict a student's performance on a future criterion-referenced task.

Prefix   Groups of letters attached to the beginning of a word to form a new word (e.g., <u>dis</u>appear, <u>pre</u>determined).

Preventive approach   An approach to intervention in which instruction is provided or the environment is modified before a deficit is observed.

Primary prevention   The elimination of the onset and development of a communication disorder by altering susceptibility or the environment for susceptible persons.

Print concepts   An individual's understanding of the uses of print and print functions needed during reading and writing.

Print referencing   An explicit teaching technique that exposes children to print and alphabetic concepts; often used during shared book reading interactions.

Private speech   Private speech occurs when children speak aloud as they are engaged in play; a term associated with Vygotskian theory.

Process-oriented measures   Measures that are dependent on psycholinguistic processes such as linguistic mental operations rather than language knowledge.

Progress monitoring   Using data that represent a student's communication progress during intervention to guide decisions and programmatic changes.

Prompts Instructions or cues that ensure that a child responds correctly (e.g., tactile, written, gestural cues).

Pullout models of service delivery The practitioner works with an individual or a small group of children in an area outside the classroom.

Punishment A negative response that makes it less likely that the unwanted behavior will occur.

Qualitative data Data describing the attributes or properties that an object possesses. Although qualitative data can be organized into categories and assigned numbers, the numbers do not have value by themselves but rather represent descriptive attributes.

Quantitative data Numeric data expressing the quantity, amount, or range of a targeted behavior.

Race A social construct based on historical and political views.

Randomized controlled trials (RCTs) Experimental studies that randomly assign individuals to an intervention group or control group to measure intervention effects; RCTs are considered the "gold standard" for evaluating the effectiveness of an intervention.

Randomized research design A research design in which individuals consent to participate in a study and then are randomly assigned to be in the treatment group or the control group.

Receptive language Refers to an individual's ability to understand and process language.

Receptive vocabulary The words a child understands, both in spoken form and written form.

Referents or referencing The speaker's/writer's ability to use specific nouns rather than nonspecific pronouns and/or the ability to make clear linkages between new and old information so that the listener/reader can comprehend linguistic output.

Reflecting feeling A strategy used in counseling, when a professional responds to a client's emotional expressions rather than to the content of a message.

Regulatory communication acts Pragmatic communication acts that indicate an individual's needs within routines of daily living.

Rehearsal strategies Learning strategies that an individual uses to self-instruct to stimulate recall; include verbalization of sequential steps and image rehearsal.

Reinforcement Behaviors following a target behavior that increase the probability that the behavior will reoccur.

Reliability The degree to which a test is free from errors of measurement across forms, raters, and time and within an instrument.

Research bias An examiner's unconscious inflation of a student's abilities based on knowledge that the student participated in a prior intervention.

Resource allocation A term from the information-processing model that suggests that the way in which energy is distributed in a cognitive system is affected by the number of parallel stages operating at one time.

Response (or responsiveness) to intervention (RTI) model A model whereby students who are identified as at risk have their progress monitored and receive increasingly intense, multi-tiered, research-based interventions.

Root word A fundamental or unmarked part of a word (e.g., *walked, walks,* and *walking* all contain the root word *walk*).

Routine A term that is used to describe times of day and/or familiar activities such as eating, bathing, bedtime, hanging out, going to the store, and traveling in the car.

Routines-based interviewing An interviewing approach in which a practitioner poses questions to family members to (a) assess a child's developmental and communication status, (b) gain information about day-to-day life, and (c) tune in to a family's feelings about their child.

Rubric A data system for qualitative behavior documentation; a set of criteria and standards used to assess an individual's performance on a specific task.

Scaffolding Graduated assistance provided to novice learners in order to help them achieve higher levels of conceptual and communicative competence; with scaffolding, adult support allows a child to engage in a challenging activity.

Scanning A process used for children with physical limitations in which a communication partner or an electronic device displays symbols in a predetermined pattern.

SCERTS approach An educational approach for children with autism that is based on social interaction, developmental, and family systems theories.

Schema A Piagetian concept that describes a concept, mental category, or cognitive structure.

Screening The initial, brief assessment process used with individuals who require formal evaluation.

Scripts Predictable patterns of interaction that facilitate the participation of language learners.

Secondary prevention The early detection and treatment of communication disorders. Early detection and treatment may lead to the elimination of a disorder or the slowing of a disorder's progress, preventing further complications.

Self-talk A modeling technique in which an adult describes what he or she is thinking, feeling, or seeing.

Semantic transparency Words or phrases in which meaning is easily observed or intuited.

Semantics The language domain that governs the meanings of words and sentences.

Sensitivity In relation to an assessment tool, how frequently an individual with a disability is identified by using the tool (i.e., whether the tool gives a positive result when the individual actually has the disability).

Sensorineural hearing loss A hearing loss that results from damage to the sensory hair cells of the inner ear or the nerves that supply them.

Sentence combining (SC) intervention An intervention in which an adult gives a student two or more simple sentences and requires the student to combine the simple sentences into a longer, more complex sentence.

Sentence recasts The adult produces sentences to target specific grammatical forms and varies the sentence modality to heighten the child's awareness of the grammar form.

Service delivery model Includes the personnel, materials, specific intervention procedure, schedule for provision of services, settings in which intervention services will be delivered, and direct or indirect roles of the practitioner as he or she provides language intervention to students with language impairments.

Shaken baby syndrome (SBS) The constellation of signs and symptoms resulting from violent shaking or from hitting the head of an infant or a small child.

Shaping A behavioral concept that describes the production of close approximations to the behavioral target prior to reinforcement; with shaping, a language trainer facilitates easy, small steps, gradually approximating the goal behavior.

Significance tests Statistical analyses that reflect the probability that the reported outcome being due to chance or random fluctuation is adequately small.

Signing Exact English (SEE, or Signed Exact English or Signed English) A system of manual communication that strives to be an exact representation of English vocabulary and grammar.

Simultaneous processing The coordination of different pieces of cognitive information into a linked system.

Single-subject research design A research design in which the subject serves as his/her own control, rather than being compared to another individual or group.

Social communication problem Limitations in an individual's social, cognitive, and language skills necessary for contextually appropriate, meaningful, and effective interpersonal communication.

Social interaction theory A theory that proposes that communication interactions play a central role in children's acquisition of language.

Social intervention An intervention that focuses on teaching specific social skill strategies and facilitating a student's use of peer communication.

Social literacy An individual's affective (i.e., emotional) response to shared literacy experiences.

Social script A repeated social interaction that is likely to occur in daily life.

Sociocultural theory Sociocultural theory states that language is learned from social and cultural interaction, not just through communicative interactions; based on the writing of Vygotsky.

Sociodramatic script training Engaging children in opportunities to role-play social scripts.

Specific language impairment (SLI) A language deficit that does not have accompanying factors such as hearing loss, low intelligence scores, or neurological damage.

Specificity The extent to which an individual without a disorder is correctly identified as such, using a screening or assessment tool.

Speech The articulation of speech sounds and the rate and quality of an individual's voice.

Speech/articulation assessment An evaluation of a child's motor ability to produce phonemes; it considers sound production in isolation, syllables, words, sentences, and running speech.

Speech chain model A basic model of communication used to explain the processes of communication from the speaker's production of words, through transmission of sound, to the listener's perception of what has been said.

Speech-motor assessment An evaluation of (a) facial symmetry; (b) structure and function of the lips, tongue, jaw, and velopharynx (i.e., the soft palate); and (c) the resonance, phonatory, and respiratory systems used for speech.

Standard deviation A statistical calculation that describes the spread of scores around the mean.

Standard error of the mean (SEM) A measure that estimates the distribution of scores for any one person; SEM is calculated because an individual's performance on a test will vary.

Standard scores or Standardized scores Transformed scores measured in standard deviation units; scores are used to interpret norm-referenced assessments.

State verbs Verbs that describe a person's "state of being" in contrast to describing an action (e.g., *knows, goes, needs, wants, loves,* or *uses*).

Stimulus overselectivity Selective response to a limited number of stimuli cues.

Story dictation A teaching technique in which an adult writes down the text of a child's dictation. Often the child then illustrates the story. The adult reads the story back while pointing to the text.

Story episode A basic narrative structure that includes an initiating event, an attempt, and a consequence.

Subjective data Data that represent an individual's opinion.

Successive processing The arrangement of incoming cognitive information in a step-by-step or linear sequence.

Suffix Groups of letters attached to the end of a word to form a new word (e.g., combust<u>ible</u>, aware<u>ness</u>).

Summative assessment An evaluation used to place a child in a particular category (e.g., language impaired versus non-impaired) or as accountability measures (e.g., state reading tests).

Surface structure A Chomskian term that describes the actual sentence a speaker produces (i.e., the words that are heard).

Surface theory A theory that proposes that morphemes' short duration and unstressed pronunciation contribute to learning difficulties for children with SLI.

Syllable recognition An individual's awareness that a word is made up of syllable subunits.

Symbolic play A Piagetian concept that describes the representational actions of a child when he or she uses one object to represent another.

Symbols Graphic, auditory, gestural, and textured or tactile representations used to represent language concepts in AAC systems.

Syntactic bootstrapping When an individual is able to glean the meaning of a novel word from the surrounding function words.

Syntax The language domain governing the order and combination of words to form sentences and the relationships among the elements within a sentence.

System for Augmenting Language (SAL) An AAC intervention consisting of (1) a speech-generating device, (2) visual-graphic symbols chosen to help the individual communicate, (3) encouragement of symbols as a means to communicate in everyday life, (4) modeling symbol use by communication, and (5) provision of feedback to family members.

T-unit One main clause, with all the subordinate clauses and nonclausal phrases attached or embedded within the sentence; T-unit analysis is completed after a child is 42 months old or when his or her MLU is greater than 4.00.

Telegraphic speech Language that typically includes only content words, such as nouns, verbs, and a few adjectives/adverbs, with few or no function words (e.g., auxiliary verbs, articles, conjunctions, and prepositions).

Tertiary prevention The reduction of a disability by attempting to restore effective functioning.

Test question The use of an obvious or known question.

Test–retest reliability The reliability index that documents that when a test is given to the same individual on different occasions, the results will be the same or very similar.

Time delay A strategy in which a language facilitator uses a nonverbal prompt and waits before providing the desired object or action.

Top-down learning Learning that is conceptually driven or guided by higher-level processes (e.g., familiarity with the context and information gained from environmental cues); also called knowledge-based learning or knowledge-based processing.

Total communication (or simultaneous communication) A mode of communication that combines spoken language with sign language.

Total number of different words (TNW) A frequently used measure of lexical diversity that is computed by counting the number of different root words in a 100-utterance language sample.

Transaction support Refers to the interpersonal support provided by a child's adult and peer communication partners and/or the environmental modifications used to promote social communication and emotional regulation.

Transactional model A theory of language learning that considers a child's utterances as the antecedent event triggering an adult response.

Transdisciplinary   An approach to assessment in which families and practitioners from different disciplines work together and make collaborative decisions; members share roles and systematically cross discipline boundaries.

Transfer of information   The ability to apply learned information to solve novel problems.

Transformational grammar   A Chomskian term that describes the grammar rules specific to each language.

Transition   Life changes that occur in the lives of young adults as well as the formal planning process that assists students with disabilities as they move from school environments to work environments.

Translocation   When a broken piece of one chromosome attaches to another; sometimes a cause of intellectual disability.

Traumatic brain injury (TBI)   An acquired injury to the brain that is caused by an external physical force and that results in total or partial functional disability or psychosocial impairment that adversely affects an individual's educational or functional performance.

Treatment efficacy   Refers to a change under highly controlled conditions; differs from treatment effectiveness, which is the extent to which an intervention results in favorable outcomes in everyday conditions.

Unaided symbol   A symbol that does not require any prosthetic or external support to convey a message.

Validity   The degree to which a test procedure accurately measures what it was designed to measure.

Verbal rehearsal   A learning strategy in which an individual self-instructs and uses verbal labels to stimulate memory and recall of information.

Vertical goal attack strategy   A strategy in which one goal at a time is targeted until some predetermined level of accuracy is achieved.

Visual scene display (VSD)   A picture, photograph, or virtual environment that depicts and represents a situation, a place, or an experience.

Writing process   The sequence of writing activities used by effective writers, including topic selection, planning, organizing, drafting, revising, editing, publishing, and presenting.

Zone of proximal development (ZPD)   A Vygotskian term that describes the competence that a child demonstrates with minimal assistance. The ZPD is the area between the zone of competence (what a child can do independently) and the zone of incompetence (what a child is unable to do, even with assistance).

AAC-Rehabilitation Engineering Research Center (RERC). (2012). *Mobile devices and communication apps: An AAC–RERC white paper.* Retrieved from http://aac-rerc.psu.edu/documents/RERC_mobiledevices_whitepaper_final.pdf.

Abbeduto, L. (2009). Forward: Language, literacy, and genetic syndromes. *Topics in Language Disorders, 29,* 109–110.

Abbeduto, L., & Murphy, M. M. (2004). Language, social cognition, maladaptive behavior, and communication in Down syndrome and fragile X syndrome. In M. L. Rice & S. F. Warren (Eds.), *Developmental language disorders: From phenotypes to etiologies.* Mahwah, NJ: Erlbaum.

Adams, C. (2002). Practitioner review: The assessment of language pragmatics. *Journal of Child Psychology and Psychiatry, 43,* 973–987.

Adams, C. (2005). Language and social competence: An integrated approach to intervention. *Seminars in Speech & Language, 26,* 181–188.

Alexander Graham Bell Association (AG Bell). (2013). Listening and spoken language. Retrieved from http://listeningandspokenlanguage.org/Document.aspx?id=525.

Alexander Graham Bell Association (AG Bell). (2011). *Statistics on hearing loss.* Retrieved from www.nidcd.nih.gov/health/statistics/Pages/quick.aspx.

Alliano, A., Herriger, K., Koutsoftas, A. D., & Bartolotta, T. E. (2012). A review of 21 iPad applications for augmentative and alternative communication purposes. *Perspectives on Augmentative and Alternative Communication, 21,* 60–71.

Alt, M., & Plante, E. (2006). Factors that influence lexical and semantic fast mapping of young children with specific language impairment. *Journal of Speech, Language, and Hearing Research, 49,* 941–954.

ALTEC, University of Kansas. (2009). RubiStar: *Creating rubrics for project-based learning.* Retrieved June 17, 2009, from http://rubistar.4teachers.org/index.php.

American Association of Intellectual and Developmental Disabilities (AAIDD). (2012). *RE: DSM-5 draft diagnostic criteria for "intellectual developmental disorder."* Retrieved from www.thearc.org/document.doc?id=3782.

American Association of Intellectual and Developmental Disabilities (AAIDD). (2013). Retrieved from www.aaidd.org/content_104.cfm.

American Psychiatric Association. (2013). *Diagnostic and statistical manual of mental disorders* (5th ed.). Arlington, VA: American Psychiatric Publishing.

American Speech-Language-Hearing Association (ASHA). (2000). *Guidelines for the roles and responsibilities of the school-based speech-language pathologist* [Guidelines]. Retrieved from www.asha.org/policy.

American Speech-Language-Hearing Association (ASHA). (2001). *Roles and responsibilities of speech-language pathologists with respect to reading and writing in children and adolescents* [Guidelines]. Rockville, MD: Author

American Speech-Language-Hearing Association (ASHA). (2004a). Admission/discharge criteria in speech-language pathology. *ASHA Supplement, 24,* 65–70.

American Speech-Language-Hearing Association (ASHA). (2004d). *Roles and responsibilities of speech-language pathologists with respect to augmentative and alternative communication* [Technical report]. Retrieved from www.asha.org/policy.

American Speech-Language-Hearing Association (ASHA). (2004e). *2004 member poll.* Rockville, MD: Author.

American Speech-Language-Hearing Association (ASHA). (2005b). *Roles and responsibilities of speech-language pathologists with respect to augmentative and alternative communication* [Position statement]. Retrieved from www.asha.org/policy.

American Speech-Language-Hearing Association (ASHA). (2006b). *2006 schools survey report: Current issues.* Rockville, MD: Author.

American Speech-Language-Hearing Association (ASHA). (2006c). *2006 schools survey report: Caseload characteristics.* Rockville, MD: Author.

American Speech-Language-Hearing Association (ASHA). (2010). *2010 Schools survey summary report: Number and type of responses, SLPs.* Rockville, MD: Author

American Speech-Language-Hearing Association (ASHA). (2012). *2012 Schools Survey report: SLP caseload characteristics.* Retrieved from www.asha.org/research/memberdata/schoolssurvey/.

American Speech-Language-Hearing Association (ASHA). (2013). *Degree of hearing loss.* Retrieved from www.asha.org/public/hearing/Degree-of-Hearing-Loss/.

Anderson, K., & Smaldino, J. (1999). Listening inventories for education: A classroom measurement tool. *The Hearing Journal, 52,* 74–76.

Anderson, P. B. (2000). *Downward causation: Minds, bodies, and matter.* Aarhus, Denmark: Aarhus University Press.

Andrews, R., Torgerson, C., Beverton, S., Freeman, A., Locke, T., Law, G., et al. (2006). The effect of grammar teaching on writing development. *British Educational Research Journal, 32,* 39–55.

Apel, K., Masterson, J. J., & Niessen, N. L. (2004). Spelling assessment frameworks. In C. A. Stone, E. R.,

Silliman, & B. J. Ehren (Eds.), *Handbook of language and literacy: Development and disorders* (pp. 644–660). New York: Guilford Press.

Armstrong, C. L. (2010). *Handbook of medical neuropsychology: Applications of cognitive neuroscience.* New York: Springer.

Bailey, J., McComas, J. J., Benavides, C., & Lovascz, C. (2002). Functional assessment in a residential setting: Identifying an effective communicative replacement response for aggressive behavior. *Journal of Developmental and Physical Disabilities, 14,* 353–369.

Baldwin, D., & Meyer, M. (2007). How inherently social is language? In E. Hoff & M. Shatz (Eds.), *Blackwell handbook of language development* (pp. 87–106). Malden, MA: Blackwell.

Ball, A. F. (2006). Teaching writing in culturally diverse classrooms. In C. A. MacArthur, S. Graham, & J. Fitzgerald (Eds.), *Handbook of writing research* (pp. 293–310). New York: Guilford.

Baranek, G. T., Parham, L. D., & Bodfish, J. W. (2005). Sensory and motor features in autism: Assessment and intervention. In F. R. Volkmar, R. Paul, A. Klin, & D. Cohen (Eds.), *Handbook of autism and pervasive developmental disorders: Vol. 2. Assessment, intervention, and policy* (3rd ed., pp. 831–862). Hoboken, NJ: Wiley & Sons.

Baron-Cohen, S., Wheelwright, S., Lawson, J., Griffin, R., Ashwin, C., Billington, J., et al. (2005). Empathizing and systemizing in autism spectrum conditions. In F. R. Volkmar, R. Paul, A. Klin, D. Cohen (Eds.), *Handbook of autism and pervasive developmental disorders: Vol. 1. Diagnosis, development, neurobiology, and behavior* (3rd ed., pp. 628–639). Hoboken, NJ: Wiley & Sons.

Baroody, A. J., Lai, J., & Mix, K. S. (2006). The development of young children's early number and operation sense and its implications for early childhood education. In B. Spodek & O. N. Saracho (Eds.), *Handbook of research on the education of young children* (2nd ed., pp. 187–222). Mahwah, NJ: Erlbaum.

Battle, D. (2009). Multiculturalism, language, and emergent literacy. In P. Rhyner (Ed.), *Emergent literacy and language development* (pp. 192–234). New York: Guilford.

Baum, W. M. (2005). *Understanding behaviorism: Behavior, culture, and evolution.* Maiden: Blackwell.

Bear, D. R., Invernizzi, M., Templeton, S., & Johnston, F. (2007). *Words their way: Word study for phonics, vocabulary, and spelling instruction* (4th ed.). Upper Saddle River, NJ: Pearson.

Beck, I. L., & McKeown, M. G. (2007). Increasing young low-income children's oral vocabulary repertoires through rich and focused instruction. *The Elementary School Journal, 10,* 251–271.

Beck, I. L., McKeown, M. G., & Kucan, L. (2002). *Bringing words to life: Robust vocabulary instruction.* New York: Guilford Press.

Beirne-Smith, M., Ittenbach, R. F., & Patton, J. R. (2002). *Mental retardation* (6th ed.). Upper Saddle River, NJ: Merrill/Prentice Hall.

Belser, R., & Sudhalter, V. (2001). Conversation characteristics of children with fragile X syndrome: Repetitive speech. *American Journal on Mental Retardation, 106,* 28–38.

Berninger, V. W., Abbott, R. D., Jones, J., Wolf, B. J., Gould, L., Anderson-Youngstrom, M., et al. (2006). Early development of language by hand: Composing, reading, listening, and speaking connections; three letter-writing modes; and fast mapping in spelling. *Developmental Neuropsychology, 29,* 61–92.

Beukelman, D. R., & Mirenda, P. (2013). *Augmentative and alternative communication: Supporting children and adults with complex communication needs* (4th ed.). Baltimore, MD: Paul H. Brookes.

Bishop, D., & Clarkson, B. (2003). Written language as a window into residual language deficits: A study of children with persistent and residual speech and language impairments. *Cortex, 39,* 215–237.

Bishop, D. V. M., Adams, C. V., & Rosen, S. (2006). Resistance of grammatical impairment to computerized comprehension training in children with specific and nonspecific language impairments. *International Journal of Language and Communication Disorders, 41,* 19–40.

Bishop, D. V. M., & Mogford-Bevan, K. (1997). *Language development in exceptional circumstances.* East Sussex, UK: Psychology Press

Bishop, D. V. M., & Snowling, M. J. (2004). Developmental dyslexia and specific language impairment: Same or different? *Psychological Bulletin, 130,* 858–886.

Bishop, D. V. M., Price, T. S., Dale, P. S., & Plomin, R. (2003). Outcomes of early language delay: II. Etiology of transient and persistent language difficulties. *Journal of Speech, Language, and Hearing Research, 46,* 561–575.

Blackstone, S. (2006). Young children: False beliefs, widely held. *Augmentative Communication News, 18*(2), 1–4.

Blackstone, S., & Hunt Berg, M. (2003). *Social networks: Communication inventory for individuals with complex communication needs and their communication partners.* Monterey, CA: Augmentative Communication, Inc.

Bland-Stewart, L. M. (2005). Difference or deficit in speakers of African American English? What every clinician should know . . . and do. *The ASHA Leader.* Retrieved from www.asha.org/Publications/leader/2005/050503/f050503a.htm.

Bloom, L., & Lahey, M. (1978). *Language development and language disorders.* New York: Wiley.

Bloom, P. (2001). Précis of "How children learn the meanings of words." *Behavioral and Brain Sciences, 24,* 1095–1103.

Blumberg, S. J., Bramlett, M. D., Kogan, M. D., et al. (2013). Changes in prevalence of parent-reported autism spectrum disorder in school-aged U.S. children: 2007 to 2011–2012. *National Health Statistics Reports; no 65.* Hyattsville, MD: National Center for Health Statistics

Boardman, A. G., Roberts, G., Vaughn, S., Wexler, J., Murray, C. S., & Kosanovich, M. (2008). *Effective instruction for adolescent struggling readers: A practice brief.* Portsmouth, NH: RMC Research Corporation, Center on Instruction.

Bodrova, E., & Leong, D. J. (2007). *Tools of the mind: The Vygotskian approach to early childhood education.* Upper Saddle River, NJ: Pearson.

Boehm, A. E. (2000). *Boehm Test of Basic Concepts– Third Edition (BTSC-3).* San Antonio, TX: The Psychological Corporation.

Bondy, A., & Frost, L. (2009). The picture exchange communication system. In P. Mirenda & T. Iacono (Eds.), *Autism spectrum disorders and AAC* (pp. 279–302). Baltimore, MD: Brookes.

Bosteels, S., Van Hove, G., & Vandenbroeck, M. (2012). The roller-coaster of experiences: Becoming a parent of a deaf child. *Disability and Society, 27,* 983–996.

Botting, N., Simkin, Z., & Conti-Ramsden, G. (2006). Associated reading skills in children with a history of specific language impairment (SLI). *Reading and Writing, 19,* 77–98.

Bowers, L., Huisingh, R., LoGiudice, C., & Orman, J. (2004). *The WORD Test-2-Elementary.* East Moline, IL: Lingua Systems.

Boyton, S. (1984). *Blue hat, green hat.* New York: Little Simon.

Bracken, B. (2007). *Bracken Basic Concept Scale— Third Edition (BBCS-3).* San Antonio, TX: Harcourt Assessment.

Brackenbury, T., & Pye, C. (2005). Semantic deficits in children with language impairments: Issues for clinical assessment. *Language, Speech, and Hearing Services in Schools, 36,* 5–16.

Bradley, R., Danielson, L., & Hallahan, D. P. (2013). *Identification of learning disabilities: Research to practice.* New York: Routledge.

Bregman, J. D. (2005). Definitions and characteristics of the spectrum. In D. Zager (Ed.), *Autism spectrum disorders: Identification, education, and treatment* (3rd ed., pp. 5–46). Mahwah, NJ: Erlbaum.

Brinton, B., & Fujiki, M. (2005). Improving peer interaction and learning in cooperative learning groups. In T. A. Ukrainetz (Ed.), *Contextualized language intervention: Scaffolding K–12 literacy achievement* (pp. 289–318). Eau Claire, WI: Thinking Publications.

Bronfenbrenner, U. (1979). *The ecology of human development: Experiments by nature and design.* Cambridge, MA: Harvard University Press.

Broun, L., & Oelwein, P. (2007). *Literacy skill development for students with special educational needs: A strength-based approach.* Port Chester, NY: National Public Resources.

Brown, C. (2006, June). *Early intervention: Strategies for public and private sector collaboration.* Paper presented at the 2006 Convention of the Alexander Graham Bell Association for the Deaf and Hard of Hearing, Pittsburgh PA.

Brown, J. D., & Hudson, T. (2002). *Criterion-referenced language testing.* New York: Cambridge University Press.

Brown, L., Sherbenou, R., & Johnsen, S. (2010). *Test of Nonverbal Intelligence–4.* San Antonio, TX: Pearson.

Brown, M. W. (2005). *Goodnight moon* [Hardcover edition]. New York: HarperCollins.

Brown, R. (1973). *A first language: The early stages.* Cambridge, MA: Harvard University Press.

Brown, V. L., Wiederholt, J. L, & Hammill D. D. (2006). *Test of reading comprehension skills* (TORC-4). Los Angeles, CA: Western Psychological Association.

Browne, M. N., & Keeley, S. (2007). *Asking the right questions: A guide to critical thinking* (8th ed.). Upper Saddle River, NJ: Prentice Hall.

Bruner, J. S. (1981). The social context of language acquisition. *Language and Communication, 1,* 155–178.

Bruner, J. S. (1982). The organization of action and the nature of adult-child transaction. In G. D'ydewalle, J. Nuttin, W. Lens, & J. W. Atkinson (Eds). *Cognition in human motivation and learning* (pp. 1–44). Mahwah, NJ: Lawrence Earlbaum Associates.

Bruner, J. S. (1983). *In search of mind: Essays in autobiography.* New York: Harper & Row.

Buehler, V. (2012, October). Treatment of (central) auditory processing disorder: Bridging the gap between the audiologist and the speech-language pathologist. *Perspectives on Hearing and Hearing Disorders in Childhood, 22,* 46–56.

Buis, K. (2004). *Making words stick: Strategies that build vocabulary and reading comprehension in the elementary grades.* Portland, ME: Stenhouse.

Cafiero, J. (2001) The effect of an augmentative communication intervention on the communication, behavior, and academic program of an adolescent with autism. *Focus on Autism and Other Developmental Disabilities, 16,* 179–193.

Calandrella, A. M., & Wilcox, M. J. (2000). Predicting language outcomes for young prelinguistic children with developmental delay. *Journal of Speech, Language, and Hearing Research, 43,* 1061–1071.

Camarata, S. M., & Nelson, K. E. (2005). Conversational recast intervention with preschool and older children. In R. J. McCauley & M. E. Fey (Eds.), *Treatment of language disorders* (pp. 237–264). Baltimore, MD: Brookes.

Cardenas-Hagan, E., Carlson, C. D., & Pollard-Durodola, S. D. (2007). The cross-linguistic transfer of early literacy skills: The role of initial L1 and L2 skills and language of instruction. *Language, Speech, and Hearing Services in Schools, 38,* 249–259.

Carle, E. (2000). *Head to toe.* New York: Scholastic.

Carlson, M. L, Driscoll, C. L., Gifford, R. H., & McMenomey, S. O. (2012). Cochlear implantation: Current and future device options. *Otolaryngologic Clinics of North America, 45*(1), 221–224.

Carr, E. G., Innis, J., Blakeley-Smith, A., & Vasdev, S. (2004). Challenging behavior: Research design and measurement issues. In E. Emerson, C. Hatton, T. Thompson, & T. R. Parmenter (Eds.), *The international handbook of applied research in intellectual disabilities* (pp. 423–441). West Sussex, UK: Wiley.

Carrow-Woolfolk, E. (1999). *Test of Auditory Comprehension of Language (TACL-3)*. Bloomington, MN: Pearson.

Carson, K. L., Gillon, G. T., & Boustead, T. M. (2012). Classroom phonological awareness instruction and literacy outcomes in the first year of school. *Language, Speech, and Hearing Services in Schools*. Published online on December, 28, 2012. doi: 10.1044/0161-1461(2012/11-0061)

Carta, J. J., & Kong, N. Y. (2009). Trends and issues for interventions for preschoolers with developmental disabilities. In S. L. Odom, R. H. Horner, M. E. Snell, & J. Blacher (Eds.), *Handbook of developmental disabilities* (pp. 181–198). New York: Guilford.

Carter, E. W., & Hughes, C. (2013). Teaching social skills and promoting supportive relationships. In P. Wehman (Ed.). *Life beyond the classroom: Transition strategies for young people with disabilities* (pp. 261–284). Baltimore, MD: Paul H. Brookes.

Casbergue, R. M., & Plauché, M. B. (2005). Emergent writing: Classroom practices that support young writers' development. In R. Indrisano & J. R. Paratore (Eds.), *Learning to write, writing to learn: Theory and research in practice* (pp. 8–25). Newark, DE: International Reading Association.

Cascella, P. W. (2006). Standardized speech-language tests and students with intellectual disability: A review of normative data. *Journal of Intellectual & Developmental Disability, 31*, 120–124.

Caselli, M. C., Casadio, P., & Bates, E. (2001). Lexical development in English and Italian. In M. Tomasello & E. Bates (Eds.), *Language development: The essential readings* (pp. 76–110). Malden, MA: Blackwell.

Catts, H. W. (2009). The narrow view of reading promotes a broad view of comprehension. *Language, Speech, and Hearing Services in Schools, 40*, 178–183.

Catts, H. W., Bridges, M., Little, T., & Tomblin, J. B. (2008). Reading achievement growth in children with language impairments. *Journal of Speech-Language-Hearing Research, 51*, 1569–1579.

Catts, H. W., Fey, M. E., Tomblin, J. B., & Zhang, Z. (2002). A longitudinal investigation of reading outcomes in children with language impairments. *Journal of Speech, Language, and Hearing Research, 45*, 1142–1157.

Catts, H., & Kahmi, A. (2005). *The connections between language and reading disabilities*. Mahwah, NJ: Erlbaum.

Centers for Disease Control and Prevention (CDC). (2007). *Prevalence of autism spectrum disorders, autism and developmental disabilities monitoring network, 14 sites, United States, 2000*, MMWR SS 2007, 56 (SS-1) (1). Retrieved February 9, 2007, from www.cdc.gov/ncbddd/autism/documents/Autism CommunityReport.pdf.

Centers for Disease Control and Prevention (CDC, 2012). *Prevalence of autism spectrum disorders — Autism and developmental disabilities monitoring network, 14 sites, United States, 2008*, 61(SS03);1–19. Retrieved November 25, 2013, from http://www.cdc.gov/mmwr/preview/mmwrhtml/ss6103a1.htm?s_cid=ss6103a1_w

Cepeda, N. J., Pashler, H., Vul, E., Wixted, J., & Rohrer, D. (2006). Distributed practice in verbal recall tasks: A review and quantitative synthesis. *Psychological Bulletin, 132*, 354–380.

Chang, F., & Burns, B. M. (2005). Attention in preschoolers: Associations with effortful control and motivation. *Child Development, 76*, 247–263.

Chapman, R. S. (2000). Children's language learning: An interactionist perspective. *Journal of Child Psychology and Psychiatry, 41*, 33–54.

Chapman, R. S. (2003). Language and communication in individuals with Down syndrome. In L. Abbeduto (Ed.), *International review of research in mental retardation: Language and communication* (pp. 1–34). New York: Academic.

Chapman, R. S., & Hesketh, L. (2000). Behavioral phenotype of individuals with Down syndrome. *Mental Retardation and Developmental Disabilities Research Reviews, 6*, 84–95.

Charity, A. H. (2008, July). African American English: An overview. *Perspectives on communication disorders and sciences in culturally and linguistically diverse populations, 15*, 33–42.

Ching, T. Y., Dillion, H., Marnane, V., Hou, S., Day, J., & Seeto, M., et al. (2013). Outcomes of early- and late-identified children at 3 years of age: Findings from a prospective population-based study. *Ear and Hearing*, doi: 10.1097/AUD.0b013e3182857718

Cheng, L. (2002). Asian and Pacific American Cultures. In D. E. Battle (Ed.), *Communication disorders in multicultural populations* (3rd ed., pp. 71–112). Boston: Butterworth- Heinemann.

Chiang, B., & Rylance, B. (2000). *Wisconsin speech-language pathologists' caseloads: Reality and repercussions*. Oshkosh, WI: University of Wisconsin–Oshkosh.

Cirrin, F. M., & Gillam, R. B. (2008). Language intervention practices for school-age children with spoken language disorders: A systematic review. *Language, Speech, and Hearing Services in Schools, 39*, 110–137.

Clegg, J., Hollis, C., Mawhood, L., & Rutter, M. (2005). Developmental language disorders: A follow-up in later adult life. Cognitive, language and psychosocial outcomes. *Journal of Child Psychology and Psychiatry, 46*, 128–149.

Cloud, N., Genesee, F., & Hamayan, E. (2000). *Dual language instruction: A handbook for enriched education*. Boston: Heinle & Heinle.

Coalition for Evidence-Based Policy. (2003). *Identifying and implementing educational practices supported by rigorous evidence: A user-friendly guide*. Washington, DC: U.S. Department of Education, Institute of Education Sciences, National Center for Education Evaluation and Regional Assistance.

Cohen, J. (1988). *Statistical power analysis for the behavioral sciences* (2nd ed.). Hillsdale, NJ: Erlbaum.

Connor, C. M., & Craig, H. K. (2006). African American preschoolers' language, emergent literacy skills, and use of African American English: A complex relation. *Journal of Speech, Language, Hearing Research, 49,* 771–792.

Conti-Ramsden, G., Botting, N., Simkin, Z., & Knox, E. (2001). Follow-up of children attending infant language units: Outcomes at 11 years of age. *International Journal of Language & Communication Disorders, 36,* 207–219.

Conti-Ramsden, G., & Durkin, K. (2012). Language development and assessment in the preschool period. *Neuropsychology Review, 22*(4), 384–401.

Cormier, S., & Nurius, P. S. (2003). *Interviewing and change strategies for helpers: Fundamental skills and cognitive behavioral interventions* (5th ed.). Pacific Grove, CA: Brooks/Cole.

Cousins, L. (2008). *Happy birthday, Maisy!* Cambridge, MA: Candlewick.

Craig, H. K., & Washington, J. A. (2000). An assessment battery for identifying language impairments in African American children. *Journal of Speech, Language, and Hearing Research, 43,* 366–379.

Craig, H. K., & Washington, J. A. (2004). Grade-related changes in the production of African American English. *Journal of Speech, Language, and Hearing Research, 47,* 450–463.

Crain-Thoreson, C., Dahlin, M. P., & Powell, T. A. (2001). Parent–child interaction in three conversational contexts: Variations in style and strategy. *New Directions for Child and Adolescent Development, 92,* 23–38

Cress, C. J., & Green, J. R. (2006). Communication disorders: Computer applications for. Communication disorders. In J. G. Webster (ed.), *Encyclopedia of medical devices and instrumentation* 2nd ed. (pp. 210–220). New York: Wiley and Sons.

Cruz, I., Quittner, A. L., Marker, C., DesJardin, J., & the CDaCI Investigative Team. (2013). Identification of effective strategies to promote language in deaf children with cochlear implants. *Child Development, 84,* 543–559.

Crystal, D. (1987). Towards a "bucket" theory of language disability: Taking account of interaction between linguistic levels. *Clinical Linguistics and Phonetics, 1,* 7–22.

Curenton, S. M., & Justice, L. M. (2004). African American and Caucasian preschoolers' use of decontexualized discourse: Literate language features in oral narratives. *Language, Speech, and Hearing Services in Schools, 35,* 240–253.

Curenton, S. M., & Lucas, T. D. (2007). Assessing narrative development. In K. L. Pence (Ed.), *Assessment in emergent literacy* (pp. 377–432). San Diego, CA: Plural.

Damico, J. S., & Nelson, R. (2010). Reading and reading impairments. In Damico, J. S., Müller, N., Ball, M. J.

(Eds.), *The handbook of language and speech disorders* (pp. 267–295). Chickchester, UK: Wiley-Blackwell.

Das Bhowmik, A., & Mukhopadhyay, K. (2012). Molecular genetics of intellectual disability with special emphasis on the idiopathic type. *International Journal of Genetics, 4,* 99–110.

Dawson G., Jones E. J., Merkle K, et al. (2012). Early behavioral intervention is associated with normalized brain activity in young children with autism. *Journal of the American Academy of Child & Adolescent Psychiatry, 51*(11), 1150–1159.

Dawson, J., Stout, C. E., & Eyer, J. A. (2003). *Structured Photographic Expressive Language Test–3 (SPELT-3).* DeKalb, IL: Janelle.

Delprato, D. (2001). Comparison of discrete-trial and normalized behavioral language intervention for young children with autism. *Journal of Autism and Developmental Disorders, 31,* 315–325.

Denes, P. B., & Pinson, E. N. (2001). *The speech chain: The physics and biology of spoken language.* New York: Macmillan.

DesJardin, J. (2006). Family empowerment: Supporting language development in young children who are deaf or hard of hearing. *The Volta Review, 106,* 275–298.

DeStefano, F., Price, C. S., & Weintraub, E. S. (2013). Increasing exposure to antibody-stimulating proteins and polysaccharides in vaccines is not associated with risk of autism. *The Journal of Pediatrics, 163,* 561–567.

Detterman, D., Gabriel, L., & Ruthsatz, J. (2000). Intelligence and mental retardation. In R. J. Sternberg, *Handbook of intelligence* (pp. 141–158). New York: Cambridge University Press.

Dinnebeil, L., Pretti-Frontczak, K., & McInerney, W. (2009). A consultative itinerant approach to service delivery: Considerations for the early childhood community. *Language, Speech, and Hearing Services in Schools, 40,* 435–445.

Dollagen, C. A. (2007). *The handbook of evidence-based practice in communication disorders.* Baltimore, MD: Brookes.

Dore, J. (1974). A pragmatic description of early language development. *Journal of Psycholinguistic Research, 3,* 343–350.

Dore, J. (1975). Holophrases, speech acts and language universals. *Journal of Child Language, 3,* 13–28.

Drager, K. D. R. (2009, *December*). Aided modeling interventions for children with autism spectrum disorders who require AAC. *Perspectives on Augmentative and Alternative Communication, 18* (4), 114–120.

Drager, K. D. R., Postal, V. J., Carrolus, L., Catellano, M., Gagliano, C., & Glynn, J. (2006). The effect of aided language modeling on symbol comprehension and production in 2 preschool children with autism. *American Journal of Speech-Language Pathology, 15,* 112–125.

Drew, C. J., & Hardman, M. L. (2004). *Mental retardation: A life-span approach to people with intellectual disabilities* (8th ed.). Upper Saddle River, NJ: Pearson.

Dubé, E., De Wals, P., & Ouakki, M. (2010). Quality of life of children and their caregivers during an AOM episode: Development and use of a telephone questionnaire. *Health Quality of Life Outcomes, 8,* 75. Retrieved from www.ncbi.nlm.nih.gov/pmc/articles/PMC2915973/.

Dube, W. V., Lombard, K. M., Farren, K. M., Flusser, D. S., Balsamo, L. M., Fowler, T. R., et al. (2003). Stimulus overselectivity and observing behavior in individuals with mental retardation. In S. Soraci Jr. & K. Murata-Soraci (Eds.), *Visual information processing* (pp. 107–123). Westport, CT: Praeger.

Dunham, G. (2011). The future at hand: Mobile devices and apps in clinical practice. *The ASHA Leader.*

Dunlap, G., & Fox, L. (2011). Function-based interventions for children with challenging behavior. *Journal of Early Intervention, 33,* 333–343.

Dunn, L. M., & Dunn, D. M. (2006) *Peabody Picture Vocabulary Test—4 (PPVT-4).* Bloomington, MN: Pearson.

Edmunds, K. M., & Bauserman, K. L. (2006). What teachers can learn about reading motivation through conversations with children. *The Reading Teacher, 59,* 414–424.

Ehren, B. J. (2007, May 8). SLPs in secondary schools: Going beyond survival to "thrival." *The ASHA Leader,* 22–23.

Ehren, B. J., Montgomery, J., Rudebusch, J., & Whitmire, K. (2006). *Responsiveness to intervention: New roles for speech-language pathologists.* American Speech-Language-Hearing Association. Retrieved June 3, 2008, from www.asha.org/members/slp/schools/prof-consult/NewRolesSLP.htm.

Eisenberg, S. L. (2006). Grammar: How can I say that better? In T. A. Ukrainetz (Ed.), *Contextualized language intervention: Scaffolding preK–12 literacy achievement* (pp. 145–194). Greenville, SC: Thinking Publications.

Eisenberg, S. L., Fersko, T. M., & Lundgren, C. (2001). The use of MLU for identifying language impairment in preschool children: A review. *American Journal of Speech-Language Pathology, 10,* 323–342.

Eisenberg, L. S., Fink, N. E., & Niparko, J. K. (2006). Childhood development after cochlear implantation: Multicenter study examines language development, *The ASHA Leader, 11,* 5, 28–29.

Eldevik, S., Hastings, R. P., Hughes, J. C., Jahr, E., Eikeseth, S., & Cross, S. (2009). Meta analysis of early intensive behavioral intervention for children with autism. *Journal of Clinical Child & Adolescent Psychology, 38*(3), 439–450.

Espin, C. A., Weissenburger, J. W., & Benson, B. J. (2004). Assessing the writing performance of students in special education. *Exceptionality, 12,* 55–66.

Evans, J. L. (2008). Emergentism and language impairment in children: It's all about change. In M. Mody & E. R. Silliman (Eds.), *Brain, behavior, and learning in language and reading disorders* (pp. 41–71). New York: Guilford.

Executive Act on Intellectual Disabilities. (2003). Executive Order No. 12994.

Fenson, L., Dale, P. S., Reznick, J. S., Thal, D., Bates, E., Hartung, J. P., Pethick, S., & Reilly, J. S. (2007). *MacArthur Communicative Development Inventories—2nd ed.* Baltimore, MD: Brookes.

Fenson, L., Marchman, V. A., Thal, D. J., Dale, P. S., Reznick, J. S., & Bates, E. (2007). MacArthur-*Bates Communicative Development inventories: User's guide and technical manual* (2nd ed.). Baltimore, MD: Brookes.

Fernald, A., Pinto, J. P., Swingley, D., Weinberg, A., & McRoberts, G. W. (2001). In M. Tomasello & E. Bates (Eds.), *Language development: The essential readings* (pp. 49–56). Malden, MA: Blackwell.

Fernald, D. (2008). *Psychology: Six perspectives.* Los Angeles: Sage.

Fey, M. E. (1986). *Language intervention with young children.* Boston: Allyn & Bacon.

Fey, M. E. (2006). Commentary on "Making evidence-based decisions about child language intervention in schools" by Gillam and Gillam. *Language, Speech, and Hearing Services in Schools, 37,* 316–319.

Fey, M. E., & Loeb, D. F. (2002). An evaluation of the facilitative effects of inverted yes-no questions on the acquisition of auxiliary verbs. *Journal of Speech, Language, and Hearing Research, 45,* 160–174.

Fey, M. E., Long, S. H., & Finestack, L. H. (2003). Ten principles of grammar facilitation for children with specific language impairments. *American Journal of Speech-Language Pathology, 12*(1), 3–15.

Fey, M. E., & Proctor-Williams, K. (2000). Recasting, elicited imitation and modeling in grammar intervention for children with specific language impairments. In D. V. M. Bishop & L. B. Leonard (Eds.), *Speech and language impairments in children: Causes, characteristics, intervention, and outcome* (pp. 177–194). East Sussex, UK: Psychology Press.

Fey, M. E., Richard, G. J., Geffner, D., Kamhi, A. G., Medwetsky, L., Paul, D., Ross-Swain, D., Wallach, G. P., Frymark, T., & Schooling, T. (2011). Auditory processing disorder and auditory/language interventions: An evidence-based systematic review. *Language, Speech, & Hearing Services in Schools, 42,* 246–264.

Gosnell, J., Costello, J., & Shane, H. (2011). Using a clinical approach to answer "What communication apps should we use?" *Perspectives on Augmentative and Alternative Communication, 20,* 87–96.

Fillmore, C. J. (1968). The case for case. In E. Bach & R. T. Harms (Ed.), *Universals in linguistic theory* (pp. 1–88). New York: Holt, Rinehart & Winston.

Fisher-Price. (2004). *Little people cars, trucks, planes, and trains.* Bath, England: Reader's Digest Children's Books.

Flexer, C., Wray, D., Sommers, R., & Schmidt-Robb, B. (2005). Early intervention for children with cochlear implants: A paradigm shift in expectations. *Hearsay, 17,* 15–27.

Forum on Educational Accountability. (2007). *Assessment and accountability for improving schools and learning: Principles and recommendations for federal law and state and local systems (Executive Summary)*. Retrieved April 6, 2007, from www.edaccountability .org/AssessmentExecSumm061207.pdf.

Fox, A. V., Dodd, B., & Howard, D. (2002). Risk factors for speech disorders in children. *International Journal of Language & Communication Disorders, 37*, 117–131.

Freitag, C. M., Kleser, C., Schneider, M., & von Gontard, A. (2007). Quantitative assessment of neuromotor function in adolescents with high functioning autism and Asperger syndrome. *Journal of Autism and Developmental Disorders, 37*(5), 948–959.

Fujiki, M., & Brinton, B. (2009). Pragmatics and social communication in child language disorders. In R. G. Schwartz (Ed.), *Handbook of child language disorders* (pp. 406–423). New York: Psychology Press.

Fulcher, A., Purcell, A., Baker, E., & Munro, N. (2012). Listen up: Children with early identified hearing loss achieve age-appropriate speech/language outcomes by 3years-of age. *International Journal of Pediatric Otorhinolaryngology, 76*(12), 1785–1794.

Frush Holt, R., Beer, J., Kronenberger, W. G., Pisoni, D. B., & LaLonde, K. (2012). Contribution of family environment to pediatric cochlear implant users' speech and language outcomes: Some preliminary findings. *Journal of Speech, Language, and Hearing Research, 55*, 848–864.

Gallaudet Research Institute (GRI). (2011). *Regional and national summary report of data from the 2009–10 annual survey of deaf and HoH children and youth*. Washington, DC: GRI, Gallaudet University.

Ganea, P. A., Bloom-Pickard, M., & DeLoache, J. S. (2008). Transfer between picture books and the real world by very young children. *Journal of Cognition and Development, 9*, 46–66.

Ganek, H., Robbins, A. M., & Niparko, J. K. (2012). Language outcomes after cochlear implantation. *Olaryngologic Clinics of North America, 45*(1), 173–185.

Gentner, D. (2006). Why verbs are hard to learn. In K. Hirsh-Pasek & R. Golinkoff (Eds.), *Action meets word: How children learn verbs* (pp. 544–564). New York: Oxford University Press.

Gillam, R. B., & Pearson, N. A. (2004) *Test of Narrative Language*. Austin, TX: PRO-ED.

Gillam, R. B., Loeb, D. F., Hoffman, L. M., Bohman, T., Champlin, C. A., Thibodeau, L., et al. (2008). The efficacy of Fast ForWord language intervention in school-age children with language impairment: A randomized controlled trial. *Journal of Speech, Language, and Hearing Research, 51*, 97–119.

Gillam, S. L., & Gillam, R. B. (2008). Teaching graduate students to make evidence-based decisions: Application of a seven-step process within an authentic learning context. *Topics in Language Disorders, 28*, 212–228.

Gillam, S. L., & Justice, L. (2010, September 21). RTI progress monitoring tools: Assessing primary-grade students in response-to-intervention programs. *The ASHA Leader*.

Gillette, Y. (2012). *Achieving communication competence: Three steps to effective intervention*. Verona, WI: Attainment Co.

Gillon, G. T. (2000). The efficacy of phonological awareness intervention for children with spoken language impairment. *Language, Speech, and Hearing Services in Schools, 31*, 126–141.

Gillon, G. T. (2002). Follow-up study investigating benefits of phonological intervention for children with spoken language impairment. *International Journal of Language and Communication Disorders, 37*, 381–400.

Gillon, G. T. (2004). *Phonological awareness: From research to practice*. New York: Guilford Press.

Gillon, G. T. (2006). Phonological awareness intervention: A preventative framework for preschool children with specific speech and language impairments. In R. J. McCauley & M. E. Fey (Eds.), *Treatment of language disorders in children* (pp. 279–308). Baltimore, MD: Brookes.

Gilman, S.R., Iossifov, I., Levy, D., et al. (2011). Rare de novo variants associated with autism implicate a large functional network of genes involved in formation and function of synapses. *Neuron, 70*(5), 898–907.

Goldman, R., & Fristoe, M. (2000). *Goldman-Fristoe Test of Articulation, 2nd ed*. Upper Saddle River, NJ: Pearson.

Goldstein, E. B. (2012). *Sensation and perception*. Independence, KY: Cengage.

Goldstein, H. (1984). Effects of modeling and corrected practice on generative language learning of preschool children. *Journal of Speech and Hearing Disorders, 49*, 389–398.

Goldstein, H. (2006). Language intervention considerations for children with mental retardation and developmental disabilities. *Perspectives on Language Learning and Education: American Speech-Language-Hearing Association, Special Interest Division 1, 13*, 21–26.

Goldstein, H., Schneider, N., & Thiemann, K. (2007). Peer-mediated social communication intervention: When clinical expertise informs treatment development and evaluation. *Topics in Language Disorders, 27*, 182–199.

Graham, S. (2005). Strategy instruction and the teaching of writing: A meta-analysis. In C. A. MacArthur, S. Graham, and J. Fitzgerald (Eds.), *Handbook of writing research* (pp. 187–207). New York: Guilford Press.

Graham, S., & Perin, D. (2007). *Writing next: Effective strategies to improve writing of adolescents in middle and high schools—A report to Carnegie Corporation of New York*. Washington, DC: Alliance for Excellent Education.

Granlund, M., Björchk-Åkesson, E., Wilder, J., & Ylvén, R. (2008). AAC interventions for children in a family environment: Implementing evidence in practice.

Augmentative and Alternative Communication, 24, 207–219.

Gray, S. (2004). Word learning by preschoolers with specific language impairment: Predictors and poor learners. *Journal of Speech, Language, and Hearing Research, 47,* 1117–1132.

Gray, S. (2005). Word learning by preschoolers with specific language impairment: Effect of phonological or semantic cues. *Journal of Speech, Language, and Hearing Research, 48,* 1452–1467.

Green, L. (2009). The nature of writing difficulties in students with language/learning disabilities. *Perspectives on Language Learning and Education, 16,* 4–8.

Greenhalgh, K. S., & Strong, C. J. (2001). Literate language features in spoken narratives of children with typical language and children with language impairments. *Language, Speech, and Hearing Services in Schools, 32,* 114–125.

Greenspan, S. (2006). Functional concepts in mental retardation: Finding the natural essence of an artificial category. *Exceptionality, 14,* 205–224.

Greenwood, C. R., Bradfield, T., Kaminski, R., Linas, M., Carta, J. J., & Nylander, D. (2011). The response to intervention (RTI) approach in early childhood. *Focus on Exceptional Children, 43,* 1–22.

Grigal, M., & Deschamps, A. (2012). Transition education for adolescents with intellectual disability. In M. L. Wehmeyer & K. W. Webb (Eds.), *Handbook of adolescent transition education for youth disabilities* (pp. 398–417). New York: Routledge.

Gutierrez-Clellen, V. F., & Pena, E. (2001). Dynamic assessment of diverse children: A tutorial. *Language, Speech, and Hearing Services in Schools, 32*(4), 212.

Haager, D., Klingner, J., & Vaughn, S. (2007). *Evidence-based reading practices for response to intervention.* Baltimore, MD: Brookes.

Halle, J. W., Ostrosky, M. M., & Hemmeter, M. L. (2006). Functional communication training: A strategy for ameliorating challenging behavior. In R. J. McCauley & M. E. Fey (Eds.), *Treatment of language disorders in children* (pp. 509–545). Baltimore, MD: Brookes.

Halliday, M. A. K. (1975). *Learning how to mean: Explorations in the development of language.* London: Edward Arnold Publishers Ltd.

Hammill, D., & Larsen, S.C. (2009). *Test of Written Language—4 (TOWL-4).* Austin, TX: PRO-ED.

Hammill, D. D., & Newcomer, P. L. (2008). *Test of Language Development Intermediate—4.* Austin, TX: PRO-ED.

Hancock, T. B., & Kaiser, A. P. (2002). The effects of trainer-implemented enhanced milieu teaching on the social communication of children who have autism. *Topics in Early Childhood Special Education, 22,* 39–54.

Hancock, T. B., & Kaiser, A. P. (2006). Enhanced milieu teaching. In R. J. McCauley & M. E. Fey (Eds.), *Treatment of language disorders in children* (pp. 203–236). Baltimore: Paul H. Brookes.

Hanselman, P., & Borman, G. D. (2012). The impacts of Success for All on reading achievement in grades 3–5: Does intervening during the later elementary grades produce the same benefits as intervening early? *Educational Evaluation and Policy Analysis.* Published online on December 20, 2012. doi: 10.3102/0162373712466940

Harris, J. C. (2006). *Intellectual disability: Understanding its development, causes, classification, evaluation, and treatment.* New York: Oxford University Press.

Hart, B., & Risley, T. R. (1995). *Meaningful differences in the everyday experience of young American children.* Paul H Brookes Publishing.

Hartley, J., & Harris, J. L. (2001). Reading the typography of text. In J. L. Harris & A. G. Kamhi (Eds.), *Literacy in African American communities* (pp. 109–126). Mawhah, NJ: Erlbaum.

Hartman, M. A. (2009). Step by step: Creating a community-based transition program for students with intellectual disabilities. *Teaching Exceptional Children, 41,* 6–11.

Hassink, J. M., & Leonard, L. B. (2010). Within-treatment factors as predictors of outcomes following conversational recasting. *American Journal of Speech-Language Pathology, 19,* 213–224.

Haynes, W. O., & Pindzola, R. H. (2008). *Diagnosis and evaluation in speech pathology* (7th ed.). Boston: Allyn & Bacon.

Hegde, M. N., & Maul, C. A. (2006). *Language disorders in children: An evidence-based approach to assessment and treatment.* Boston: Allyn & Bacon.

Heilmann, J., Nockerts, A., & Miller, J. F. (2010). Language sampling: Does the length of the transcript matter? *Language, Speech, and Hearing Services in Schools, 41,* 393–404.

Henry, L. A., & MacLean, M. (2003). Relationships between working memory, expressive vocabulary and arithmetical reasoning in children with and without intellectual disabilities. *Educational and Child Psychology, 20,* 51–64.

Hickson, L., Murdoch, B., Houston, T., & Constantinescu, G. (2010). Is auditory-verbal therapy effective for children with hearing loss? *Volta Review, 110*(3), 361–387.

Hodapp, R. M., & Dykens, E. M. (2004). Genetic and behavioral aspects: Application to maladaptive behavior and cognition. In J. A. Rondal, R. M. Hodapp, S. Soresi, E. M. Dykens, & L. Nota (Eds.), *Intellectual disabilities: Genetics, behavior, and inclusion* (pp. 13–49). London: Whurr.

Hodson, B. W. (2004). *Hodson Assessment of Phonological Patterns, 3rd ed.* Austin, TX: PRO-ED.

Hoff, E. (2006). How social contexts support and shape language development. *Developmental Review, 26,* 55–88.

Hogan, T. P., Catts, H. W., & Little, T. D. (2005). The relationship between phonological awareness and reading: Implications for the assessment of phonological awareness. *Language, Speech, and Hearing Services in Schools, 36,* 285.

Howlin, P., Magiati, I., & Charman, T. (2009). Systematic review of early intensive behavioral interventions for children with autism. *American Journal of Intellectual and Developmental Disabilities, 114*(1), 23–41.

Howlin, P., Mawhood, L., & Rutter, M. (2000). Autism and developmental receptive language disorder—A follow-up comparison in early adult life. II: Social, behavioral, and psychiatric outcomes. *Journal of Child Psychology and Psychiatry, 41,* 561–578.

Huber, M., & Kipman, U. (2012). Cognitive skills and academic achievement of deaf children with cochlear implants. *Otolaryngology—Head and Neck Surgery, 14,* 763–774.

Hughes, C., & Carter, E. W. (2012). *The new transition handbook: Strategies secondary high school teachers use that work.* Baltimore, MD: Paul H Brookes.

Hughett, K., Kohler, F. W., & Raschke, D. (2013). The effects of a buddy skills package on preschool children's social interactions and play. *Topics in Early Childhood Special Education, 32,* 246–254.

Hwa-Froelich, D. A. (2000). *Frameworks of education: Perspectives of Asian parents and Head Start staff.* Unpublished doctoral dissertation, Wichita State University, Wichita, KS.

Hwa-Froelich, D., & Vigil, D. C. (2004). Three aspects of cultural influence on communication: A literature review. *Communications Disorders Quarterly, 25,* 107–118.

IDEA. (2004). *Reauthorization of the Individuals with Disabilities Education Act: Guidance with Respect to State and Federal Regulations Implementing the Individuals with Disabilities Education Act of 2004.* Retrieved November 17, 2007, from www.ed.gov/policy/speced/guid/idea/idea2004.html.

Idol, L. (2006). Toward inclusion of special education students in general education: A program evaluation of eight schools. *Remedial and Special Education, 27,* 77–94.

Ingersoll, B., & Schreibman, L. (2006). Teaching reciprocal imitation skills to young children using a naturalistic behavioral approach: Effects on language pretend play and joint attention. *Journal of Autism and Developmental Disorders, 36,* 487–505.

Invernizzi, M., Sullivan, A., Meier, J., & Swank, L. (2004). *Phonological Awareness Literacy Screening—Pre-Kindergarten.* Charlottesville: University of Virginia.

Jones, M. C., Walley, R. M., Leech, A., Paterson, M., Common, S., & Metcalf, C. (2006). Using goal attainment scaling to evaluate a needs-led exercise program for people with severe and profound intellectual disabilities. *Journal of Intellectual Disabilities, 10,* 317–335.

Justice, L. M. (2002). *The syntax handbook: Everything you learned about syntax . . . but forgot.* Eau Claire, WI: Thinking Publications.

Justice, L. M. (2006). Evidence-based practice, response to intervention, and the prevention of reading difficulties. *Language, Speech, and Hearing Services in Schools, 37,* 284–297.

Justice, L. M., Bowles, R., Eisenberg, S. L., Kaderavek, J. N., Ukrainetz, T. A., & Gillam, R. B. (2006). The index of narrative micro-structure (INMIS): A clinical tool for analyzing school-aged children's narrative performance. *American Journal of Speech-Language Pathology, 15,* 177–191.

Justice, L. M., Bowles, R., Pence, K., & Gosse, C. (2010). A scalable tool for assessing children's language abilities within a narrative context: The NAP (Narrative Assessment Protocol). *Early Childhood Research Quarterly, 25,* 218–234.

Justice, L. M., Chow, S. M., Capellini, C., Flanigan, K., & Colton, S. (2003). Emergent literacy intervention for vulnerable preschoolers: Relative effects of two approaches. *American Journal of Speech-Language Pathology, 12,* 1–14.

Justice, L. M., & Ezell, H. K. (2002). Use of storybook reading to increase print awareness in at-risk children. *American Journal of Speech-Language Pathology, 11,* 17–29.

Justice, L. M., & Fey, M. E. (2004, September 21). Evidence-based practice in schools: Integrating craft and theory with science and data. *The ASHA Leader,* pp. 4–5, 30–32.

Justice, L. M., Invernizzi, M. A., & Meier, J. D. (2002). Designing and implementing an early literacy screening protocol: Suggestions for the speech-language pathologist. *Language, Speech, and Hearing Services in Schools, 33,* 84–101.

Justice, L. M., & Kaderavek, J. N. (2004). Embedded-explicit emergent literacy intervention I: Background and description of approach. *Language, Speech, and Hearing Services in Schools, 35,* 201–211.

Kaderavek, J. N., & Justice, L. M. (2002). Shared storybook reading as an intervention context: Practices and potential pitfalls. *American Journal of Speech-Language Pathology, 11,* 101–110.

Kaderavek, J. N., & Justice, L. M. (2004). Embedded-explicit emergent literacy intervention II: Goal selection and implementation in the early childhood classroom. *Language, Speech, and Hearing Services in Schools, 35,* 212–228.

Kaderavek, J. N., Laux, J. M., & Mills, N. H. (2004). A counseling training module for students in speech-language pathology training programs. *Contemporary Issues in Communication Science & Disorders, 31,* 153–163.

Kaderavek, J. N., & Pakulski, L. M. (2007). Facilitating literacy development in young children with hearing loss. *Seminars in Speech and Language, 28,* 69–78.

Kaderavek, J. N., & Rabidoux, P. (2004). Interactive to independent literacy: A model for designing literacy goals for children with atypical communication. *Reading and Writing Quarterly, 20,* 237–260.

Kaderavek, J. N., & Sulzby, E. (2000). Issues in emergent literacy for children with specific language impairments: Language production during storybook reading, toy play and oral narratives. In L. R. Watson, T. L. Layton, & E. R. Crais (Eds.), *Handbook of early language impairment in children: Assessment and treatment* (pp. 199–244). New York: Delmar.

Kahmi, A. G. (2009). The case for the narrow view of reading. *Language, Speech, and Hearing Services in Schools, 40,* 174–177.

Kaiser, A. P., & Hancock, T. B. (2003). Teaching parents new skills to support their young children's development. *Infants & Young Children, 16,* 9–21.

Kaiser, A. P., Hancock, T. B., & Nietfeld, J. P. (2000). The effects of parent-implemented enhanced milieu teaching on the social communication of children who have autism. *Early Education and Development, 11,* 423–446.

Kaiser, A. P., & Roberts, M. Y. (2013). Parent-implemented enhanced milieu teaching with preschool children who have intellectual disabilities. *Journal of Speech, Language and Hearing Research, 56*(1), 295.

Kaiser, A. P., & Trent, J. A. (2007). Communication intervention for young children with disabilities: Naturalistic approaches to promoting development. In S. Odom, R. Horner, M. Snell, & J. Blacher (Eds.), *Handbook of developmental disabilities* (pp. 224–246). New York: Guilford Press.

Kanner, L. (1943). Autistic disturbances of affective contact. *Nervous Child, 2,* 217–250.

Kasari, C., Rotheram-Fuller, E., Locke, J., & Gulsrud, A. (2012). Making the connection: Randomized controlled trial of social skills at school for children with autism spectrum disorders. *Journal of Child Psychology & Psychiatry, 53*(4): 431–439.

Katims, D. (2000). *The quest for literacy: Curriculum and instructional procedures for teaching reading and writing to students with mental retardation and developmental disabilities.* Reston, VA: The Council for Exceptional Children.

Kearney, P. M., & Griffin, T. (2001). Between joy and sorrow: Being a parent or a child with developmental disability. *Issues and Innovations in Nursing Practice, 34,* 582–592.

Kellogg, S. (1997). *Jack and the beanstalk.* New York: Harper Collins.

Kennedy Krieger Institute and American Academy of Pediatrics. (2013). *Bringing the Early Signs of Autism Spectrum Disorders Into Focus.* Retrieved from www.youtube.com/watch?v=YtvP5A5OHpU&feature=youtu.be.

Kim, Y. S., Leventhal, B. L., Koh, Y. J., Fombonne, E., Laska, E., Lim, E. C., et al. (2011). Prevalence of autism spectrum disorders in a total population sample. *American Journal of Psychiatry, 168*(9), 904–912.

King, J. M. (2013). Supporting communication with technology. In N. Simmons-Mackie, J. King, & D. Beukelman (Eds.), *Supporting communication for adults with acute and chronic aphasia.* Baltimore, MD: Paul H. Brookes.

Klin, A., McPartland, J., & Volkmar, F. R. (2005). Asperger syndrome. In F. R. Volkmar, R. Paul, A. Klin, & D. Cohen (Eds.), *Handbook of autism and pervasive developmental disorders: Vol. 1. Diagnosis, development, neurobiology, and behavior* (3rd ed., pp. 88–125). Hoboken, NJ: Wiley.

Klingner, J. K., & Edwards, P. A. (2006). Cultural considerations with Response to Intervention models. *Reading Research Quarterly, 41,* 108–17.

Koegel, R. L., & Koegel, L. K. (2006). *Pivotal response treatments for autism: Communication, social, and academic development.* Baltimore, MD: Brookes.

Kong, A., Frigge, M. L., Masson, G., et al. (2012). Rate of de novo mutations and the importance of father's age to disease risk. *Nature, 488*(7412), 471–475.

Koshino, H., Carpenter, P. A., Minshew, N. J., Cherkassky, V. L., Keller, T. A., & Just, M. A. (2005). Functional connectivity in an fMRI working memory task in high functioning autism. *Neuroimage, 24*(3), 810–821.

Kumin, L. (2001). Speech intelligibility in individuals with Down syndrome: A framework for targeting specific factors for assessment and treatment. *Down Syndrome Quarterly, 6,* 1–8.

Kral, A., & Sharma, A. (2012). Developmental neuroplasticity after cochlear implantation. *Trends in Neurosciences, 35,* 111–122.

Lahey, M. (1988). *Language disorders and language development.* New York: Macmillan.

Lahey, M. (1990). Who shall be called language disordered? Some reflections and one perspective. *Journal of Speech and Hearing Disorders, 55,* 612–620.

Landau, B., & Zukowski, A. (2003). Objects, motions, and paths: Spatial language of children with Williams Syndrome. *Developmental Neuropsychology, 23,* 105–138.

Larkin, R. F., & Snowling, M. J. (2008). Comparing phonological skills and spelling abilities in children with reading and language impairments. *International Journal of Language and Communication Disorders, 43,* 111–124.

Larsen, S., Hammill, D., & Moats, L. (1999). *Test of written spelling* (4th ed.). Austin, TX: PRO-ED.

Law, J., Campbell, C., Roulstone, S., Adams, C., & Boyle, J. (2008). Mapping practice onto theory: The speech and language practitioner's construction of receptive language impairment. *International Journal of Language & Communication Disorders, 43,* 245–263.

Layton, T. (2000). Young children with Down syndrome. In T. Layton, E. Crais, & L. Watson (Eds.), *Handbook of early language impairment in children: Nature* (pp. 193–232). Albany, NY: Delmar Publishers.

Lederberg, A. R., Schick, B., & Spencer, P. E. (2013). Language and literacy development of deaf and hard-of-hearing children: Successes and challenges. *Developmental Psychology, 49,* 15–30.

Leonard, L. B. (1998). *Children with specific language impairment*. Cambridge, MA: MIT Press.

Leonard, L. B., Camarata, S. M., Pawtowska, M., & Camarata, M. N. (2006). Tense and agreement morphemes in the speech of children with specific language impairment during intervention: Phase 2. *Journal of Speech Language and Hearing Research, 49*, 749–770.

Lepola, J., Salonen, P., & Vauras, M. (2000). The development of motivation orientations as a function of divergent reading careers from preschool to second grade. *Learning and Instruction, 10*, 153–177.

Lidz, C. S., & Pena, E. D. (2009). Responsiveness to intervention: New opportunities and challenges for the speech-language pathologist. *Seminars in Speech & Language 3*, 121–133.

Light, J. (2012). *Effects of AAC systems with "just in time" programming for children with complete communication needs*. Presentation at the annual American Speech-Language-Hearing Association, Atlanta, GA.

Light, J., & Drager, K. (2006). Beginning communicators: Improving AAC outcomes. *Augmentative Communication News, 18*(1), 8–10.

Light, J., & Drager, K. (2007). AAC technologies for young children with complex communication needs: State of the science and future research directions. *Augmentative and Alternative Communication, 23*, 204–216.

Light, J., & McNaughton, D. (2012). Supporting the communication, language, and literacy development of children with complex communication needs: State of the science and future research priorities. *Assistive Technology, 24*(1), 34–44.

Light, J., Drager, K., McCarthy, J., Mellott, S., Millar, D., Parrish, C., et al. (2004). Performance of typically developing four- and five-year-old children with AAC systems using different language organization techniques. *Augmentative and Alternative Communication, 20*, 63–88.

Lin, F. R., Niparko, J. K., & Ferrucci, L. (2011). Hearing loss prevalence in the United States. *Archives of Internal Medicine, 171*, 1851–1853.

Lindamood, P. C., & Lindamood, P. (2004). *Lindamood Auditory Conceptualization Test—Third Edition (LAC-3)*. Austin, TX: PRO-ED.

Ling, D. (1989). *Foundations of spoken language for hearing-impaired children*. Washington, DC: Alexander Graham Bell Association for the Deaf.

Ling, D. (2002). *Speech and the hearing-impaired child: Theory and practice* (2nd ed.). Washington, DC: Alexander Graham Bell Association for the Deaf.

Lord, C., & Corsello, C. (2005). Diagnostic instruments in autistic spectrum disorders. In F. R. Volkmar, R. Paul, A. Klin, D. Cohen (Eds.), *Handbook of autism and pervasive developmental disorders. Vol. 2: Assessments, interventions, and policy* (3rd ed., pp. 730–771). Hoboken, NJ: Wiley.

Losardo, A., & Notari-Syverson, A. (2001). *Alternative approaches to assessing young children*. Baltimore, MD: Brookes.

Lovaas, O. I. (2003). *Teaching individuals with developmental delays: Basic intervention techniques*. Austin, TX: PRO-ED.

Lovelace, S., & Stewart, S. R. (2009). Effects of robust vocabulary instruction and multicultural text on the development of word knowledge among African American children. *American Journal of Speech-Language Pathology, 18*, 168–179.

MacDonald, J. D. (2004). *Communicating partners: 30 years of building responsive relationships with late talking children including autism, Asperger's syndrome (ASD), Down syndrome, and typical development*. London: Jessica Kingsley Publishers.

Machalicek, W., Davis, T., O'Reilly, M. F., Beretvas, N., Sigafoos, J., Lancioni, G., Green, V., & Edrisinha, C. (2008). Teaching social skills in school settings. In J. K. Luiselli, D. C. Russo, W. P., & S. M. Wilcyznski (Eds.), *Effective practices for children with autism: Educational and behavior support interventions that work* (pp. 269–298). New York: Oxford.

MacKall, D. D. (1997). *Picture me with Jonah and the whale*. Akron, OH: Playhouse Publishing.

MacWhinney, B. (1998). Models of the emergence of language. *Annual Review of Psychology, 49*, 199–227.

MacWhinney, B. (2010). A tale of two paradigms. In M. Kail & M. Hickman (Eds.), *Language acquisition across linguistic and cognitive systems* (pp. 17–32). New York: John Benjamins.

Marcus, G. F., & Fisher, S. E. (2003). FOXP2 in focus: What can genes tell us about speech and language? *Trends in Cognitive Sciences, 7*, 257–262.

Margolis, H., & McCabe, P. P. (2006). Improving self-efficacy and motivation: What to do, what to say. *Intervention in School and Clinic, 41*, 218–227.

Martin, N. A., & Brownell, R. (2010). *Receptive One-Word Picture Vocabulary Test—4 (ROWPVT-4)*. Novato, CA: Academic Therapy Publications.

Martin, B., & Carle, E. (2008). *Brown bear, brown bear, what do you see?* [40th anniversary edition]. New York: Henry Holt.

Maryland School for the Deaf (MSD). (2009). *Handbook for Parents and Students*. Retrieved from www.msd.edu/forms/cc_handbook.pdf.

Mashburn, A. J., Justice, L. M., Downer, J. T., & Pianta, R. C. (2009). Peer effects on children's language achievement during pre-kindergarten. *Child Development, 80*, 686–702.

Masterson, J. J., & Apel, K. (2000). Spelling assessment: Charting a path to optimal intervention. *Topics in Language Disorders, 20*, 50–65.

Masterson, J. J., Apel, K., & Wasowicz, J. (2002). *Spelling Performance Evaluation for Language & Literacy, 2nd ed.* (SPELL-2). Evanston, IL: Learning by Design.

Mattie, H. D. (2001). Generalization effects of cognitive strategies conversation training for adults with moderate to severe disabilities. *Education and Training in Mental Retardation and Developmental Disabilities, 36*, 178–187.

Mayes, S. D., Calhoun, S. L., Murray, M. J., Morrow, J. D., Yurich, K. K., Mahr, F., et al. (2009). Comparison of scores on the checklist for Autism Spectrum disorder, Childhood Autism Rating Scale, and Gilliam Asperger's Disorder Scale for children with low functioning autism, high functioning autism, Asperger's disorder, ADHD, and typical development. *Journal of Autism and Developmental Disorders, 39*(12), 1682–1693.

McCabe, A., & Bliss, L. S. (2003). *Patterns of narrative discourse: A multicultural, life-span approach.* Boston: Allyn & Bacon.

McCord, M. S., & Soto, G. (2004). Perceptions of AAC: An ethnographic investigation of Mexican-American families. *Augmentative and Alternative Communication, 20,* 209–227.

McDuffie, A., Kover, S. T., Hagerman, R., & Abbeduto, L. (2012). Investigating word learning in fragile X syndrome: A fast-mapping study. *Journal of Autism and Developmental Disorders,* pp. 1–16. DOI 10 .1007/s10803-012-1717-3

McGinty, A. S., & Justice, L. M. (2007). Classroom-based versus pull-out interventions: A review of the experimental evidence. *EBP Briefs, 1,* 1–14.

McGregor, K. (2009). Semantics in child language disorders. In R. G. Schwartz (Ed.), *Handbook of child language disorders* (pp. 365–387). New York: Psychology Press.

McKenna, M. C., & Stahl, S. A. (2003). *Assessment for reading instruction.* New York: Guilford Press.

McLaren, E. M., & Nelson, C. M. (2009). Using functional behavior assessment to develop behavior interventions for students in head start. *Journal of Positive Behavior Interventions, 11,* 3–21.

McTigue, E. M., Beckman, A. R., & Kaderavek, J. N. (2007). Assessing literacy motivation and orientation. In K. Pence (Ed.), *Assessment in emergent literacy* (pp. 481–518). San Diego, CA: Plural.

McWilliam, R. A., & Casey, A. M. (2007). *Engagement of every child in the preschool classroom.* Baltimore, MD: Brookes.

McWilliam, R. A., & Clingenpeel, B. (2003, August). *Functional intervention planning: The routines-based interview.* National Individualizing Preschool Inclusion Project, Vanderbilt Medical Center. Retrieved June 15, 2008, from www.collaboratingpartners.com/docs /R_Mcwilliam/RBI%20Flyer%20April%202005.pdf.

McWilliam, R. A., Scarborough, A. S., & Kim, H. (2003). Adult interactions and child engagement. *Early Education & Development, 14,* 7–28.

Millar, D. C., Light, J., & Schlosser, R. W. (2006). The impact of augmentative and alternative communication intervention on the speech production of individuals with developmental disabilities: A research review. *Journal of Speech, Language, and Hearing Research, 49,* 248–264.

Miller, C. A., & Wagstaff, D. A. (2011). Behavioral profiles associated with auditory processing disorder and specific language impairment. *Journal of Communication Disorders, 44,* 745–763.

Miller, J. (2006). Language and communication development in children with Down syndrome. *Perspectives on Language Learning and Education: American Speech-Language Hearing Association, Special Interest Division 1, 13,* 17–20.

Mintz, T. H., & Gleitman, L. R. (2002). Adjectives really do modify nouns: The incremental and restricted nature of early adjective acquisition. *Cognition, 84,* 267–293.

Mitchell, R., & Karchmer, M. (2004). Chasing the mythical ten percent: Parental hearing status of deaf and hard of hearing students in the United States. *Sign Language Studies, 4,* 138–163.

Miyamoto, R. T., Hay-McCutcheon, M. J., Kirk, K. I., Houston, D. M., & Bergeson-Dana, T. R. (2007, August). *Speech and language skills of profoundly deaf children implanted under 12 months of age: Preliminary results.* Oral presentation at the Collegium Oto-Rhino-Laryngologicum Amicitiae Sacrum, Seoul, Korea.

Moerk, E. L. (2004). The guided acquisition of first language skills. Westport, CT: Greenwood Publishing Group.

Moog, J. S. (2002). Changing expectations for children with cochlear implants. *The Annals of Otology, Rhinology, and Laryngology, 111,* 138–142.

Moore, A. (2012). *Teaching and learning: Pedagogy, curriculum and culture.* New York: Routledge.

Morrow, L. M. (2005). *Literacy development in the early years* (5th ed.). Boston: Allyn & Bacon.

Morrow, L. M. (2007). *Developing literacy in preschool.* New York: Guildford.

Naess, K., Melby-Lervag, M., Hulme, C., & Lyster, S. (2012). Reading skills in children with Down syndrome: A meta-analytic review. *Research in Developmental Disabilities, 33,* 737–747.

Nail-Chiwetalu, B. J., & Ratner, N. B. (2006). Information literacy for speech-language pathologists: A key to evidence-based practice. *Language, Speech, and Hearing Services in Schools, 37,* 157–167.

National Institute of Child Health and Human Development (NICHD). (2000). *Report of the National Reading Panel. Teaching children to read: An evidence-based assessment of the scientific research literature on reading and its implications for reading instruction: Reports of the subgroups* (NIH Publication No. 00–4754). Washington, DC: U.S. Government Printing Office.

National Institute on Deafness and Communication Disorders (NIDCD). (2013). *Statistics about hearing, balance, ear infections, and deafness.* Retrieved from www.nidcd.nih.gov/health/statistics/Pages/Default.aspx.

National Reading Panel. (2000). *Report of the National Reading Panel: Teaching children to read.* Washington, DC: National Academy Press.

National Research Council. (2001). *Educating children with autism.* Committee on Educational Interventions for Children with Autism. Division of Behavioral and Social Sciences and Education. Washington, DC: National Academy Press.

Neale B. M., Kou, Y., Liu, L., et al. (2012). Patterns and rates of exonic de novo mutations in autism spectrum disorders. *Nature, 485*(7397), 242–245.

Nelson, N. W. (2010). *Language and literacy disorders: Infancy through adolescence.* Upper Saddle River, NJ: Pearson.

Nelson, N. W. (2011). Questions about certainty and uncertainty in clinical practice. *Language, Speech, and Hearing Services in Schools, 42,* 81–87.

Nelson, N. W., Bahr, C. M., & Van Meter, A. M. (2004*). The writing lab approach to language instruction and intervention.* Baltimore, MD: Brookes.

Nelson, N. W., & Van Meter, A. M. (2006a). Finding the words: Vocabulary development for young authors. In T. A. Ukrainetz (Ed.), *Contextualized language intervention: Scaffolding PreK–12 literacy achievement* (pp. 95–143). Greenville, SC: Thinking Publications.

Nelson, N. W., & Van Meter, A. M. (2006b). The writing lab approach for building language, literacy, and communication abilities. In R. J. McCauley & M. E. Fey (Eds.), *Treatment of language disorders in children* (pp. 383–422). Baltimore, MD: Brookes.

Niccols, A., Atkinson, L., & Pepler, D. (2003). Mastery motivation in young children with Down's syndrome: Relations with cognitive and adaptive competence. *Journal of Intellectual Disability Research, 47,* 121–133.

Nicholas, J. G., & Geers, A. E. (2006). Effects of early auditory experience on the spoken language of deaf children at 3 years of age. *Ear and Hearing, 27,* 286–298.

Nilsson, P. (2008). Teaching for understanding: The complex nature of pedagogical content knowledge in pre-service education. *International Journal of Science Education, 30*(10), 1281–1299.

Numminen, H., Service, E., Ahonen, T., Korhonen, T., Tolvanen, A., Patja, K., et al. (2000). Working memory structure and intellectual disability. *Journal of Intellectual Disability Research, 44,* 579–590.

Ochs, E., & Schieffelin, B. (2001). Language acquisition and socialization: Three developmental stories and their implications. In A. Duranti (Ed.), *Linguistic anthropology: A reader* (pp. 263–301). Oxford, UK: Blackwell.

Odom, S. L., Boyd, B. A., Hall, L. J., & Hume, K. (2010). Evaluation of comprehensive treatment models for individuals with autism spectrum disorders. *Journal of autism and developmental disorders, 40*(4), 425–436.

Oelwein, P. L. (2002). Liberation from traditional reading and math teaching methods and measurements. In W. I. Cohen, L. Nadel, & M. E. Madnick (Eds.), *Down syndrome* (pp. 421–436). New York: Wiley-Liss.

Oetting, J. B., & Hadley, P. (2009). Morphosyntax in child language disorders. In R. G. Schwartz (Ed.), *Handbook of child language disorders* (pp. 341–364). New York: Psychological Press.

Oross, S., & Woods, C. B. (2003). Exploring visual perception abilities in individuals with intellectual disabilities: Assessment and implications. In S. Soraci Jr. & D Murata-Soraci (Eds.), *Visual information processing* (pp. 35–79). Westport, CT: Praeger.

Paradis, J., Emmerzael, K., & Sorenson Duncan, T. (2010). Assessment of English language learners: Using parent report on first language development. *Journal of Communication Disorders, 43,* 474–497.

Paradis, J., Schneider, P., Duncan, T. S. (2013). Discriminating children with language impairment among English-language learners from diverse first-language backgrounds. *Journal of Speech, Language, and Hearing Research, 56,* 971–981.

Parette, H. P., Brotherson, M. J., & Huer, M. B. (2000). Giving families a voice in augmentative and alternative communication decision-making. *Education and Training in Mental Retardation and Developmental Disabilities, 35*(2), 177–190.

Parette, P., Chung, S.-J. L., & Huer, M. B. (2004). First-generation Chinese American families' attitudes regarding disability and educational interventions, *Focus on Autism and Other Developmental Disabilities, 19,* 114–123.

Parisier, S. C. (2003). Cochlear implants: Growing pains. *Laryngoscope, 113,* 1470–1472.

Paul, D. (2013). A quick guide to DSM-5. *The ASHA Leader, 18,* 52–54.

Paul, R., & Cascella, P. W. (2006). *Introduction to clinical methods in communication disorders.* Baltimore, MD: Brookes.

Paul, R., & Elder, L. (2008). *Critical thinking: Concepts and tools* (5th ed.). Dillon Beach, CA: Foundation for Critical Thinking.

Paul, R., & Norbury, C. F. (2012). *Language disorders from infancy through adolescence: Assessment and intervention* (4th ed.). St. Louis: Mosby.

Paul, R., & Sutherland, D. (2005). Enhancing early language in children with autism spectrum disorders. In Volkmar, F. R., Paul, R., Klin, A., & Cohen, D. (Eds.), *Handbook of autism and pervasive developmental disorders* (Vol. 2, 3rd ed., pp. 946–976). New York: Wiley & Sons.

Peets, K. F. (2009). The effects of context on the classroom discourse skills of children with language impairment. *Language, Speech, and Hearing Services in Schools, 40,* 5–16.

Pelios, L. V., MacDuff, G. S., & Axelrod, S. (2003). The effects of a treatment package in establishing independent academic work skills in children with autism. *Education and Treatment of Children, 26,* 1–21.

Penagarikano, O., Mulle, J. G., & Warren, S. T. (2007). The pathophysiology of fragile X syndrome. *Annual Review of Genomics and Human Genetics, 8,* 109–129.

Pence, K. L., Bojczyk, K. E., & Williams, R. S. (2007). Assessing vocabulary knowledge. In K. L. Pence (Ed.), *Assessment in emergent literacy* (pp. 431–480). San Diego, CA: Plural.

Phelps-Terasaki, D., & Phelps-Gunn, T. (2007). *Test of Pragmatic Language—Second Edition.* Austin, TX: PRO-ED.

Phillips, N., & Duke, M. (2001). The questioning skills of clinical teachers and preceptors: A comparative study. *Journal of Advanced Nursing, 33,* 523–532.

Poll, G. H. (2011). Increasing the odds: Applying emergentist theory in language intervention. *Language, Speech, and Hearing Services in Schools, 42,* 580–591.

Powell, D. R., Burchinal, M. R., File, N., & Kontos, S. (2008). An eco-behavioral analysis of children's engagement in urban public school preschool classrooms. *Early Childhood Research Quarterly, 23,* 108–123.

Prizant, B. M., & Wetherby, A. M. (2006). Critical issues in enhancing communication abilities for persons with autism spectrum disorders. In F. R. Volkmar, R. Paul, A. Klin, & D. Cohen (Eds.), *Handbook of autism and pervasive developmental disorders: Vol. 2. Assessment, interventions, and policy* (3rd ed., pp. 925–945). New York: Wiley.

Prizant, B. M., Wetherby, A. M., & Rydell, P. J. (2000). Communication intervention issues for children with autism spectrum disorders. In A. M. Wetherby & B. M. Prizant, *Autism spectrum disorders: A transactional developmental perspective* (pp. 193–224). Baltimore, MD: Brookes.

Prizant, B. M., Wetherby, A. M., Rubin, E., Laurent, A. C., & Rydell, P. J. (2006a). *The SCERTS™ model: A comprehensive educational approach for children with autism spectrum disorders: Vol. 1. Program planning and intervention.* Baltimore, MD: Brookes.

Prizant, B. M., Wetherby, A. M., Rubin, E., Laurent, A. C., & Rydell, P. J. (2006b). *The SCERTS™ model: A comprehensive educational approach for children with autism spectrum disorders: Vol. 1: Assessment.* Baltimore, MD: Brookes.

Proctor-Williams, K., Fey, M. E., & Loeb, D. F. (2001). Parental recasts and production of copulas and articles by children with specific language impairment and typical language. *American Journal of Speech-Language Pathology, 10,* 155–168.

Puranik, C. S., & Lonigan, C. J. (2012). Name-writing proficiency, not length of name, is associated with preschool children's emergent literacy skills. *Early Childhood Research Quarterly, 27,* 284–294.

Puranik, C. S., Petscher, Y., Al Otaiba, S., Catts, H. W., & Lonigan, C. J. (2008). Development of oral reading fluency in children with speech or language impairments: A growth curve analysis. *Journal of Learning Disabilities, 41,* 545–560.

Quittner, A. L., Cruz, I., Barker, D. H., Tobey, E., Eisenberg, L. S., Niparko, J. K., & Childhood Development after Cochlear Implantation Investigative Team. (2013). Effects of maternal sensitivity and cognitive and linguistic stimulation on cochlear implant users' language development over four years. *The Journal of Pediatrics, 162,* 343–348.

Rabidoux, P. C., & MacDonald, J. D. (2000). An interactive taxonomy of mothers and children during storybook interactions. *American Journal of Speech-Language Pathology, 9,* 331–344.

Rafferty, Y., Piscitelli, V., & Boettcher, C. (2003). The impact of inclusion on language development and social competence among preschoolers with disabilities. *Exceptional Children, 69,* 467–479.

Ratner, N. B. (2006). Evidence-based practice: An examination of its ramifications for the practice of speech-language pathology. *Language, Speech, and Hearing Services in Schools, 37,* 257–267.

Ravid, D., Levie, R., & Avivi Ben-zvi, G. (2003). The role of language typology in linguistic development: Implications for the study of language disorders. In Y. Levy & J. Schaeffer (Eds.), *Language competence across populations: Towards a definition of specific language impairment* (pp. 171–196). Mahwah, NJ: Erlbaum.

Rehabilitation Engineering Research Center on Communication Enhancement (AAC-RERC) (2011). *Mobile devices and communication apps: An AAC-RERC white paper.* Retrieved December 4, 2013 from http://aac-rerc.psu.edu/documents/RERC_mobiledevices_ whitepaper_final.pdf

Reichow, B., & Wolery, M. (2009). Comprehensive synthesis of early intensive behavioral interventions for young children with autism based on the UCLA young autism project model. *Journal of Autism & Developmental Disorders, 39*(1), 23–41.

Rescorla, L. (2009). Age 17 language and reading outcomes in late-talking toddlers: Support for a dimensional perspective on language delay. *Journal of Speech, Language, and Hearing Research, 52,* 16–30.

Rescorla, L., & Lee, E. (2000). Language impairment in young children. In T. Layton, E. Crais, & L. Watson (Eds.). *Handbook of early language impairments in children: Nature* (pp. 1–55). Albany, NY: Delmar.

Rescorla, L., & Lee, E. (2001). Language impairment in young children. In T. Layton, E. Crais, and L. Watson (Eds.). *Handbook of early language impairments in children: Nature* (pp. 1–55). Albany, NY: Delmar.

Rey, M., & Rey, H. A. (1985). *Curious George and the Pizza.* Boston: Houghton Mifflin Books for Children.

Rice, M. L. (2000). Grammatical symptoms of specific language impairment. In D. V. M. Bishop & L. B. Leonard (Eds.), *Speech and language impairments in children: Causes, characteristics, intervention, and outcome* (pp. 17–34). East Sussex, UK: Psychology Press.

Rice, M. L., Redmond, S. M., & Hoffman, L. (2006). MLU in children with SLI and younger control children shows concurrent validity, stability, and parallel growth trajectories. *Journal of Speech, Language, and Hearing Research, 49,* 793–808.

Rice, M. L., Smith, S. D., & Gayán, J. (2009). Convergent genetic linkage and associations to language, speech and reading measures in families of probands with specific language impairment. *Journal of Neurodevelopmental Disorders, 1*(4), 264–282.

Rice, M. L., Smolik, F., Perpich, D., Thompson, T., Rytting, N., & Blossom, M. (2010). Mean length of utterance levels in 6-month intervals for children 3 to 9 years with and without language impairments. *Journal of Speech, Language, and Hearing Research, 53,* 333–349.

Rice, M. L., Warren, S. F., & Betz, S. K. (2005). Language symptoms of developmental language disorders: An overview of autism, Down syndrome, fragile x, specific language impairment, and William syndrome. *Applied Psycholinguistics, 26,* 7–27.

Roach, A. T., & Elliott, S. N. (2005). Goal attainment scaling: An efficient and effective approach to monitoring student progress. *Teaching Exceptional Children, 37,* 8–17.

Robbins, A. M., Koch, D. B., Osberger, M. J., & Zimmerman-Philips, S. (2004). Effect of age at cochlear implantation on auditory skill development in infants and toddlers. *Archives of Otolaryngology—Head & Neck Surgery, 130,* 570–574.

Robins, D. L., Fein, D., Barton, M. L., & Green, J. A. (2001). The Modified Checklist for Autism in Toddlers: An initial study investigating the early detection of autism and pervasive developmental disorders. *Journal of Autism & Developmental Disorders, 31*(2), 131–144.

Roberts, J. E., Mirrett, P. L, & Burchinal, M. (2001). Receptive and expressive communication development of young males with fragile X syndrome. *American Journal on Mental Retardation, 106,* 216–230.

Rogers, S. J., Cook, I., & Meryl, A. (2005). Imitation and play in autism. In F. R. Volkmar, R. Paul, A. Klin, & D. Cohen (Eds.), *Handbook of autism and pervasive developmental disorders: Vol. 1. Diagnosis, development, neurobiology, and behavior* (3rd ed., pp. 382–405). Hoboken, NJ: Wiley.

Rogers, S. J., & Dawson, G. (2010). *Early start Denver model for young children with autism: Promoting language, learning, and engagement.* New York: Guilford.

Rogers, S. J., & Vismara, L. A. (2008). Evidence-based comprehensive treatments for early autism. *Journal of Clinical Child & Adolescent Psychology, 37*(1), 8–38.

Rogoff, B. (2001). Becoming a cooperative parent in a parent co-operative. In B. Rogoff, C. Turkanis, & L. Bartlett (Eds.), *Learning together: Children and adults in a school community* (pp. 145–155). Oxford: Oxford University Press.

Romski, M. A., & Sevcik, R. A. (1996). Breaking the speech barrier: Language development through augmented means. Baltimore, MD: Brookes.

Romski, M. A., Sevcik, R. A., Adamson, L. B., & Bakeman, R. A. (2005). Communication patterns of individuals with moderate or severe cognitive disabilities: Interactions with unfamiliar partners. *American Association on Mental Retardation, 110*(3), 226–238.

Romski, M., Sevcik, R. A., Adamson, L. B., Cheslock, M., Smith, A., Barker, R. M., & Bakeman, R. (2010). Randomized comparison of augmented and nonaugmented language interventions for toddlers with developmental delays and their parents. *Journal of Speech, Language, and Hearing Research, 53,* 350–364.

Rondal, J. A. (2004). Intersyndrome and intrasyndrome language differences. In J. A. Rondal, R. M. Hodapp, S. Soresi, E. M. Dykens, & L. Nota (Eds.), *Intellectual disabilities: Genetics, behavior, and inclusion* (pp. 49–113). London: Whurr.

Roseberry-McKibben, C., & Brice, A. (2013). *Acquiring English as a second language: What's "normal," what's not.* Retrieved from www.asha.org/public/speech /development/easl/.

Rosemary, C. A., & Roskos, K. A. (2002). Literacy conversations between adults and children at child care: Descriptive observations and hypotheses. *Journal of Research in Childhood Education, 16,* 212–231.

Roseti, S., Tellis, G. M., & Gabel, R. (2001, November). *African-American middle and high school students' perceptions about stuttering.* Seminar presented at ASHA Convention, New Orleans, LA.

Rosin, P. (2006). *Communication skills and challenges of young children with Down syndrome: Bridging research to practice.* Presentation made to The Alberta Early Years Conference, Alberta, Canada.

Rosin, P., & Miolo, G. (2005). *Improving communication skills in children with Down syndrome using performance and literacy-based activities.* Presentation made to 4th International Conference on Developmental Issues in Down Syndrome, Portsmouth, England.

Roth, F., & Paul, R. (2007). Communication intervention: Principles and procedures. In R. Paul & P. W. Cascella (Eds.), *Introduction to clinical methods in communication disorders* (2nd ed., pp. 157–178). Baltimore, MD: Brookes.

Saddler, B., & Graham, S. (2005). The effects of peer-assisted sentence-combining instruction on the writing performance of more and less skilled young writers. *Journal of Educational Psychology, 97,* 43–54.

Sandall, S., Giacomini, J., Smith, B. J., & Hemmeter, M. L. (2006). *DEC recommended practices toolkits: Interactive tools to improve practices for young children with special needs and their families* [CD-ROM]. Missoula, MT: Division for Early Childhood.

Schalock, R. L. (2004). The emerging disability paradigm and its implications for policy and practice. *Journal of Disability Policy Studies, 14,* 204–215.

Schalock, R. L., & Luckasson, R. (2005). American Association on Mental Retardation's definition, classification, and system of supports and its relation to international trends and issues in the field of intellectual disabilities. *Journal of Policy and Practice in Intellectual Disabilities, 1,* 136–146.

Schalock, R. L., Luckasson, R. A., & Shogren, K. A. (2007). The renaming of "mental retardation": Understanding the change to the term "intellectual disability." *Intellectual and Developmental Disabilities, 45,* 116–124.

Schirmer, B. R. (2000). *Language and literacy development in children who are deaf* (2nd ed.). Boston: Allyn & Bacon.

Schlosser, R. W. (2004). Goal attainment scaling as a clinical measurement technique in communicative disorders: A critical review. *Journal of Communication Disorders, 37,* 217–239.

Schlosser, R. W., & Wendt, O. (2007, November). *Effects of the Picture Exchange Communication System: A systematic review.* Poster session presented at the annual meeting of the American Speech-Language-Hearing Association, Boston.

Schmidt, C., & Stichter, J. P. (2012). The use of peer-mediated interventions to promote the generalization of social competence for adolescents with high-functioning autism and Asperger's syndrome. *Exceptionality, 20,* 94–113.

Schooling, T., Venediktov, R., & Leech, H. (2010). Evidence-based systematic review: Effects of service delivery on the speech and language skills of children from birth to 5 years of age. *ASHA's National Center for Evidence-Based Practice in Communication Disorders.* Retrieved from www.asha.org/uploadedFiles/EBSR-Service-Delivery.pdf.

Schopler, E., Reichler, R. J., & Renner, B. R. (1988). *Childhood Autism Rating Scale (CARS).* Los Angeles, CA: Western Psychological Services.

Schuele, C. M., & Justice, L. M. (2006). The importance of effect sizes in the interpretation of research. *The ASHA Leader, 11*(10), 14–15, 26–27.

Scott, C. M. (2002). A fork in the road less traveled: Writing intervention based on language profile. In K. G. Butler & E. R. Silliman (Eds.), *Speaking, reading, and writing in children with language learning disabilities* (pp. 219–237). Mahwah, NJ: Erlbaum.

Scott, C. M., & Nelson, N. W. (2009). Sentence combining: Assessment and intervention applications. *Perspectives on language learning and education, 16,* 14–20.

Scott, C. M., & Windsor J. (2000). General language performance measures in spoken and written narrative and expository discourse of school-age children with language learning disabilities. *Journal of Speech, Language, and Hearing Research, 43,* 324–339.

Seal, B. (2010, November). About baby signing. *The ASHA Leader.* Retrieved from www.asha.org/publications /leader/2010/101102/about-baby-signing.htm.

Segal, E. F. (1975). Psycholinguistics discovers the operant: A review of Roger Brown's "A first language: The early stages." *Journal of the experimental analysis of behavior, 23,* 149–158.

Seligman, L. (2004). *Techniques and conceptual skills for mental health professionals.* Upper Saddle River, NJ: Prentice Hall.

Semel, E., Wiig, E. H., & Secord, W. A. (2004). *Clinical Evaluation of Language Fundamentals—Preschool—2nd ed. (CELF-P-2).* San Antonio, TX: Pearson.

Semel, E., Wiig, E. H., & Secord, W. A. (2013). *Clinical Evaluation of Language Fundamentals-5th Ed.* San Antonio, TX: Pearson.

Seung, H. (2013). Cultural considerations in serving children with ASD and their families: Asian American perspective. *Perspectives on Language Learning and Education, 20,* 14–19.

Seymour, H., Roeper, T., & deVilliers, J. (2005). *The diagnostic evaluation of language variation.* San Antonio, TX: Harcourt.

Seymour, H. N. (2004). The challenge of language assessment for African American English-speaking children: A historical perspective. *Seminars in Speech and Language, 25,* 3–12.

Shames, G. H. (2000). *Counseling the communicatively disabled and their families: A manual for clinicians.* Boston: Allyn & Bacon.

Shane, H. C., Blackstone, S., Vanderheiden, G., Williams, M., & DeRuyter, F. (2012). Using AAC technology to access the world. *Assistive Technology, 24*(1), 3–13.

Sharma, A. (2007). *Central auditory development and plasticity in infants and children with hearing aids and cochlear implants.* Presented at the AG Bell conference, July 2007, Washington, DC.

Sharma, A., Dorman, M., & Spahr, A. (2002). A sensitive period for the development of the central auditory system in children with cochlear implants: Implications for age of implantation. *Ear & Hearing, 23,* 532–539.

Sharma, M., Purdy, S. C., & Kelly, A. S. (2009). Comorbidity of auditory processing, language, and reading disorders. *Journal of Speech, Language, and Hearing Research, 52,* 706–722.

Shattuck, P., Durkin, M., Maenner, M., et al. (2009). Timing of identification of children with Autism Spectrum Disorder: Findings from a population-based surveillance study. *Journal of the American Academy of Child and Adolescent Psychiatry, 48,* 474–483.

Shea, V., & Mesibov, G. B. (2005). Adolescents and adults with autism. In F. R. Volkmar, R. Paul, A. Klin, & D. Cohen (Eds.), *Handbook of autism and pervasive developmental disorders: Vol. 1. Diagnosis, development, neurobiology, and behavior* (3rd ed., pp. 288–311). Hoboken, NJ: Wiley.

Sherer M., Pierce K.I., Paredes S., Kisacky K.L., Ingersoll B., & Schreibman L. (2001). Enhancing conversation skills in children with autism via video technology: Which is better, "self" or "other" as a model. *Behavior Modification, 25,* 140–158.

Singleton, R. J., Holman, R. C., Plant, R., Yorita, K. L., Holve, S., Paisano, E. L., & Cheeck, J. E. (2009). Trends in otitis media and myringotomy with tube placement among American Indian/Alaska native children and the US general population of children. *The Pediatric Infectious Disease Journal, 28,* 102–107.

Sininger, Y. S., Grimes, A., & Christensen, E. (2010). Auditory development in early amplified children: Factors influencing auditory-based communication outcomes in children with hearing loss. *Ear and Hearing, 31,* 166–185.

Skinner, B. F. (1957). *Verbal behavior.* Englewood Cliffs, NJ: Prentice Hall.

Slobin, D. I. (1973). Cognitive prerequisites for the development of grammar. In C. A. Ferguson & D. I. Slobin (Eds.), *Studies of child language development* (pp. 175–208). New York: Holt, Reinhart & Winston.

Smedley, A., & Smedley, B. D. (2005). Race as biology is fiction, racism as a social problem is real: Anthropological and historical perspectives on the social construction of race. *American Psychologist, 60,* 16–26.

Smith, T., Groen, A. D., & Wynn, J. W. (2000). A randomized trial of intensive early intervention for children with pervasive developmental disorder. *American Journal of Mental Retardation, 5,* 269–285

Solomon, R., Necheles, J., Ferch, C., & Bruckman, D. (2007). Pilot study of a parent training program for young children with autism: The PLAY Project Home Consultation program. *Autism, 11,* 205–224.

Soto, G. (2012). Training partners in AAC in culturally diverse families. *Perspectives on Augmentative and Alternative Communication, 21,* 144–150.

Soto, G., & Zangari, C. (Eds.) (2009). *Practically speaking: Language, literacy, and academic development for students with AAC needs.* Baltimore, MD: Brookes.

Spencer, L. J., Barker, B. A., & Tomblin, J. B. (2003). Exploring the language and literacy outcomes of pediatric cochlear implant users. *Ear and Hearing, 24,* 236–247.

Strain, P. S., Schwartz, I. S., & Bovey, E. (2008). Social competence interventions for young children with autism. In W. H. Brown, S. L. Odom, & S. R. McConnell (Eds.), *Social competence of young children: Risk, disability, and intervention* (pp. 253–272). Baltimore, MD: Brookes.

Stanovich, K. (2000). *Progress in understanding reading: Scientific foundations and new frontiers.* New York: Guilford Press.

Stanovich, K. E. (1986). Matthew effects in reading: Some consequences of individual differences in the acquisition of literacy. *Reading Research Quarterly, 21,* 360–407.

Steppling, M., Quattlebaum, P., & Brady, D. E. (2007). Toward a discussion of issues associated with speech-language pathologists' dismissal practices in public school settings. *Communication Disorders Quarterly, 28,* 179–187.

Stout, C. E., & Hayes, R. A. (2004). *The evidence-based practice: Methods, models, and tools for mental health professionals.* Hoboken, NJ: Wiley.

Strauss, S. L. (2003). Challenging the NICHD reading research agenda. *Phi Delta Kappan, 84,* 38–42.

Strock, M. (2004). *Autism spectrum disorders (Pervasive developmental disorders).* NIH Publication No. NIH 04–5511, National Institute of Mental Health, National Institutes of Health, U.S. Department of Health and Human Services, Bethesda, MD. Retrieved from www.hnimh.nih.gov/publicat/autism.cfm.

Spreckley, M., & Boyd, R. (2009). Efficacy of applied behavioral intervention in preschool children with autism for improving cognitive, language, and adaptive behavior: A systematic review and meta-analysis. *Journal of Pediatrics, 154*(3), 338–344.

Strain, P. S., & Bovey, E. (2008). LEAP preschool. In J. Handleman & S. Harris (Eds.), *Preschool education programs for children with autism* (pp. 249–280). Austin, TX: PRO-ED.

Strain, P. S., & Bovey, E. H. (2011). Randomized, controlled trial of the LEAP model of early intervention for young children with autism spectrum disorders. *Topics in Early Childhood Special Education, 31,* 133–154.

Svirsky, M. A., Robbins, A. M., Kirk, K. I., Pisoni, D. B., & Miyamoto, R. T. (2000). Language development in profoundly deaf children with cochlear implants. *Psychological Science, 11*–153–158.

Swanson, L. A., Fey, M. E., Mills, C. E., & Hood, L. S. (2005). Use of narrative-based language intervention with children who have specific language impairment. *American Journal of Speech-Language Pathology, 14,* 131–141.

Sylva, K., Chan, L. L., Melhuish, E., Sammons, P., Siraj-Blatchford, I., & Taggart, B. (2011). Emergent literacy environments: Home and preschool influences on children's literacy development. In S. B. Neuman & D. K. Dickinson (Eds.), *Handbook of early literacy research* (Vol. 3, pp. 97–115). New York: Guilford.

Thompson, C. K. (2007). Complexity in language learning and treatment. *American Journal of Speech and Language Pathology, 16,* 3–5.

Thompson, J. R., Bryant, B. R., Campbell, E. M., Craig, E. M., Hughes, C. M., Rotholz, D. A., Schalock, R., Silverman, W., Tasse, M., & Wehmeyer, M. (2004). *The Supports Intensity Scale (SIS): Users manual.* Washington, DC: American Association on Mental Retardation.

Timler, G. R., Olswang, L. B., & Coggins, T. E. (2005b). Social communication interventions for preschoolers: Targeting peer interactions during peer group entry and cooperative play. *Seminars in Speech and Language, 26,* 170–180.

Tomblin, J. (1996). Genetic and environmental contributions to the risk for specific language impairment. In M. Rice (Ed.), *Toward a genetics of language* (pp. 191–210). Hillsdale: Erlbaum.

Tomblin, J., Records, N., Buckwalter, P., Zhang, X., Smith, E., & O'Brian, M. (1997). Prevalence of specific language impairment in kindergarten children. *Journal of Speech, Language, and Hearing Research, 40,* 1245–1260.

Tomlinson, C. (2003). *Fulfilling the promise of the differentiated classroom: Strategies and tools for responsive teaching.* Alexandria, VA: Association for Supervision and Curriculum Development.

Torgesen, J. K. (1998). Catch them before they fall. *American Educator, 22,* 32–41.

Torgesen, J. K., & Bryant, B. R. (2004). *Test of Phonological Awareness—Second Edition: PLUS.* Austin, TX: PRO-ED.

Treiman, R., & Bourassa, D. C. (2000). The development of spelling skills. *Topics in Language Disorders, 20,* 1–18.

Tsatsanis, K. D. (2005). Neuropsychological characteristics in autism and related conditions. In F. R. Volkmar, R. Paul, A. Klin, & D. Cohen (Eds.), *Handbook of autism and pervasive developmental disorders: Vol. 1. Diagnosis, development, neurobiology, and behavior* (3rd ed., pp. 365–381). Hoboken, NJ: Wiley.

Tyler, A., Lewis, K., Haskill, A., & Tolbert, L. (2003). Outcomes of different speech and language goal attack strategies. *Journal of Speech, Language, and Hearing Research, 46,* 1077–1094.

Ucles, P., Alonso, M. F., Aznar, E., & Lapresta, C. (2012). The importance of right otitis media in childhood language disorders. *International Journal of Otolaryngology.* Retrieved from www.hindawi.com/journals/ijol/2012/818927/abs/.

Ukrainetz, T. (2006). The many ways of exposition: A focus on discourse structure. In T. Ukrainetz (Ed.), *Contextualized language intervention: Scaffolding preK–12 literacy achievement* (pp. 247–288). Eau Claire, WI: Thinking Publications.

Ukrainetz, T. A. (2005). What to work on how: An examination of the practice of school-age language intervention. *Contemporary Issues in Communication Sciences and Disorders, 32,* 108–119.

Ukrainetz, T. A. (2009) How much is enough? The intensity evidence in language intervention foreword. *Topics in Language Disorders, 29,* 291–293.

Ukrainetz, T. A., Justice, L. M., Kaderavek, J. N., Eisenberg, S. L., Gillam, R. B., & Harm, H. M. (2005). The development of expressive elaboration in fictional narratives. *Journal of Speech, Language, and Hearing Research, 48,* 1363–1377.

U.S. Department of Education. (2002). *Twenty-fourth annual report to Congress on the implementation of the Individuals with Disabilities Education Act.* Washington, DC: Government Printing Office.

van Kleeck, A., Schwarz, A. L., Fey, M., Kaiser, A., Miller, J., & Weitzman, E. (2010). Should we use telegraphic or grammatical input with children in the early stages of language development? Evidence from research and experts. *American Journal of Speech-Language Pathology, 19,* 3–21.

Vigil, D. C., Hodges, J., & Klee, T. (2005). Quantity and quality of parental language input to late-talking toddlers during play. *Child Language Teaching and Therapy, 21,* 107–122.

Volk, H. E, Lurmann, F., Penfold, B., Hertz-Picciotto, I., & McConnell, R. (2013). Traffic-related air pollution, particulate matter, and autism. *JAMA Psychiatry, 70*(1), 71–77.

Vygotsky, L. (1934). *Thought and language.* Cambridge, MA: MIT Press.

Vygotsky, L. S. (1978). *Mind in society: The development of higher psychological processes.* Cambridge, MA: Harvard University Press.

Vygotsky, L. S. (1987). *The collected works of L. S. Vygotsky,* Vol. 1. New York: Plenum.

Wacker, D. P., Berg, W. K., Harding, J. W., Anjali, B., Rankin, B., & Ganzer, J. (2005). Treatment effectiveness, stimulus generalization, and acceptability to parents of functional communication training. *Educational Psychology, 25,* 233–256.

Wadman, R., Durkin, K., & Conti-Ramsden, G. (2008). Self-esteem, shyness, and sociability in adolescents with specific language impairment. *Journal of Speech, Language, and Hearing Research, 51,* 938–952.

Wagner, N., L, Cameto, R., Levine, P., & Garza, N. (2005). *An overview of findings from wave 2 of the national longitudinal transition study—2 (NLTS-2).* (NCSER 2006-3004). Menlo Park: CA: SRI International.

Wagner, R. K., Torgesen, J. K., & Rashotte, C. A., & Pearson, N. A. (2013). *Comprehensive Test of Phonological Processing—2nd ed. (CTOPP-2).* Austin, TX: PRO-ED.

Walker, E. A., Spratford, M., Moeller, M. P., Oleson, J., Hua, O., Roush, P., & Jacobs, S. (2013). Predictors of hearing aid use time in children with mild-to-severe hearing loss. *Language, Speech, and Hearing Services in Schools, 44,* 73–88.

Wallace, D., & Hammill, D. D. (2013) *Comprehensive Receptive and Expressive Vocabulary Test-Third Edition.* Austin, TX: PRO-ED.

Walpole, S., & McKenna, M. C. (2004). *The literacy coach's handbook: A guide to research-based practice.* New York, Guilford Press.

Warren, S. F., Brady, N. C., & Fey, M. E. (2004). Communication and language: Research design and measurement. In E. Emerson, C. Hatton, T. Thompson, & T. R. Parmenter (Eds.), *The international handbook of applied research in intellectual disabilities* (pp. 385–405). West Sussex, UK: Wiley.

Warren, S. F., Fey, M. E., & Yoder, P. J. (2007). Differential treatment intensity research: A missing link to creating optimally effective communication interventions. *Mental Retardation and Developmental Disabilities Research Reviews, 13,* 70–77.

Wasik, B. A., Bond, M. A., & Hindman, A. (2006). The effects of a language and literacy intervention on Head Start children and teachers. *Journal of Educational Psychology, 98,* 63–74.

Wayman, M. M., Wallace, T., Wiley, H. I., & Renáta, T., & Espin, C. A. (2007). Literature synthesis on curriculum-based measurement in reading. *Journal of Special Education, 41,* 85–120.

Webb, N. M., Shavelson, R. J., & Haertel, E. H. (2007). Reliability coefficients and generalizability theory. In C. R. Rao & S. Sinharay (Ed.), *Handbook of statistics* (Vol. 26, pp. 81–124). Radarweg, Amsterdam: Elsevier.

Wehman, P. (2013). *Life beyond the classroom: Transition strategies for young people with disabilities* (5th ed., pp. 3–41). Baltimore, MD: Paul H. Brookes.

Wieder, S., & Greenspan, S. I. (2003). Climbing the symbolic ladder in the DIR model through floor time/interactive play. *Autism, 7*(4), 425–435.

Weismer, S. E., & Robertson, S. (2006). Focused stimulation approach to language intervention. In R. J. McCauley & M. E. Fey (Eds.), *Treatment of language disorders in children* (pp. 267–278). Baltimore, MD: Brookes.

Weismer, S. E., & Thordardottir, E. T. (2002). Cognition and language. In P. J. Accardo, B. T. Rogers, & A. J. Capute (Eds.), *Disorders of language development* (pp. 21–37). Baltimore, MD: York.

Weiss, A. L. (2001). *Preschool language disorders resource guide: Specific language impairment*. San Diego, CA: Singular.

Weitzman, E., & Greenberg, J. (2002). *Learning language and loving it: A guide to promoting children's social, language, and literacy development in early childhood settings* (2nd ed.). Toronto, ON: Hanen Centre.

Wendt, O. (2008, November). *A systematic review of AAC interventions applying graphic symbols for Autism Spectrum Disorders*. Poster session presented at the annual meeting of the American Speech-Language-Hearing Association, Chicago, IL.

Westby, C. (2005). Assessing and facilitating text comprehension problems. In H. Catts & A. Kahmi (Eds.), *Language and reading disabilities* (2nd ed., pp. 157–232). Boston: Allyn & Bacon.

Westby, C. E. (2008). Children's play: Reflections of social competence. *Seminars in Speech and Language, 9,* 1–14.

Whitmire, K. (2002). The evolution of school-based speech-language services: A half-century of change and a new century of practice. *Communication Disorders Quarterly, 23,* 68–76.

Wiederholt, J. L., & Bryant, B. R (2012). *Gray Oral Reading Tests-Fifth Edition* (GORT-5). Austin, TX: Pro-Ed.

Wiig, E. H., & Secord, W. A. (2006, Feb. 7). Clinical measurement and assessment: A 25-year retrospective. *The ASHA Leader, 11*(2), 10–11.

Wiig, E. H., Secord, W., & Semel, E. (2004). *Clinical Evaluation of Language Fundamentals—Preschool—2*. San Antonio, TX: The Psychological Corporation.

Wilkes, E. M., & Sunshine Cottage for Deaf Children. (1999). *Cottage Acquisition Scales for Listening, Language, and Speech*. San Antonio, TX: Sunshine Cottage School for Deaf Children.

Williams, A. L. (2000). Multiple oppositions: Case studies of variables in phonological intervention. *American Journal of Speech and Language Pathology, 9,* 289–299.

Wilson, K., & Chapman, J. (2001). *Bear snores on*. New York: Simon & Schuster Children's Publishing.

Winsler, A. (2003). Introduction to the special issue: Vygotskian perspectives in early childhood education. *Early Education and Development, 14,* 253–269.

Wood, A. J., & Pledger, M. (2001). *In the ocean*. Berkeley, CA: Silver Dolphin Books.

Woodcock, R. W. (2011). *Woodcock reading mastery tests—3rd ed. (WRMT-3)*. San Antonio, TX: Pearson.

World Health Organization (WHO). (2001). *World Health Report, Mental Retardation*. Retrieved December 4, 2006, from www.who.int/mediacentre/factsheets/fs265/en/.

World Health Organization (WHO). (2002). *Towards a common language for functioning, disability, and health: The international classification of functioning, disability and health*. Retrieved August, 22, 2007, from www.who.int/classifications/icf/site/beginners/bg.pdf.

World Health Organization (WHO). (2013). *Disabilities*. Retrieved from www.who.int/topics/disabilities/en/.

Wright, H. H., & Newhoff, M. (2001). Narration abilities of children with language-learning disabilities in response to oral and written stimuli. *American Journal of Speech-Language Pathology, 10,* 308–319.

Yeargin-Allsopp, M., Rice, C., Karapurkar, T., Doernberg, N., Boyle, C., & Murphy, C. (2003). Prevalence of autism in a US metropolitan area. *JAMA: The Journal of the American Medical Association, 289*(1), 49–55.

Yew, S. G. K., & O'Kearney, R. (2013). Emotional and behavioral outcomes later in childhood and adolescence for children with specific language impairments: Meta-analyses of controlled prospective studies. *Journal of Child Psychology and Psychiatry, 54,* 516–524.

Yoder, P. J., & Warren, S. F. (2002). Effects of prelinguistic milieu teaching and parent responsivity education on dyads involving children with intellectual disabilities. *Journal of Speech, Language, and Hearing Research, 45,* 1158–1174.

Yoshinaga-Itano, C., & de Uzcategui, A. C. (2001). Early identification and social-emotional factors of children with hearing loss and children screened for hearing loss. In E. Kurtzer-White & D. Luterman (Eds.), *Early childhood deafness* (pp. 13–28). Timonium, MD: York Press.

Ypsilanti, A., & Grouios, G. (2008). Linguistic profile of individuals with Down syndrome: Comparing the linguistic performance of three developmental disorders. *Child Neuropsychology, 14,* 148–170.

Zeidner, M. (2001). Invited forward and introduction. In J. J. W. Andrews, D. H. Saklofske, & H. L. Janzen (Eds.), *Handbook of psychoeducational assessment: Ability, achievement, and behavior in children* (pp. 1–10). San Diego: Academic Press.

Zimmerman, I. L., Steiner, V. G., & Pond, R. E. (2002). *Preschool Language Scale—4th ed. (PLS-4)*. San Antonio, TX: Pearson.

Zimmerman, I. L., Steiner, V. G., & Pond, R. E. (2011). *Preschool Language Scale* (5th ed.; PLS-5). San Antonio, TX: Pearson.

Zipoli, R. P., & Kennedy, M. (2005). Evidence-based practice among speech-language pathologists: Attitudes, utilization, and barriers. *American Journal of Speech-Language Pathology, 14,* 208–222.